W0105752

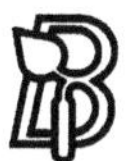

Respiratory
Pharmacology and
Pharmacotherapy

Series Editors:

Dr. David Raeburn
Discovery Biology
Rhône-Poulenc Rorer Ltd
Dagenham Research Centre
Dagenham
Essex RM10 7XS
England

Dr. Mark A. Giembycz
Department of Thoracic Medicine
National Heart and Lung Institute
Imperial College of Science, Technology and Medicine
London SW3 6LY
England

Molecular Biology of the Lung
Volume I: Emphysema and Infection

Edited by
R. A. Stockley

Springer Basel AG

Editor:

Prof. Robert A. Stockley
University Hospital Birmingham
Department of Respiratory Medicine
Edgbaston, Birmingham B15 2TH
UK

Library of Congress Cataloging-in-Publication Data

Molecular biology of the lung / edited by
R.A. Stockley
p. cm. – (Respiratory pharmacology and pharmacotherapy)
Contents: V. 1. Emphysema and infection – V. 2. Asthma and cancer.
ISBN 978-3-0348-9791-4 ISBN 978-3-0348-8831-8 (eBook)
DOI 10.1007/978-3-0348-8831-8

1. Lungs–Diseases–Molecular aspects. I. Stockley, Robert A. II. Series.
[DNLM: 1. Lung Diseases, Obstructive–immunology. 2. Pulmonary Emphysema. 3. Asthma. WF 600M719 1998]
RC756.M67 1998
616.2' 407 – dc21
DNLM/DLC
for Library of Congress 98–36983
CIP

Die Deutsche Bibliothek – CIP-Einheitsaufnahme

Molecular biology of the lung / ed by R. A. Stockley. – Basel ; Boston ; Berlin : Birkhäuser
(Respiratory pharmacology and pharmacotherapy)
ISBN 978-3-0348-9791-4

Vol. 1 Emphysema and infection. – 1999
ISBN 978-3-0348-9791-4

Originally published by Birkhäuser Verlag in 1999
Printed on acid-free paper produced from chlorine-free pulp. TCF ∞

Cover design: Markus Etterich

ISBN 978-3-0348-9791-4

9 8 7 6 5 4 3 2 1

Contents

List of Contributors

Eric W.F.W. Alton, Imperial College School of Medicine at the National Heart & Lung Institute, Manresa Road, London SW3 6LR, UK; e-mail: e.alton@ic.ac.uk

Eleonora Cavarra, Institute of General Pathology, University of Siena, via Aldo Moro, I-53100 Siena, Italy

Gerd Döring, Department of General and Environmental Hygiene, Hygiene-Institute, University of Tübingen, Wilhelmstrasse 31, D-72074 Tübingen, Germany; e-mail: gerd.doering@uni-tuebingen.de

Jack Gauldie, Department of Pathology, McMaster University, Hamilton, Ontario L8N 3Z5, Canada

Duncan Geddes, Royal Brompton Hospital, Sydney Street, London SW3 6NP, UK

Uta Griesenbach, Imperial College School of Medicine at the National Heart & Lung Institute, Manresa Road, London SW3 6LR, UK

Pieter S. Hiemstra, Leiden University Medical Centre, Department of Pulmonology (C3-P), P.O. Box 9600, NL-2300 Leiden, The Netherlands

John R. Hoidal, Division of Respiratory, Critical Care and Occupational Pulmonary Medicine, University of Utah School of Medicine, 50 North Medical Drive, Salt Lake City, UT 84132-1001, USA; e-mail: jhoidal@med.utah.edu

Noor Kalsheker, Division of Clinical Chemistry, School of Clinical Laboratory Sciences, Faculty of Medicine, Queen Medical Centre, Nottingham NG7 2UH, UK; e-mail: Noor.Kalsheker@nottingham.ac.uk

Karin L. Klingman, State University of New York at Buffalo, Erie County Medical Center, 462 Grider St., Buffalo, NY 14215, USA

Giuseppe Lungarella, Institute of General Pathology, University of Siena, via Aldo Moro, I-53100 Siena, Italy; e-mail: lungarella@unisi.it

Piero A. Martorana, Institute of General Pathology, University of Siena, via Aldo Moro, I-53100 Siena, Italy

Timothy J. Mitchell, Division of Infection and Immunity, Joseph Black Building, University of Glasgow, Glasgow G12 8QQ, UK; e-mail: t.mitchell@bio.gla.ac.uk

Kevin Morgan, Division of Clinical Chemistry, School of Clinical Laboratory Sciences, Faculty of Medicine, Queen Medical Centre, Nottingham NG7 2UH, UK

Timothy F. Murphy, State University of New York at Buffalo, Buffalo VAMC, Medical Research 151, 3495 Bailey Avenue, Buffalo, NY 14215, USA; e-mail: murphyt@acsu.buffalo.edu

Joel Rosenbloom, Department of Anatomy and Histology, School of Dental Medicine, University of Pennsylvania, 4001 Spruce Street, Philadelphia, PA 19104, USA; e-mail: jrosen@biochem.dental.upenn.edu

Jean-Michel Sallenave, Rayne Laboratory, Department of Medicine, Edinburgh Medical School University, Teviot Place, Edinburgh EH8 9AG, Scotland, UK

Neil W. Schluger, Division of Pulmonary, Allergy, and Critical Care Medicine, College of Physicians and Surgeons, Columbia University, 630 West 168th Street, New York, NY 10032, USA; e-mail: ns311@columbia.edu

Steven D. Shapiro, Department of Pediatrics, Medicine, and Cell Biology (North Campus), Washington University School of Medicine, 216 South Kingshighway, St. Louis, MO 63110, USA;
e-mail: sshapiro@imgate.wustl.edu

Robert A. Stockley, Department of Medicine, Queen Elizabeth Hospital, Edgbaston, Birmingham B15 2TH, UK

Jan Stolk, Leiden University Medical Centre, Department of Pulmonology (C3-P), P.O. Box 9600, NL-2300 RC Leiden, The Netherlands;
e-mail: jstolk@pulmonology.azl.nl

Anne B. Sturrock, Divison of Respiratory, Critical Care and Occupational Pulmonary Medicine, University of Utah School of Medicine, 50 North Medical Drive, Salt Lake City, UT 84132-1001, USA

Molecular Biology of the Lung
Vol. 1: Emphysema and Infection
ed. by R.A. Stockley

CHAPTER 1
Application of Transgenic and Gene-Targeted Mice to Dissect Mechanisms of Lung Disease

Steven D. Shapiro

Department of Pediatrics, Medicine, and Cell Biology, Washington University School of Medicine St. Louis MO 673110, USA

1. Introduction

By just after the beginning of the next millenium, the sequence of all human genes should be known. The function of the proteins encoded by most of these genes will, however, remain a mystery. Transgenic and gene-targeted mice provide powerful techniques to determine protein function *in vivo* [1]. In fact, these models have recently led to new insight into the function of many proteins that have been extensively studied for decades. "One invariable lesson of biological research has been the difficulty, virtual impossibility, of reliably predicting the properties of intact organisms from the properties of their constituent tissues, cells and molecules" [2]. Thus, hypotheses need to be confirmed in intact, complex biological organisms – not prokaryotes or lower eukaryotes, but mammals.

"Gain of function" models may be achieved by overexpression of proteins in transgenic mice, and "loss of function" models achieved by targeted mutagenesis. These techniques, particularly targeted mutagenesis, allow investigators to change single variables and in essence perform controlled experiments in mammals. These models may help both to determine the physiologic function of proteins and to dissect mechanisms of disease. For example, overexpression or deletion of specific proteins may result in features that resemble human disease. Alternatively, application of established models of disease to gene-deficient mice may determine the contribution of individual proteins to the disease state.

Why the mouse? Just over a decade ago, techniques to achieve germline transmission of genetic material in mice drastically changed our ability to approach biological questions. Introduction of a linear DNA fragment (transgene) into the pronucleus of one-celled embryos (or more recently into embryonic stem cells) allows study of either the pattern of expression of that gene or the biological consequences of overexpression of the protein encoded by the gene in specific tissues. More recently, targeted mutagenesis by homologous recombination in embryonic stem cells has allowed investigators to generate strains of mice that lack individual proteins, providing specific "loss of function" models.

Advantages of the mouse over other experimental animals include the capacity to manipulate germline transmission of genetic information, a rapid reproductive cycle, and large litter sizes. In addition, knowledge of mouse biology is extensive, antibody and cDNA probes for the mouse are abundant, and mice are relatively cheap compared with other experimental animals. Most importantly, evolutionary conservation has shown us that mice and other mammals are, on the whole, genetically similar to humans. In the future, transgene expression in larger animals will allow large-scale production of recombinant proteins. The possibility of targeted mutagenesis in rat embryonic stem cells might allow investigators to study models of disease requiring surgical techniques that cannot be applied to mice.

2. Methods for Generating Transgenic Mice [3–6] (Fig. 1)

2.1. DNA Construct

For protein overexpression, the gene of interest or cDNA is linked to either a strong non-specific promoter or a cell-specific promoter for more precise targeting of gene expression. If a cDNA is used, inclusion of intronic sequences and a polyadenylation signal (often from growth hormone or other genes) is helpful [7, 8]. If the goal is to test promoter sequences required for gene regulation, promoter fragments are linked to reporter genes such as β-galactosidase. "Humanized" green fluorescent protein (GFP) may prove to be a promising marker, but data are limited to date [9].

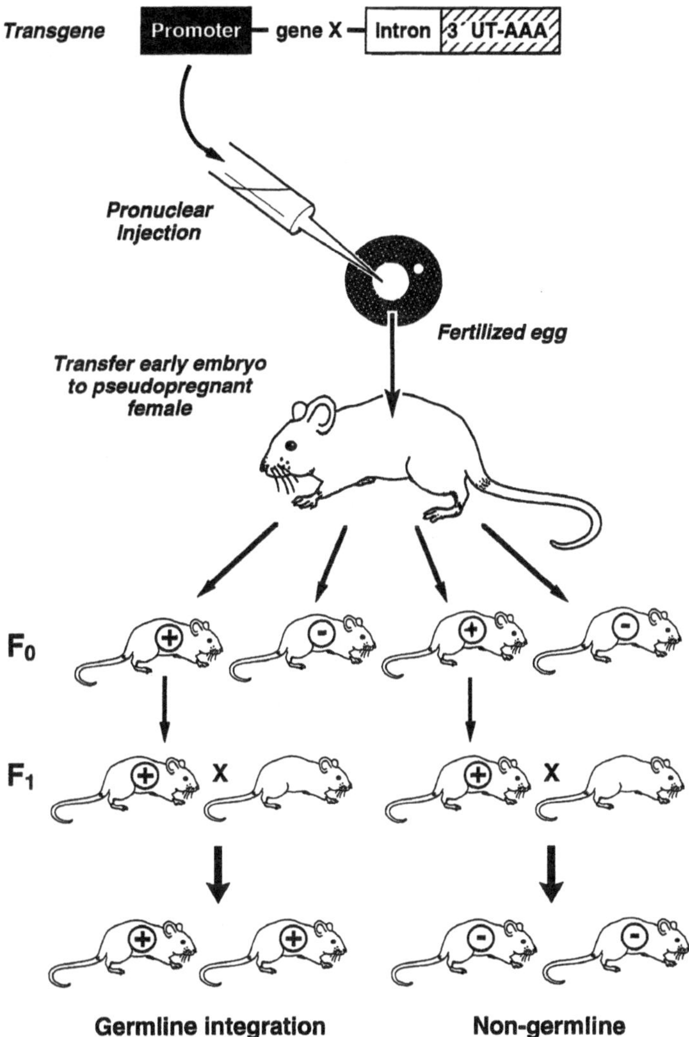

Figure 1. Generating transgenic mice: the transgene construct carrying the DNA required to generate a functional protein is microinjected into the (male) pronucleus of a fertilized egg. Eggs are placed in the uterine horns of "pseudopregnant" females. Founder line (F0) offspring carrying the transgene genomic are identified (+). F0 matings determine whether the transgene has been incorporated into the germline, and those transgenic +F1 mice are used for further studies.

2.2. Egg Microinjection

The goal of pronuclear microinjection of double-stranded DNA into fertilized mammalian eggs is to integrate the DNA into the genome, allowing transfer of the genetic material to offspring [10]. For this reason DNA is introduced into the zygote as early as possible, i. e. at the pronuclear stage soon after fertilization. Females are often treated with hormones (PMS and human chorionic gonadotropin or hCG) for superovulation upon fertilization with a fertile male. Eggs are harvested and small amounts of DNA (1–2 pl at 200 ng/μl) are injected directly into eggs which are then reimplanted into pseudopregnant females (which were mated with vasectomized males on the previous day). Of the eggs 15–20 are implanted into each oviduct; 20 days later gestation is complete. Offspring from this mating are termed founders (F0).

2.3. Generation of Lines of Transgenic Mice

Litter sizes vary depending upon strains of mice used and mothering abilities. Generally, if the gene is not fatal, about 15% of the offspring should carry the transgene DNA. Often the DNA is inserted from one to hundreds of copies as concatamers in a single random site within the genome. If the transgene has been stably incorporated into the genome of the germ cells, then F0 mice should transmit the transgene to all future offspring. As a result of the random nature of integration, several lines of transgenic mice should be bred to insure that the phenotype is independent of integration site. Although transgenic mice are easier to generate than gene-targeted mice, lack of reproducible cell-specific targeting has led some investigators to pursue "knock-in" strategies for targeted transgenesis as discussed below.

3. Generation of Gene-Targeted Mice

3.1. Targeting Constructs

The general general strategy is to isolate isogenic genomic DNA and either insert or replace exonic DNA of the gene of interest with a selectable marker, such as the neomycin phosphotransferase gene driven by the phosphoglycerol kinase promoter (PGK-neo). This will cause a mutation that prevents the generation of a functional protein, and it often results in loss of stable mRNA as well. Moreover, use of a positive selection marker will allow the selection of clones that allowed integration of the construct into chromosomal DNA as described below. Thymidine kinase (TK) is often included at the 5′- and/or 3′-end as a negative selection marker to prevent non-homologous recombination in the presence of gancyclovir.

Large fragments of isogenic genomic DNA are isolated and subcloned into plasmids for further manipulation. Many strategies are available to introduce selectable markers and generate mutations. A general rule of thumb is to have at least a couple of kilobases of native genomic sequence flanking both sides of the mutation: the longer the sequence, the greater

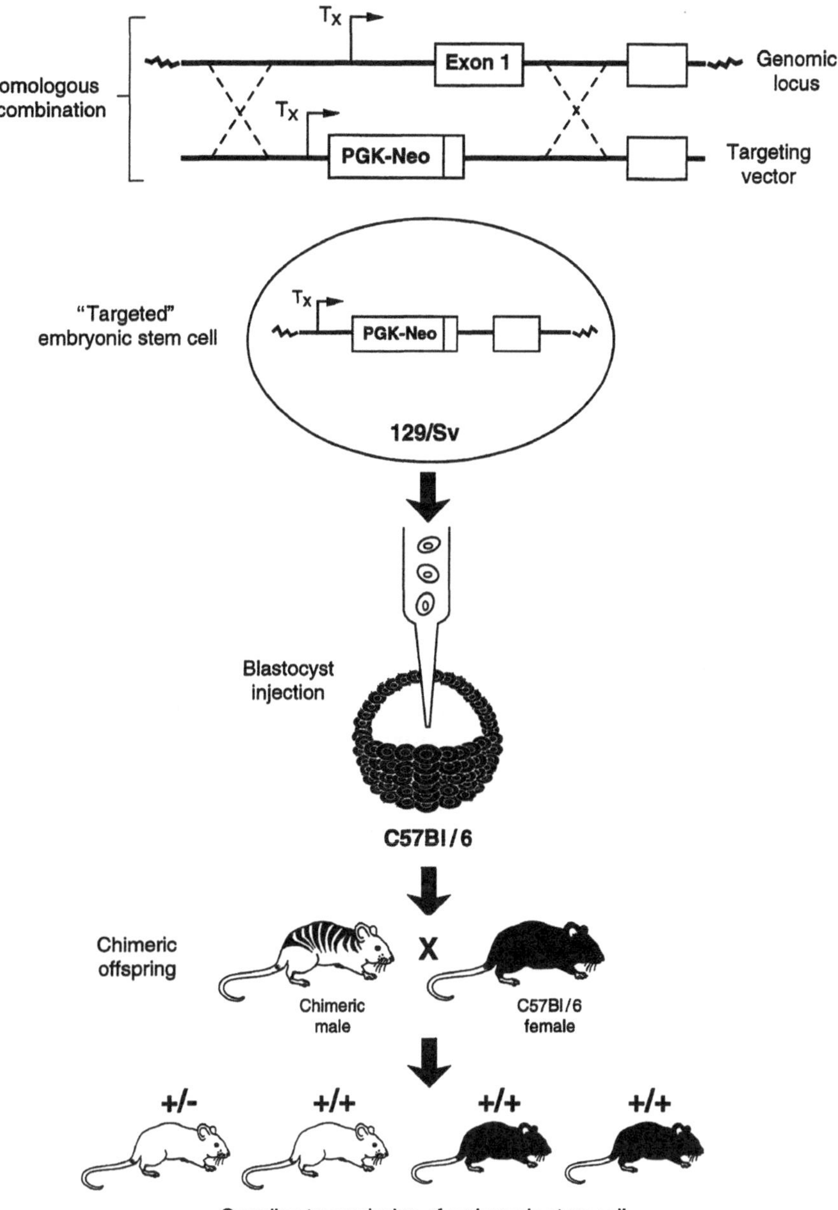

Figure 2. Generating gene-targeted mice: the targeting construct carrying a mutation with a positive selection marker, such as PGK-neo shown here inserted distal to the transcription start site (Tx) replacing part of exon 1, is transfected into embryonic stem (ES) cells (here of 129/Sv origin with agouti pigment). ES cells that have homologously incorporated the mutation are identified, injected into blastocysts (from C57B1/6 mice, black coat color), and implanted into receptive females. Chimeric offspring (i.e. agouti on black) are bred initially to C57B1/6, and germline transmission is determined by pure agouti mice resulting from this breeding. Heterozygotes are identified (one-half of agouti mice) and bred to generate mice homozygous deficient in the gene of interest.

the recombination frequency [11, 12]. A limit is the amount of DNA that can be subcloned into convenient plasmids. Sequence information and detailed restriction enzyme mapping are critical; however, strategies involving introduction of restriction enzyme site by *in vitro* mutagenesis are becoming a popular way for quickly generating constructs with less information. This strategy also allows the placement of mutations in precise areas of interest. For example, replacement of a sequence near (and including) the ATG translation-initiation codon for PGK-neo and another gene of interest should create both a knock-in and a knock-out mouse, i.e. in addition to deleting expression of the target tene, it is possible to achieve expression of the reporter gene in the genomic locus of the native gene. Thus, the reporter is now expressed under regulation, of the original gene which has been deleted. This may require subsequent deletion of the PGK-neo cassette using Lox P technology (see section 7. *The Next Generation*) because the PGK promoter might interfere with native gene regulation.

3.2. Gene Targeting in Embryonic Stem Cells

The targeting vectors are transfected into embryonic stem cells (ES cells) by electroporation [13]. ES cells are cultured in the presence of G418 to select only colonies that incorporated the neomycin-resistance gene by homologous recombination. Gancyclovir is often used for negative selection, killing clones that have undergone non-homologous recombination incorporating thymidine kinase. Clones that underwent appropriate homologous recombination are identified and confirmed by Southern analyses (using probes outside of the construct). Targeting frequency is highly variable, but generally ranges between 1% and 15%, i.e. of clones that underwent appropriate selection, only 1–15% will have undergone homologous recombination in the single site of integration.

3.3. Generation of Gene-Deficient Mice

Targeted ES clones (e.g. from 129/Sv mice that are agouti, i.e. have yellow coat pigment) are injected into blastocysts derived, for example, from C57B1/6 females (black color) and inserted into receptive females (often Swiss-Webster). Highly chimeric male pups, i.e. showing a significant amount of agouti, are raised and bred with C57B1/6 (and later 129/Sv) females. Pure agouti mice resulting from these matings demonstrate that the ES cell has been incorporated into the germline, one-half of which should carry the mutant allele. These heterozygous mice are then bred to obtain homozygous "knock outs", i.e. animals in which both alleles have been disrupted. It is also possible to breed chimeras that show a tendency to transmit the ES cell to the germline, to mice in the background of the ES cell to obtain mice in a pure genetic background quickly without laborious backcrossing.

4. Application of Transgenic and Gene-Targeted Mice to Pulmonary Disease

Mouse models have been used to duplicate diseases caused by simple single genetic mutations with varying success. For example, mutations in surfactant B are lethal in both mice and humans [14]. Decreased surfactant B levels in heterozygous mice led to disrupted lamellar body formation and abnormal lung function, similar to partial surfactant B deficiency that has recently been observed in infants [14]. In contrast, although CFTR–/– mice demonstrate severe gastrointestinal toxicity, pulmonary abnormalities were mild. CFTR–/– mice did, however, have increased numbers of goblet cells and inspissated eosinophilic secretions with gland obstruction [15]. As these mice age, there are some reports (unpublished) that they develop more severe pulmonary disease and poor response to infections. Others believe that mice have additional chloride transporters which may negate the results [16]. The identity and knock-out of these other proteins are under investigation.

Gene deletion has also resulted in surprising phenotypes, for example, the loss of granulocyte-macrophage colony-stimulating factor (GM-CSF) resulted in alveolar proteinosis in mice [17]. Transgenic mice expressing GM-CSF in the lung under the control of the surfactant C promoter in the background of GM-CSF–/– corrected surfactant homeostasis, leading to the conclusion that GM-CSF regulates clearance or catabolism of surfactant proteins and lipids [18].

Alternatively, application of transgenic mice to established murine models of disease may allow dissection of the pathogenesis of disease. Application of transgenic mice to specific diseases requires murine models of disease that replicate the human condition. Studies on emphysema will be used as an example.

4.1. Pulmonary Emphysema

This is defined as enlargement of terminal airspaces, accompanied by destruction of their walls. Typically, cigarette smoke induces a chronic inflammatory response with accumulation of macrophages and, to a much lesser extent, neutrophils in respiratory bronchioles and alveolar space. Release of inflammatory cell proteinases, in excess of inhibitors, coupled to abnormal matrix repair lead to emphysema. Inherited deficiency of α_1-antitrypsin, the primary inhibitor of neutrophil elastase – a serine proteinase –, predisposes individuals to early onset emphysema; in addition, intrapulmonary instillation of elastolytic enzymes such as neutrophil elastase in experimental animals causes lung destruction that is characteristic of emphysema. Together, these findings have led to the hypothesis that emphysema results from proteolytic injury, presumably by neutrophil elastase directed against elastin [19]. Subsequently, other elastolytic proteinases of neutrophil and macrophage origin have been found in the lungs of smokers. If mice develop emphysema in response to chronic cigarette smoke in a similar way to humans, in a reasonable time frame, then it would be possible to use targeted mutagenesis to determine the contribution of these proteinases to emphysema.

On long-term exposure to cigarette smoke, mice develop inflammation within a month and airspace enlargement characteristic of human centriacinar emphysema within 6 months [20]. Application of mice deficient in macrophage elastase (MME–/–) by targeted mutagenesis [21] to this exposure demonstrated that, in contrast to wild-type littermates, mice deficient in macrophage elastase (MME-12) failed to recruit macrophages and did not develop pulmonary emphysema in response to cigarette smoke exposure [20] (Figure 3). Whether human emphysema is also dependent on this single MMP is of course uncertain. At the very least, this study demonstrates a critical role of macrophages in the development of emphysema and unmasks a proteinase-dependent mechanism of inflammatory cell recruitment which may have broader biological implications.

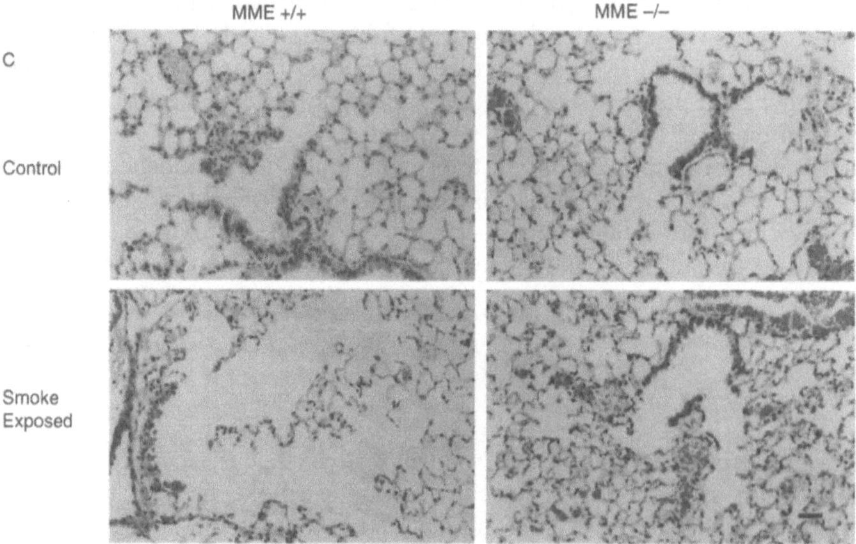

Figure 3. Wild-type (MME+/+) mice, but not MME-deficient (MME–/–) mice, develop emphysema in response to cigarette smoke. Lungs from MME+/+ and MME–/– mice exposed to cigarette smoke for 6 months and age-matched controls were inflated by intratracheal administration of 10% formalin under constant pressure (25 cmH_2O). After fixation, hematoxylin and eosin-stained midsagittal sections were prepared. Note, the MME+/+ smoke-exposed lung has centriacinar dilatation of alveolar ducts compared with the control. MME–/– lungs of smoke-exposed mice resemble control lungs. (Bar = 48 μm).

Alternatively, overexpression of interstitial collagenase, another matrix metalloproteinase, also led to airspace enlargement in transgenic mice [22]. In this study a human collagenase-1 (MMP-1) transgene driven by the haptoglobin reporter unexpectedly resulted in lung-specific expression in several independent founder lines. These mice developed enlarged airspaces characteristic of emphysema. Also, as MMP-1 is inactive against mature elastin, this result suggested that collagen degradation was sufficient to cause emphysema. However, it is not certain whether the alveolar pathology in these animals was the result of destruction of collagen in mature lung tissue or whether expression of the transgene during growth and development interfered with normal elastic fiber assembly, perhaps through destruction of the elastic fiber microfibrillar scaffold. Also, as opposed to application of a disease model to gene-deficient mice, this type of study demonstrated that a particular protein, when overexpressed, can result in pathology similar to the disease of interest, but it cannot necessarily be concluded that this particular protein is involved in disease pathogenesis.

5. Limitations of Transgenic Technology

5.1. Transgenic Mice

Successful application of classic pronuclear microinjection of transgenes presumes that cell-specific expression will be directed by regulatory sequences within the transgene, independent of the site of chromosomal integration. Multiple founder lines are required to verify integration-independent expression. Occasionally, unexpected findings, such as the haptoglobin promoter specifically directing expression in the lung, can yield interesting results, at the expense of negating the original aim. Another limitation of transgenics is the uncontrolled expression of the transgene during development, a particular problem for toxic proteins such as proteinases, unless embryonic development is the focus of study.

5.2. Targeted Mutagenesis

Lack of expression of a critical protein during embryonic development may be lethal, confirming the importance of the protein, but limiting further studies. Alternatively, gene deletion may fail to result in a phenotype. Several explanations have been proposed to explain the lack of an expected phenotype [23]:

1. Loss of a gene could upregulate a *compensatory* pathway regulated by a common feedback mechanism.

2. *Redundancy* or co-expression of proteins with overlapping function as a means of guarding against loss of an individual protein.
3. The protein may have a modest but non-vital function, thus providing a small reproductive advantage and becoming fixed in the genome, although undetectable by gene deletion.
4. Economics of gene control: a protein may be expressed in tissue where it has no function at all. Although this appears to be a waste of energy, perhaps the price of individual gene regulation is greater than maintaining common control elements.

This last explanation seems unlikely for proteinases and other proteins where expression could be harmful at inappropriate sites.

5.3. Of Mice and Men

The capacity to extrapolate findings from transgenic/gene-disrupted mice to human biology is limited by differences in protein profiles between the two species. Knowledge of protein expression in mice is only now emerging for many protein families, making detailed comparison with humans premature. The more were appreciate the similarities and differences between mice and humans, the better use we can make of transgenic technology to understand human biology. Nevertheless, findings in mice may teach us much about biological mechanisms regardless of whether identical proteins subserve these functions in humans.

Another potential limitation in extrapolating transgenic results to the human condition relates to the differences between mouse and human biology. Although general biological principles are maintained among all mammals, differences clearly exist. With respect to pulmonary emphysema for example, mouse lungs differ subtly from humans. Rodents do have few mucous glands in the larger airways, and they lack respiratory bronchioles. Nevertheless, in response to chronic exposure to cigarette smoke, they develop characteristic inflammation followed by acinar enlargement that characterizes the human disease.

6. Know Your Mouse

The considerations above represent inherent limitations of transgenic technology. There are other factors that can lead to erroneous interpretation of results which the investigator can control. One should be aware of the following.

6.1. Strain Differences

Many null mutations are generated using 129/Sv embryonic stem cells injected into C57B1/6 blastocysts. This strategy allows investigators to follow coat pigment to assess, targeting. These strains, which are both derived from the same major histocompatibility complex (MHC) background, are quite similar. However, they differ in response to several stimuli and in several disease models, such as susceptibility to certain infectious agents. Transgenic mice may be obtained in many genetic backgrounds, usually chosen on the basis of breeding and mothering capabilities. To complicate matters further, some disease models are strain specific, such as the experimental autoimmune encephalomyelitis model of multiple sclerosis in SJL/J mice or the collagen-induced arthritis model in DBA1 mice. Strategies are available to generate mice with these backgrounds initially or to breed genetically engineered mice laboriously into the appropriate strains. One should also be aware of breeding strategies employed in studies. If a mixed background is used, wild-type (or heterozygous) littermates are ideal controls for knock-out mice. This will limit the "genetic drift" which may occur over time.

6.2. "Neighborhood Knockouts"

An interesting yet disturbing problem is the finding that standard gene-targeting techniques many influence expression of linked genes. Targeting of the myogenic basic helix-loop-helix gene and some *Hox* gene family members, for example, resulted in decreased expression of neighboring genes [24]. With respect to proteinases, a targeted mutation in the T cell serine proteinase granzyme B demonstrated that this proteinase was critial for T cell cytotoxicity [25]. Subsequent sequencing of the granzyme B genomic locus, combined with S1 nuclease protection assays of neighboring granzymes, demonstrated decreased expression of neighboring granzymes (within about 75 kilobases or kb) in activated T cells of –/– mice compared with wild type (Ley, unpublished data).

One potential explanation for neighborhood knockouts is that the PGK promoter, often inserted to drive an antibiotic resistance gene and disrupt native genomic sequences (see Figure 1), interacts with long-range locus control elements, acting as a transcriptional "sink" and interfering with expression of the linked genes. Whatever the mechanism, one must interpret results of knockout studies with some caution, because in most cases the genomic loci are not well defined, and expression of linked genes is rarely tested. Techniques to remove these promoter elements in ES cells are available and may be required in some circumstances (see below).

7. The Next Generation

Techniques are rapidly being developed to make mutations specifically when and where desired (Figure 4). Making use of the bacteriophage Cre recombinase, which lines up and removes sequences bracketed by Lox P sites, Rajewsky and colleagues developed "conditional knockouts" that deleted the DNA polymerase β gene (flanked by Lox P sites) specifically in T cells that were engineered to express the Cre recombinase [26]. Subsequently, they developed "inducible knockouts" [27]. Again, mice were

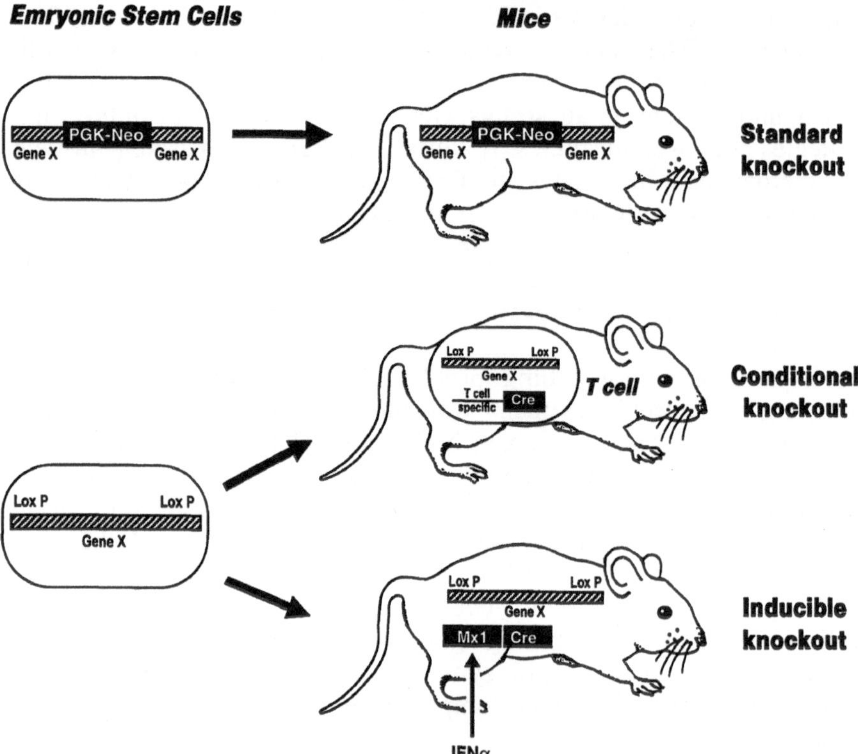

Figure 4. Strategies to delete genes in mice: to perform standard targeted mutagenesis, an antibiotic resistance gene, such as the neomycin resistance gene driven by the phosphoglycerate kinase (PGK) promoter is often inserted or used to replace native exonic sequences of the gene of interest (gene X). This mutation in embryonic stem cells renders the gene inactive in all cells throughout development and adult life. Conditional knockouts achieve cell-specific gene deletion by flanking the native gene (gene X) with Lox P sites which should not interfere with expression of the gene of interest. When these mice are crossed with a transgenic mouse expressing Cre recombinase under cell-specific control, the gene is excised only in those cells expressing Cre (such as the T cell shown above). Inducible knockouts use the same strategy as conditional knockouts, but instead these mice are crossed with transgenic mice expressing an inducible promoter driving Cre – in this case the IFN-α inducible promoter Mx1 [27]. (Reproduced with permission from Shapiro [1]).

targeted with intact polymerase β flanked by Lox P sites and crossed with transgenic mice expressing interferon-α (IFN-α)-inducible Mx1 sequences linked to Cre recombinase. Upon treatment with IFN-α, Cre was produced, deleting the gene of interest. Use of Cre/Lox P in ES cells will also allow investigators to "knock-in" virtually any gene into the genomic locus and put it under regulatory control of any other gene [29]. This technology may also be used to remove potentially troublesome PGK-neo from traditional knockouts.

Other methods include use of the FLP recombinase (a yeast enzyme similar to Cre) which removes sequences flanked by "frt" . Although this system does not appear to work well in ES cells, it may offer an effective way to remove repressor sequences, allowing inducible overexpression of genes in transgenic mice. Inducible transgenes may also be achieved using ecdysone, an insect steroid hormone, which, when bound to its (transgenic) hormone receptor, translocates to the nucleus and binds to *cis*-acting DNA sequences, inducing expression of a transgene. Tetracycline is widely used to induce transgenes as well. Use of inducible, cell-specific expression may overcome inherent problems associated with transgene overexpression during development, making studies on mature mice more feasible. In summary, methods are rapidly being developed to overexpress and delete genes under both spatial and temporal control. Unlimited possibilities will soon be practical, limited only by the investigator's imagination and resources.

8. Future Challenges

Before long, all human genes will be identified. Use of transgenic technology will be important to determine protein function in physiology and pathology. Lack of an obvious phenotype upon gene deletion may be secondary to redundancy and multiple knockouts may be required for the expected phenotype; however, the mice may have to be "stressed" to bring out the function of a particular protein. Lethal phenotypes confirm the importance of a particular protein but currently negate further investigation. Conditional knockouts late in postnatal development will overcome this limitation. Murine models of disease will be required to test the putative roles of proteins in various disease states. For the best application of the findings from these studies to human physiology and pathology, we must appreciate the similarities and differences between mice and humans. Nevertheless, transgenic and gene-deficient mice offer unique opportunities to perform controlled experimens in complex biological organisms. These studies will certainly lead to more unexpected findings and definitively demonstrate many exciting functions of individual proteins thereby dissecting mechanisms of lung disease.

References

1 Shapiro SD (1997) Mighty mice: transgenic technology "knocks out" questions of matrix metalloproteinase function. *Matrix Biol* 15: 527–533
2 Piagen K (1995) A miracle enough: the power of mice. *Nature Med* 1: 215–220
3 Hogan B, Constantini F, Lacy E (1986) *Manipulating the Mouse Embryo*, A Laboratory Manual. Cold Spring Harbor Laboratory, Plainview, NY
4 Green EL (ed) and the Jackson Laboratory Staff (1975) *Biology of the Laboratory Mouse*. Dover Publications, Dover, NY
5 *Handbook of Genetrically Standardized Jax Mice*, The Jackson Laboratory, Bar Harbor Maine, 1987
6 Rafferty RA (1970) *Methods in experimental embryology of the mouse*. The Johns Hopkins Press, Baltimore
7 Brinster RL, Chen HY, Trunbauer ME, Yagle MK, Palmiter RD (1985) Factors affecting the efficiency of introducing foreign DNA into mice by microinjecting eggs. *Proc Natl Acad Sci USA* 82: 4438–4442
8 Brinster RL, Allen JM, Behringer RR, Gelinas RE, Palmiter RD (1988) Introns increase transcriptional efficiency in transgenic mice. *Proc Natl Acad Sci USA* 85: 836–840
9 Chiocchetti A, Tolosano E, Hirsch E, Silengo L, Altruda F (1977) Green fluorescent protein as a reporter of gene expression in transgenic mice. *Biochem Biophys Acta* 1352: 193–202
10 Gordon JW, Ruddle FH (1981) Integration and stable germline transmission of genes injected into mouse pronuclei. *Science* 214: 1244–1246
11 Bradley A (1991) Modifying the mammalian genome by gene targeting. *Curr Opin Biotechnol* 2: 823–829
12 Thomas KR, Deng C, Capecchi MR (1992) High-fidelity gene targeting in embryonic stem cells by using sequence replacement vectors. *Mol Cell Biol* 12: 2919–2923
13 Robertson EJ (ed) (1987) *Tetratocarcinomas and Embryonic Stem Cells: A Practical Approach*. IRL Press, Oxford
14 Clark JC, Wert SE, Bachurski CJ, Stahlman MT, Stripp BR, Weaver TE, Whitsett JA (1995) Targeted disruption of the surfactant protein B gene disrupts surfactant homeostasis, causing respiratory failure in newborn mice. *Proc Natl Acad Sci USA* 92: 7794–7798
15 Dorin JR, Dickenson P, Alten EW, Smith SN, Gelles DM, Stevenson BJ, Kimber WL, Fleming S, Clarke AR, Hooper ML (1992) Cystic fibrosis in the mouse by targeted insertional mutagenesis. *Nature* 359: 211–215
16 Clarke LL, Grubb BR, Yankaskas JR, Cotton CU, McKenzie A, Boucher RC (1994) Relationship of a non-cystic fibrosis transmembrane conductance regulator-mediated chloride conductance to organ-level disease in Cftr(–/–) mice. *Proc Natl Acad Sci USA* 91: 479–483
17 Dranoff G, Crawford AD, Sadelain M, Ream B, Rashid A, Bronson RT, Dickersin GR, Bachurski CJ, Mark EL, Whitsett JA (1994) Involvement of granulocyte-macrophage colony-stimulating factor in pulmonary homeostasis. *Science* 264: 713–716
18 Huffman JA, Hull WM, Dranoff G, Mulligan RC, Whitsett JA (1996) Pulmonary epithelial cell expression of GM-CSF corrects the alveolar proteinosis in GM-CSF-deficient mice. *J Clin Invest* 97: 649–655
19 Snider GI (1992) Emphysema: the first two centuries – and beyond: a historical overview with suggestions for future research: Parts 1 and 2. *Am Rev Respir Dis* 146: 1334–1344; 1615–1622
20 Hautamaki RD, Kobayashi DK, Senior RM, Shapiro SD (1977) Macrophage elastase is required for cigarette smoking induced emphysema in mice. *Science* 277: 2002–2004
21 Shipley JM, Wesselschmidt RL, Kobayashi DK, Ley TJ, Shapiro SD (1996) Metalloelastase is required for macrophage-mediated proteolysis and matrix invasion in mice. *Proc Natl Acad Sci USA* 93: 3942–3946
22 D'Armiento J, Dalal SS, Okada Y, Berg RA, Chada K (1992) Collagenase expression in the lungs of transgenic mice causes pulmonary emphysema. *Cell* 71: 955–961
23 Erickson HP (1993) Gene knockouts of c-src, transforming growth factor β1, and tenascin suggest superfluous, nonfunctional expression of proteins. *J Cell Biol* 120: 1079–1081
24 Olson EN, Arnold HH, Rigby PWJ, Wold BJ (1996) Know your neighbors: Three phenotypes in null mutants of the myogenic bHLH gene MRF4. *Cell* 85: 1–4

25 Heusel JW, Wesselschmidt RL, Shresta S, Russell JH, Ley TJ (1994) Cytotoxic lymphocytes require granzyme B for the rapid induction of DNA fragmentation and apoptosis in allogeneic target cells. *Cell* 76: 989–1000
26 Gu H, Marth JD, Orban PC, Mossmann H, Rajewsky K (1994) Deletion of a DNA polymerase β gene segment in T cells using cell type-specific gene targeting. *Science* 265: 103–106
27 Kuhn R, Schwenk F, Auguet M, Rajewsky K (1995) Inducible gene targeting in mice. *Science* 269: 1427–1429
28 Wang Y, Schnegelsberg PN, Dausman J, Jaenisch R (1996) Functional redundancy of the muscle-specific transcription factors and myogenin. *Nature* 379: 823–825
29 Barinaga M (1994) Knockout mice: Round two. *Science* 265: 26–28

Emphysema

Molecular Biology of the Lung
Vol. 1: Emphysema and Infection
ed. by R. A. Stockley

CHAPTER 2
Models of Genetic Emphysema: The C57Bl/6J Mice and their Mutants: Tight-Skin, Pallid and Beige

Giuseppe Lungarella, Eleonora Cavarra and Piero A. Martorana

Institute of General Pathology, University of Siena, Siena, Italy

1. Introduction

Emphysema is a slow progressive disease which is defined in anatomical terms as “a condition of the lung characterized by abnormal, permanent enlargement of airspaces distal to the terminal bronchiole, accompanied by the destruction of their walls, and without obvious fibrosis” [1]. A generally accepted hypothesis for the pathogenesis of emphysema is that the lung destruction results from an imbalance between elastolytic proteases (particularly neutrophil elastase) released by inflammatory cells in the peripheral lung, and their naturally occurring inhibitors (i.e. α_1-proteinase inhibitor (α_1-PI)). In humans, this imbalance is usually the result of a deficiency in antiprotease screen, which can be either genetic (α_1-PI deficiency) or acquired (i.e. inactivation of α_1-PI by cigarette smoke) in origin [2–4].

The most common means of producing experimental emphysema consists of an instillation of a large dose of a protease with elastolytic activity into the lungs of laboratory animals. This alters the protease/antiprotease balance in the peripheral lung in favour of the protease, and results in anatomical emphysema [5, 6]. Although this model has provided significant biochemical, morphological, and physiological data, it has limited usefulness [7].

There is thus the need for an animal model of genetic serum α_1-PI deficiency. In the mouse, the two major serum proteinase inhibitors are α_1-PI and contrapsin. The former inhibits neutrophil elastase and cathepsin G; the latter, which does not correspond to any of the known serum protease inhibitors characterized in humans, inhibits only trypsin. Both these two inhibitors are synthesized and secreted by hepatocytes. The α_1-PI and contrapsin genes are members of two different multigene families, each containing at least three genes, closely linked on chromosome 12 [8–11].

Recently, the mouse strain C57Bl/6J and three of its mutants – the tight-skin, pallid and beige mice – have been reported to have a deficiency in serum α_1-PI and to develop spontaneous emphysema. However, the time course for the development of emphysema is very different in these strains of mice, and the factors that participate in the development of this lesion are not fully known. Investigation of the development of the lung lesion in these strains of mice may provide helpful information for the study of the pathogenesis of emphysema and/or for testing therapeutic interventions. The present work is a review of the literature on these mouse models of genetic emphysema.

2. The C57Bl/6J Mouse

2.1. Background

Mice of the strain C57Bl/6J are highly inbred and known to be weaned at 3 weeks, to have initial fertile mating at 6–10 weeks and to have a mean lifespan of 22.8 months [12]. The phenotype has a black coat with black eyes. Compared with other inbred strains, C57Bl/6J mice have a low incidence of spontaneous tumours, and no tendency to die with a particular type of gross pathology [12]. This strain is widely used in many fields of biological research.

2.2. *Antiprotease Screen*

In a study investigating the mouse antiprotease screen, α_1-PI was isolated from mouse serum by a series of electrophoretic and chromatographic steps. Using an immunological quantification, it was found that α_1-PI concentration in serum differed among inbred strains, and that female mice always had lower concentrations than male mice. Among the strains tested, α_1-PI had the highest serum concentration in DBA/2J mice (males 8.5 ± 0.87; females 4.09 ± 0.51 mg/ml) and the lowest in C57Bl/6J mice (males 5.58 ± 0.71; females 3.02 ± 0.39 mg/ml) [13]. In another study, Gardi et al., using single radial immunodiffusion, found, in serum of various strains of male mice, high values in the NMRI (5.7 ± 0.5 mg/ml) and Balb/c (5.9 ± 12 0.5 mg/ml) mice, and low values in the C57Bl/6J (4.4 ± 0.3 mg/ml) mice. The serum elastase inhibitory capacity (EIC) values in these animals correlated highly with the α_1-PI data, whereas the serum trypsin inhibitory capacity (TIC) values did not [14].

These studies confirm that in the mouse α_1-PI is mainly responsible for the serum EIC and show that females have lower serum α_1-PI values than males. Also female C57Bl/6J mice have 26% less serum α_1-PI than females of other strains. The deficiency of the male C57Bl/6J mice ranges between – 23% and – 34%.

2.3. *Neutrophil Lysosomal Functions and Lung Elastase Burden*

Elastase has been localized in neutrophils of NMRI, Balb/c and C57Bl/6J mice using electron microscopy and an immunogold-labelling technique with rabbit anti-mouse leukocyte elastase (MLE) IgG. No apparent difference in gold particle density was observed between C57Bl/6J mice and the other two strains of mice [14]. Also, similar levels of elastase and cathepsin G activites were found in lysosomal neutrophil extracts from C57Bl/6J, NMRI and Balb/c mice [14]. In addition, when neutrophils from these strains of mice were tested for their ability to release lysosomal enzymes after stimulation with N-formyl-L-methionyl-L-leucyl-L-phenylalanine (FMLP)/cytochalasin b, no difference in elastase, cathepsin G and β-glucuronidase activities was found among the strains [14]. Thus, neutrophil lysosomal functions are similar in C57Bl/6J mice and in mice with normal serum levels of α_1-PI.

The lung neutrophil elastase burden was investigated in another study by means of an immunogold method, in thin lung sections prepared for electron microscopy using anti-MLE antibodies. Very few colloidal gold particles were found in association with the connective tissue of the alveolar walls of α_1-PI-deficient (C57Bl/6J) as well as of non-α_1-PI-deficient (NMRI) mice (0.6 ± 0.8 and 0.7 ± 0.8 particles/µm^2 respectively) [15]. Thus, the deficiency in α_1-PI in C57Bl/6J mice does not result in an increase in lung elastase burden.

2.4. Lung Elastin Content

There is one report that compares lung elastin content in C57Bl/6J mice and in mice that are not deficient in serum α_1-PI. The content, assessed as micrograms of elastin per lung, was found to be similar in C57Bl/6J and NMRI mice (166±7 and 170±12 µg/lung respectively) [15].

2.5. Emphysema

To our knowledge there is only one study, presented in abstract form, about the appearance of spontaneous emphysema in C57Bl/6J mice. The lungs of six male and six female, 30 month-old, C57Bl/6J mice were compared with those of DBA/2N mice (a strain with high serum levels of α_1-PI) of the same age and sex. A pathological score showed a definite trend towards emphysematous changes in the lungs of the C57Bl/6J mice. Also, measurement of the mean linear intercept (*L*m) revealed a small, but significant, increase in the lungs of the male C57Bl/6J mice compared with the corresponding controls (46.2±5.4 and 39.0±4.3 µm, respectively) [16]. In another study in which the lungs of C57Bl/6J mice were investigated by means of light microscopy and scanning electron microscopy, at 1, 12, and 24 months of age, no emphysema was seen at any time in life [17] (Figure 1a). The difference in age of the mice, and possible bouts of infections occurring in senescent animals, may explain the discrepancy between these two studies.

The role played by the polymorphonuclear leukocytes (PMN) in the development of emphysema in C57Bl/6J mice was investigated by Cavarra et al. [15]. C57Bl/6J and NMRI mice had FMLP instilled intratracheally. Both strains of mice showed a similar influx of PMNs in alveolar spaces with an increase (about four- to five-fold) in bronchoalveolar lavage total cell count, which peaked at 24–48 hours. At this time, differential cell count in both strains revealed an approximately 40-fold increase in neutrophils. Fourteen days after FMLP treatment, a significant increase in neutrophil elastase burden in the alveolar interstitium (assessed by the immunogold technique) was seen in both strains of mice. However, the value found in the C57Bl/6J mice was almost three times greater than that of the NMRI mice (9.9±1.2 *vs.* 3.8±1.5 particles/µm^2). This was followed in the C57Bl/6J, but not in the NMRI mice, by a decrease in lung elastin content (−17%), and by the development of significant emphysema (*L*m +28%). Similarly, Starcher and Williams [18], instilled endotoxin intratracheally in C57Bl/6J mice once a week for 10 weeks. Endotoxin caused a rapid influx of neutrophils into the lungs, reaching a maximum after 18 hours and remaining elevated for another 30 hours. After 10 weeks there were histological signs of alveolar wall damage and the *L*m was increased by 30%.

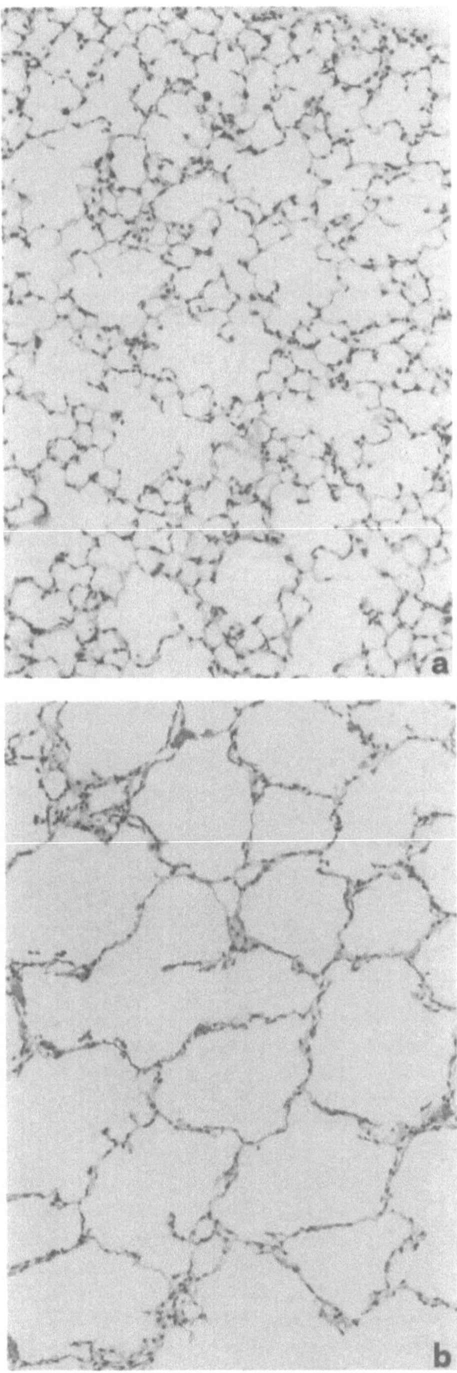

Figure 1. (**a**) Well-fixed normal lung parenchyma of a 24-month-old C57Bl/6J mouse. Haematoxylin and eoxin (H & E), original magnification × 32. (**b**) Marked diffuse emphysema of a 24-month-old-tight-skin mouse. H & E, original magnification × 32.

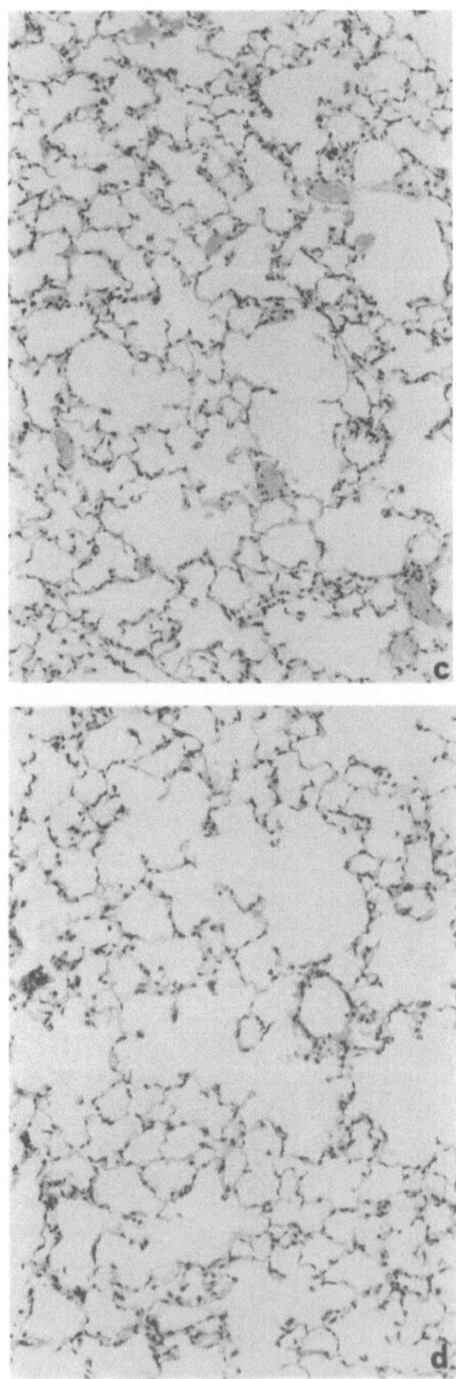

Figure 1. (**c**) Patchy areas of emphysema in a 24-month-old pallid mouse. H & E, original magnification × 32. (**d**) Loose lung parenchymal net of a 24-month-old beige mouse. H & E, original magnification × 32.

These studies indicate that the C57Bl/6J mice, probably as a result of their partial deficiency in serum α_1-PI, develop emphysema after recruitment and activation of PMNs into their lungs. In addition, they may develop spontaneous emphysema at a very advanced age.

3. The Tight-Skin Mouse

3.1. Background

The tight-skin (*Tsk)* mutation was discovered in the inbred B10.D2 (58N)/Sn strain at the Jackson Laboratory in 1976 by Bunker [19], who recognized that the mice were abnormal by the tightness of the skin over the shoulders when she attempted to pick them up. The *Tsk* mutation is caused by an autosomal dominant gene. Homozygous *Tsk*/*Tsk* embryos die *in utero* at approximately 8 days of gestation, whereas *Tsk*/+ heterozygous mice have a normal survival rate. The *Tsk* gene is located on chromosome 2 very close (about 2 cM) to the visible parker *pa* (pallid). This allowed the construction of a stock with a genetic C57Bl/6J background by mating *Tsk*/+ with *pa*/*pa* (C57Bl/6J *Tsk*+/+*pa*). The phenotype of the C57Bl/6J *Tsk*+/+*pa* mice has black coat, black eyes, tightness of the skin, increased thoracic size with a hunchback position, and enlarged lungs [19].

The *Tsk* gene is associated with a tandem duplication of the fibrillin I (*FbnI*) gene which results in a larger than normal in-frame *FbnI* transcript. As the FbnI protein participates in microfibril assembly and provides a structural basis for microfibril formation, the *FbnI* mutation may be responsible for the connective tissue alterations seen in these mice [20].

The *Tsk* mouse has been proposed as a model for various human diseases associated with abnormalities of the connective tissue. It has been used as a model for scleroderma [21, 22], congenital fascial dystrophy (stiff skin syndrome) [23], abnormal wound healing [24, 25] and myocardial fibrosis [26, 27]. The *Tsk* mouse is also used as a model for autoimmune diseases [28, 29]. However, the autoimmune abnormalities appear to occur subsequent to the development of the connective tissue alterations [30].

3.2. Antiprotease Screen

The serum of *Tsk* mice has a low EIC against the homologous elastase (– 66% compared with either NMRI or Balb/c mice) [14, 31]. This is probably the result of the low levels of serum α_1-PI (–53% *vs.* either NMRI or Balb/c mice) found in these mice [14].

3.3. Neutrophil Lysosomal Functions and Lung Elastase Burden

Abnormally high levels of elastase and cathepsin G have been found in neutrophils of *Tsk* mice. When neutrophils of *Tsk* and control (NMRI and Balb/c) mice were stimulated with FMLP/cytochalasin b, the highest enzyme activities for elastase and cathepsin G (in the presence of normal levels of β-glucuronidase) were found in the incubation medium for *Tsk*. This feature may be accounted for by the high levels of elastase and cathepsin G in neutrophil lysosomes of this strain [14].

The high neutrophil elastase levels correlate well with the high elastase burden (9.6 ± 2.0 gold particles/μm^2) found in the alveolar septa of these mice (Figure 2). This is 16 times the value found in control mice (0.6 ± 0.8 gold particles/μm^2) [32].

3.4. Lung Elastin Content

This parameter was investigated in *Tsk* and control mice at 4 days, and at 1 and 2 months of life. At 4 days after birth no changes were seen. At 1 month of age there was a marked decrease in lung insoluble elastin content (–48% *vs.* controls), with a further slight decrease at 2 months (–58%) [33].

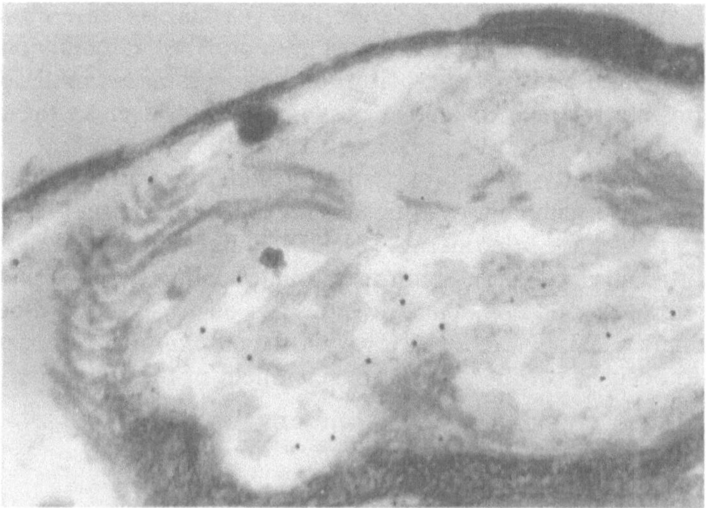

Figure 2. Alveolar wall from a 2-month-old *Tsk* mouse after immunolocalization with anti-mouse leukocyte elastase antibodies. Colloidal gold particles are present on lung interstitium. Uranyl acetate and lead citrate, original magnification × 34000.

3.5. Emphysema

In their original description of this mutant, Green et al. reported that the lungs of the *Tsk* mice were enlarged [19]. A few years later Szapiel et al. [34] and Rossi et al. [35] made a morphological investigation of the *Tsk* lungs. They observed a generalized enlargement of airspaces, with markedly thinned or broken alveolar walls, and an increase in size of the pores of Kohn. These morphological changes were accompanied by increases in total lung capacity and static compliance. On the basis of these findings the *Tsk* mouse was proposed as a model of genetically determined emphysema. Martorana et al. [36], in a morphometric study, reported three main phases in the evolution of emphysema in *Tsk* mice. The first phase, from 4 days to 2 months after birth, included enlargement of the peripheral lung units, evident at 4 and 15 days, and destruction of the lung parenchyma, which occurred between 15 days and 1 month and rapidly progressed up to 2 months. A second phase of stabilization or of mild progression of the emphysematous lesion occurred between 2 and 8 months of age. A third phase, between 8 and 16 months of age, included a further exacerbation of the parenchymal destruction (Figure 1 b).

A scanning electron microscopic study of the lungs 1-, 12-, and 24-month-old *Tsk* mice revealed that at all ages the parenchyma was distorted with enlargement of alveolar ducts and sacs, and with alveoli with a large number of pores. These changes increased with age. The number of alveolar pores was larger than the controls at all ages (+59% at 1 month, +119% at 12 months, and +80% at 24 months) [17].

Biochemical analysis of the lungs of 4-day-old and 1- and 2-month-old *Tsk* mice revealed no changes at 4 days but a significant increase of salt-extractable collagen at 1 and 2 months of age [33]. In a subsequent study, the values of lung collagen at 6 and 12 months of age were only moderately but significantly increased with respect to those observed at 2 months. As a consequence, because of the ongoing parenchymal destruction, a progressive accumulation of lung collagen was observed in the residual septa. The increase in collagen deposition was accompanied by a relative increase in type I collagen. The authors interpreted these data to indicate that a change in lung collagen metabolism may be part of a remodelling process taking place during and after lung destruction [37].

In the literature there has been a controversy over the role played by an elastolytic process in the development of emphysema. Starcher and James [38] crossed *Tsk* mice with beige (*bg*) mice that were thought to lack neutrophil elastase and cathepsin G. As the cross *Tsk*+/+*bg* developed emphysema, it was concluded that these two proteases could not be the cause of the lesion. On the other hand, Keil et al. [17] and Cavarra et al. [39] argued that because (1) heterozygous mice from a cross between *bg* and various strains do not show intermediate but rather normal levels of elastase and cathepsin G [40], (2) normal amounts of cathepsin G are secreted by *bg* neutrophils and elastase, present in a latent form in *bg* neutrophils, undergoes spontaneous activation when released *in vivo* [39], and (3) in the *bg* mice themselves develop spontaneous emphysema [17, 18], the results obtained with the *Tsk+/+bg* cross could not be used to rule out a role for an elastolytic process.

Probably, both an elastolytic process and the inborn defect of connective tissue play a role in the development of emphysema in *Tsk* mice [31] which may help to explain its very rapid appearance.

In *Tsk* mice, emphysema is followed by the development of right ventricular hypertrophy. This starts to develop in mature to senescent animals between 8 and 16 months of age and progresses thereafter. At 24 months of age the right ventricle left ventricle weight ratio is 60% greater than in control mice [41, 42]. A parallel study indicated a dynamic role for cardiac collagen both before and during the development of right ventricular hypertrophy secondary to emphysema [43].

4. The Pallid Mouse

4.1. Background

The pallid (*pa*) mutation was first discovered in a wild mouse [44] and was placed on a C57Bl/6J background by repeated crossing [45]. The only difference between the congenic C57Bl/6J *pa/pa* mouse and a normal C57Bl/6J+/+ is the *pa* gene on chromosome 2 [19, 46, 47]. The mutation is inherited in an autosomal recessive fashion and the *pa/pa* phenotype has a very light colour coat (pallid), red eyes, a defect of kidney and neutrophil lysosomal enzyme secretion [14, 47], and platelet granule defects [47].

4.2. Antiprotease Screen

The EIC of *pa*, C57Bl/6J and BALB/c mice was investigated against MLE. At 4 days of age the mice of the BALB/s strain had the highest EIC value. The serum of the C57Bl/6J mice exhibited a significantly lower value (–26%), whereas that of the *pa* mice had the lowest value of all (–71% compared with the value for the BALB/c mice, and –60% compared with the C57Bl/6J mice). Similar results were obtained at 2 months of age. In all strains of mice serum EIC levels did not change significantly during the course of their life [49]. On the other hand, serum TIC showed similar values in all strains [14]. As mentioned at the start of this chapter, the presence in the mouse of two distinct inhibitors, one active against elastase (α_1-PI) and the other against trypsin (contrapsin), explains why TIC levels did not correlate with EIC values [14].

Serum α_1-PI concentrations were also determined in these strains of mice at 2 months of age. The values obtained were: 2.7 ± 0.4, 4.4 ± 0.3 and 5.9 ± 0.5 mg/ml for *pa*, C57Bl/6J and BALB/c, respectively. The values for each animal group correlated highly with the EIC serum levels. However, the differences in serum α_1-PI levels in these mice were not matched by different expressions of α_1-PI mRNA in the liver as there was no difference in α_1-PI (or contrapsin) expression between *pa* and the other two strains of mice [49].

In about 1–2% of *pa* mice of our colony, no serum levels of α_1-PI could be measured (unpublished results). It would be of great interest to breed these null mutants successfully.

4.3. Neutrophil Lysosomal Functions and Lung Elastase Burden

Similar levels of elastase specific activity were found in neutrophils from *pa* and control (NMRI) mice. However, when *pa* neutrophils were tested for their ability to release lysosomal enzymes after stimulation with FMLP/cytochalasin b, only moderate amounts of elastase, cathepsin G and β-glucuronidase were detected in the degranulation assay medium. This suggests that a defective degranulation process is present in neutrophils of *pa* mice [14].

Using an immunogold-electron microscopic method, a positive reaction for MLE was observed on elastin within the alveolar walls of *pa* mice from 2 months of age onwards. The average gold particle density increased progressively with age, reaching high values at 12 and 16 months of age [50].

4.4. Lung Elastin Content

Lung elastin content of *pa* mice had normal values at 2, 4 and 8 months of age. However, it was significantly lower at 12 and 16 months of age. The values of the lung elastin content correlated inversely with the immunogold values of the elastase burden [49].

4.5. Emphysema

At ultrastructural examination, disruption of alveolar septa was first seen at 8 months of age. At histological examination, some patchy areas of airspace enlargement with destruction of alveolar septa were seen from 12 months of age onward [36, 49] (Figure 1c). In another study, the lungs of 24-month-old *pa* mice showed a mild but generalized enlargement of the airspaces associated in some cases with distortion of the alveolar septa [17]. This means that, in these mice, an α_1-PI deficiency may lead to both patchy and generalized changes. In a scanning electron microscopy study, the lung parenchyma of *pa* mice did not differ significantly from that of the controls at 1 month of age. At 12 months the alveoli appeared to be larger. At 24 months, in some fields alveolar ducts were enlarged; the alveoli were also enlarged and very shallow. The number of interalveolar pores was not different from controls at 1 month but greater at 12 (+49%) and 24 (+26%) months. The lower increase in the number of pores at 24 months, compared with that at 12 months, was thought to result from a coalescence of two or more pores because these, at 24 months, appeared to be larger than at 12 months [17].

In *pa* mice, intratracheal instillation of FMLP resulted in a massive neutrophil recruitment into the lungs and in the development of a marked emphysema (*L*m +56% *vs.* NMRI, non-α_1-PI-deficient mice). In comparison, in C57Bl/6J mice with a moderate α_1-PI deficiency, the *L*m increased by 28% [15].

In conclusion, *pa* mice with a marked deficiency of α_1-PI develop a very mild form of emphysema spontaneously late in life. This is probably caused by the degranulation defect present in the neutrophils of this mutant. However, after a large influx of neutrophils into the lungs (i.e. induced by substances such as FMLP) significant emphysema develops.

Of interest as a possible marker of the spontaneously developing emphysema is the finding that, in *pa* mice from 8 months age onwards, pulmonary macrophages contain intracytoplasmatic crystalloid inclusions, which are electrodense and bounded by a single membrane. Using electron microscopy and an immunogold-labelling technique with anti-mouse I–III collagen IgG, these inclusions were identified as collagen-derived products [50] (Figure 3).

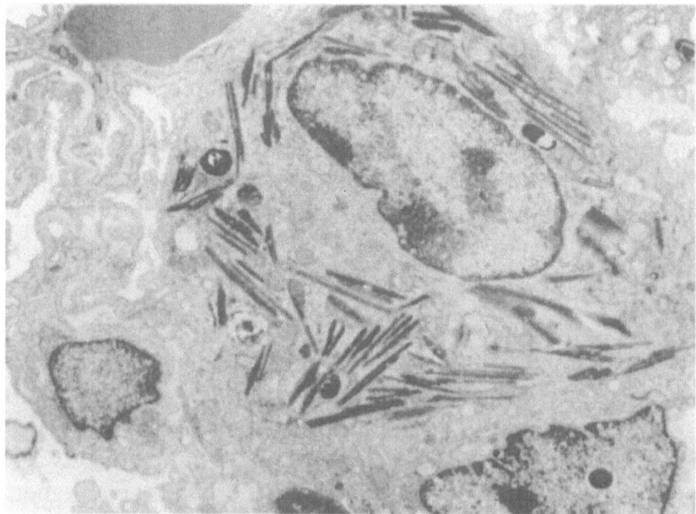

Figure 3. Electron micrograph of an alveolar macrophage from a 12-month-old pallid mouse. Several crystalloid intracytoplasmic inclusions are evident. Uranyl acetate and lead citrate, original magnification × 8000.

5. The Beige Mouse

5.1. Background

The beige (*bg*) mutation is available on three different inbred genetic backgrounds. Most studies, however, have utilized the spontaneous mutation of the C57Bl/6J line (C57Bl/6J *bg*/*bg*). The phenotype is characterized by a coat colour lighter than the parental strain (this is more evident on the abdominal area) and black eyes [51, 52]. The *bg* mutation is caused by an autosomal recessive gene located at the centromeric end of chromosome 13. *Lyst* (lysosomal trafficking regulator), a candidate gene for *bg*, has recently been identified [53].

The *bg* mutant expresses some of the phenotypic characteristics of a human disorder, the Chédiak-Higashi syndrome, such as giant lysosomes, platelet storage disease and increased susceptibility to infections [48, 51]. The last has been ascribed to a deficiency of neutrophil elastase and cathepsin G, and to a defective degranulation of neutrophils [51, 54]. Consequently the *bg* mouse has been widely used as a model of elastase and cathepsin G deficiency.

Two recent studies, however, show that neutrophils of *bg* mice secrete normal amounts of cathepsin G and a 46-kDa latent form of elastase that is activated extracellularly by proteolytic activity [14, 39]. Thus, the validity of the *bg* mouse as a model of neutrophil elastase and cathepsin G deficiency has been seriously questioned.

5.2. Antiprotease Screen

We reported a few years ago that *bg* mice have normal serum levels of α_1-PI [14]. In subsequent testing of a larger number of animals we found that serum levels of α_1-PI show wide variations in *bg* mice, and that their mean value is low and corresponds to that of the parent strain C57Bl/6J (G. Lungarella et al., unpublished results).

5.3. Neutrophil Lysosomal Functions and Lung Elastase Burden

As mentioned above, *in vitro* the level of cathepsin G activity in neutrophils of *bg* mice was found to be similar to that of control mice (NMRI, Balb/c). Only the extraction time, necessary to obtain this level of activity, was three times longer in *bg* mice. It was concluded that cathepsin G is probably bound to lysosomal membranes of *bg* mice, so that current methodology used for the extraction of neutrophil lysosomal enzymes is ineffective in this strain [14]. A latent form of elastase was found in *bg* neutrophil lysosomes. It was proposed that this may undergo spontaneous activation by a proteolytic mechanism [14]. Similar effects were obtained (*in vivo*), with the additional information of a normal neutrophil migration in *bg* mice [39]. In addition, the presence of normal amount of cathepsin G in beige mice has been reported "*in vivo*" in a model of granulomatous inflammation [55].

There are no data available on constitutive elastase burden in *bg* mice.

5.4. Lung Elastin Content

No difference in lung elastin content was reported between *bg* and control mice [18].

5.5. Emphysema

In one study, lungs of *bg* and control mice were morphometrically assessed from 4 days after birth to about 4 months of age. In control animals, during the early neonatal period (4–18 days), there was a marked decrease of the *L*m, which reached a constant value before they were aged 20 days. In *bg* mice, the *L*m was similar to that of the controls shortly after birth, but did not decrease afterwards to the same extent as the controls. The lungs of adult *bg* mice appeared to have enlarged alveolar ducts with fewer and perhaps larger alveoli, and there were no obvious areas of lung destruction. Their *L*m was significantly larger than that of the controls (+46%). This emphysematous lesion was considered to result from a defect of alveolarization during neonatal development [18].

In another study the lungs of *bg* and control mice were assessed histologically at 1, 12 and 24 months of age. The lungs of the *bg* mice showed, at all ages, a generalized enlargement of the airspaces, which was not accompanied by changes of the alveolar septa. In control animals, the *L*m remained constant between 1 and 12 months of age; however, it increased by 16% between 12 and 24 months. In *bg* mice, the *L*m was larger than that of the controls at 1 month (+27%), but remained practically constant at all ages (Figure 1 d). As a consequence, the difference between their *L*m values and those of the controls decreased with age [17]. In the same study, scanning electron microscopic examination of the lungs of *bg* mice revealed, at 1 month, enlarged alveolar ducts and alveolar sacs throughout the parenchyma. The alveoli were also enlarged and shallow with flattened alveolar septa. These changes deteriorated with age [17].

The effect of an influx of neutrophils into the lung was also investigated in *bg* mice. In one study, neutrophil recruitment was induced by intratracheal instillation of endotoxin once a week for 10 weeks. No exacerbation of the emphysematous changes was found [18]. In another study, neutrophil influx was induced by FMLP given once intratracheally. This procedure resulted in significant worsening of the emphysema accompanied by a decrease in lung elastin content [56].

In conclusion, *bg* mice with a moderate deficiency in serum α_1-PI develop a form of emphysema which, however, is probably the result of a defect of alveolar formation. There is a discrepancy in whether substances capable of recruiting and activating neutrophils into the lungs can induce an exacerbation of the pre-existent emphysematous changes. The difference in the results obtained may depend on the severity of the pre-existing lesion.

6. Conclusions

We have reviewed here the literature about four mouse models of genetic deficiency of serum α_1-PI deficiency.

In C57Bl/6J mice the deficiency is mild (about −25%), and spontaneous emphysema does not develop unless the mice are senescent (30 months of age). C57Bl/6J mice, however, show a susceptibility to develop significant emphysema after administration of substances capable of recruiting and activating PMNs into their lungs. This is not observed in mouse strains with normal serum levels of α_1-PI.

Beige mice have a serum α_1-PI deficiency similar to that of the C57Bl/6J mice. They develop moderate emphysema at 2–4 weeks after birth. A defect in alveolar formation is probably responsible for the development of the emphysema. Substances inducing PMN influx into and activation of the lungs can either exacerbate or have no effect on the pre-existing emphysema.

Pallid mice have a marked deficiency in serum α_1-PI (about −55%). However, their neutrophils have a degranulation defect. As a consequence, *pa* mice develop only a very mild form of emphysema late in life (at about 12 months of age). However, marked emphysema can be induced with substances that induce recruitment into and activation of PMNs in their lungs.

Tight-skin mice have a similar deficiency in serum α_1-PI as *pa* mice. Additionally, *Tsk* mice have elevated elastase levels in their neutrophils. Extensive emphysema develops very rapidly at about 2–4 weeks of age. A genetic defect of connective tissue probably plays a role in the development of emphysema. These mice develop cor pulmonale late in life, at about 16 months.

Thus, each mouse model has its own characteristics and limitations. They may all contribute to the understanding of the development of emphysema in humans, because the various factors that play a role in the pathogenesis of this disease are not fully understood. They may also be used in investigations concerning substitution/pharmacological interventions aimed at limiting the extent the emphysematous lesion. These studies should be carried out with substances capable of inhibiting MLE. It should be remembered that human α_1-PI is a poor inhibitor of this enzyme.

Acknowledgements

Supported by a grant from MURST (Rome, Italy) (Fondi 60%) and by the grant BMH4-CT96-0152 from Biomed 2 (Brussels, Belgium).

References

1 Snider GL, Kleinerman J, Thurlbeck WM, Bengali ZH (1985) The definition of emphysema. Report of a National Heart, Lung, and Blood Institute, Division of Lung Disease Workshop. *Am Rev Respir Dis* 132: 182–185
2 Eriksson S (1965) Studies in α_1-antitrypsin deficiency. *Acta Med Scand* 177 (suppl 432): 1–85
3 Snider GL, Ciccolella DE, Morris SM, Stone PJ Lucey E (1991) Putative role of neutrophil elastase in the pathogenesis of emphysema. *Ann NY Acad Sci* 624: 45–59
4 Ogushi F, Hubbard RC, Vogelmeier C, Fells GA, Crystal RG (1991) Risk factors for emphysema. Cigarette smoking is associated with a reduction in the association rate constant of lung α_1-antitrypsin for neutrophil elastase. *J Clin Invest* 87: 1060–1065
5 Karlinsly JB, Snider GL (1978) Animal models of emphysema. *Am Rev Respir Dis* 117: 1109–1133
6 Snider GL, Lucey E, Stone PJ (1986) Animal models of emphysema. *Am Rev Respir Dis* 133: 149–169
7 Cambell EJ (1986) Preventing therapy of emphysema. Lessons from the elastase model. *Am Rev Respir Dis* 134: 435–437
8 Nathoo S, Rasmus A, Katz J, Ferguson WS, Finlay TH (1982) Purification and properties of 2 different α_1-protease inhibitors from mouse plasma. *Arch Biochem Biophys* 219: 306–315
9 Takahara H, Sinohara H (1982) Mouse plasma trypsin inhibitors. *J Biol Chem* 257: 2438–2446
10 Baumann H, Jahreis GP, Gaines (1983) Synthesis and regulation of acute phase plasma proteins in primary culture of mice hepatocytes. *J Cell Biol* 97: 866–876
11 Hill RE, Shaw PH, Barth RK, Hastie ND (1985) A genetic locus closely kinked to a protease inhibitor gene complex controls the level of multiple RNA transcripts. *Mol Cell Biol* 5: 2114–2122
12 Store JV (1966) Longevity and gross pathology at death of 22 inbred mouse strains. *J Gerontol* 21:404–409
13 Minnich M, Kueppers F, James H (1984) α_1-antitrypsin from mouse serum isolation and characterisation. *Comp Biochem Physiol* B 78: 413–419
14 Gardi C, Cavarra E, Calzoni P, Marcolongo P, de Santi M, Martorana PA, Lungarella G (1994) Neutrophil lysosomal dysfunctions in mutant C57Bl/6J mice: interstrain variations in content of lysosomal elastase, cathepsin G and their inhibitors. *Biochem J* 299: 237–245
15 Cavarra E, Martorana PA, Gambelli F, de Santi M, van Even P, Lungarella G (1996) Neutrophil recruitment into the lungs is associated with increases lung elastase burden, decreased lung elastin, and emphysema in α_1-proteinase inhibitor-deficient mice. *Lab Invest* 75: 273–280
16 Kueppers F, Edmonds P, Williams JC (1994) Pulmonary emphysema in age mice. *Am J Respir Crit Care Med* 149 (part 2): A366
17 Keil M, Lungarella G, Cavarra E, van Even P, Martorana PA (1996) A scanning electron microscopic investigation of genetic emphysema in tight-skin, pallid, and beige mice, three different C57Bl/6J mutants. *Lab Invest* 74: 353–362
18 Starcher B, Williams (1989) The beige mouse: role of neutrophil elastase in the development of pulmonary emphysema. *Exp Lung Res* 15: 785–800
19 Green MC, Sweet HO, Bunker LE (1976) Tight-skin, a new mutation of the mouse causing excessive growth of connective tissue and skeleton. *Am J Pathol* 82: 493–512
20 Siracusa LD, McGrath R, Ma Q, Moskow JJ, Manne J, Christner PJ, Buchberg AM, Jimenez SA (1996) A tandem duplication within the fibrillin 1 gene is associated with the mouse thight-skin mutation. *Genome Res* 6: 300–313

21 Jimenez SA, Millan A, Bashey RI (1984) Scleroderma-like alterations in collagen metabolism occurring in the Tsk (tight-skin) mouse. *Arthritis Rheum* 27: 180–185
22 Kasturi KN, Shibata S, Muroy T, Bona CA (1994) Tight-skin mouse as an experimental model of scleroderma. *Int Rev Immunol* 11: 253–271
23 Jablonska S, Scubert H, Kikuchi I (1989) Congenital fascial dystrophy: stiff skin syndrome – a human counterpart of the tight-skin mouse. *J Am Acad Dermatol* 21: 943–950
24 Ehrlich HP, Needle AL (1983) Wound healing in tight-skin mice: delayed closure of excised wounds. *Plast Reconstr Surg* 72: 190–198
25 Agren MS, Mertz PM (1994) Are excessive granulation tissue formation and retarded wound contraction due to decreased collagenase activity in wounds in tight-skin mice? *Br J Dematol* 131: 337–340
26 Osborn TG, Bashey RI, Moore TL, Fischer VW (1987) Collagenous abnormalities in the heart of the tight-skin mouse. *J Mol Cell Cardiol* 19: 581–587
27 Chapman D, Eghbali M (1990) Expression of fibrillar types I and III and basement membrane collagen type IV genes in myocardium of tight-skin mouse. *Cardiovasc Res* 24: 578–583
28 Bocchieri MH, Henriksen PD, Kasturi KN, Muroy T, Bona CA, Jimenez SA (1991) Evidence for autoimmunity in the tight-skin mouse model of systemic sclerosis. *Arthritis Rheum* 34: 599–605
29 Bona CA, Rothfield N (1994) Autoantibodies in scleroderma and tight-skin mice. *Curr Opin Immunol* 6: 931–937
30 Boros P, Chen J, Bona CA, Unkeless JC (1990) Autoimmune mice make anti-Fcy receptor antibodies. *J Exp Med* 171: 1581–1595
31 Gardi C, Martorana PA, van Even P, de Santi MM, Lungarella G (1990) Serum antielastase deficiency in tight-skin mice with genetic emphysema. *Exp Mol Pathol* 52: 46–53
32 de Santi MM, Gardi C, Martorana PA, van Even P, Lungarella G (1989) Immunoelectronmicroscopic demonstration of elastase in emphysematous lungs of tight-skin mice. *Exp Mol Pathol* 51: 18–30
33 Gardi C, Martorana PA, de Santi MM, van Even P, Lungarella G (1989) A biochemical and morphological investigation of the early development of genetic emphysema in tight-skin mice. *Exp Mol Pathol* 50: 398–410
34 Szapiel SV, Fulmer JD, Hunninghake GW, Elson NA, Kawanami O, Ferrans VJ, Crystal RG (1981) Hereditary emphysema in the tight-skin (Tsk/+) mouse. *Am Rev Respir Dis* 123: 680–685
35 Rossi GA, Hunninghake GW, Gadek JE, Szapiel SV, Kawanami O, Ferrans VJ, Crystal RG (1984) Hereditary emphysema in the tight-skin mouse. Evaluation of pathogenesis. *Am Rev Respir Dis* 129: 850–855
36 Martorana PA, van Even P, Gardi C, Lungarella G (1989) A 16-month study of the development of genetic emphysema in tight-skin mice. *Am Rev Respir Dis* 139: 226–232
37 Gardi C, Martorana PA, Calzoni P, van Even P, de Santi MM, Cavarra E, Lungarella G (1992) Lung collagen synthesis and deposition in tight-skin mice with genetic emphysema. *Exp Mol Pathol* 56: 163–172
38 Starcher B, James H (1991) Evidence that genetic emphysema in tight-skin mice is not caused by neutrophil elastase. *Am Rev Respir Dis* 143: 1365–1368
39 Cavarra E, Martorana PA, Cortese S, Gambelli F, Di Simplicio P, Lungarella G (1997) Neutrophils in beige mice secrete normal amounts of cathepsin G and a 46 kDa latent form of elastase that can be activated extracellularly by proteolytic activity. *Biol Chem* 378: 417–423
40 Takeuchi K, Wood H, Swank RT (1986) Lysosomal elastase and cathepsin G in beige mice. Neutrophils of beige (Chediak–Higashi) mice selectively lack lysosomal elastase and cathepsin G. *J Exp Med* 163: 665–677
41 Martorana PA, Wilkinson M, van Even P, Lungarella G (1990) Tsk mice with genetic emphysema. Right ventricular hypertrophy occurs without hypertrophy of muscular pulmonary arteries or muscularization of arterioles. *Am Rev Respir Dis* 142: 333–337
42 Martorana PA, Wilkinson M, de Santi MM, van Even P, Gardi C, Lungarella G (1991) Development of cor pulmonale in tight-skin mice with genetic emphysema. *Ann NY Acad Sci* 624: 345–347
43 Gardi C, Martorana PA, Calzoni P, Cavarra E, Marcolongo P, van Even P, de Santi MM, Lungarella (1994) Cardiac collagen changes during the development of right ventricular hypertrophy in tight-skin mice with genetic emphysema. *Exp Mol Pathol* 60: 100–107

44 Roberts E (1931) A new mutation in the house mouse (mus musculus). *Science* 74: 569
45 Lane PW, Lyon MF (1989) In: Lyon MF, Searle AG (eds): Genetic variants and strains of the laboratory mouse. New York, Oxford University Press, 825–842
46 White RA, Peters LL, Adkison LR, Korsgren C, Cohen CM, Lux SE (1992) The murine pallid mutation is a platelet storage pool disease associated with the protein 4.2 (pallidin) gene. *Nature Genetics* 2: 80–83
47 Gwynn B, Korsgren C, Cohen CM, Ciciote SL, Peters LL (1997) The gene encoding protein 4.2 is distinct from the mouse platelet storage pool deficiency mutation pallid. *Genomics* 42: 532–535
48 Novak EK, Hui S, Swank RT (1984) Platelet storage pool deficiency in mouse pigment mutations associated with seven distinct genetic loci. *Blood* 63: 536–544
49 Martorana PA, Brand T, Gardi C, van Even P, de Santi MM, Calzoni P, Marcolongo P, Lungarella G (1993) The pallid mouse. A model of genetic α_1-antitrypsin deficiency. *Lab Invest* 68: 233–241
50 de Santi MM, Martorana PA, Cavarra E, Lungarella G (1995) Pallid mice with genetic emphysema. Neutrophil elastase burden and elastin loss occur without alteration in the bronchoalveolar lavage cell population. *Lab Invest* 73: 1–8
51 Brandt EJ, Swank RT, Nowak EK (1981) The murine Chediak-Higashi mutation and other murine pigmentation mutations. In: Gershwin ME, Merchant B (eds): *Immunological Defects in Laboratory Animals*. New York, Plenum Press, 99–117
52 Lane PW, Murphy ED (1972) Susceptibility to spontaneous pneumonitis in an inbred strain of beige and satin mice. *Genetics* 72: 451–460
53 Barbosa MDFS, Nguyen QA, Tchernev VT, Ashley JA, Detter JC, Blaydes SM, Brandt SJ, Chotai D, Hodgman C, Solari RCE, Lovett M, Kingsmore SK (1996) Identification of the homologous beige and Chediak–Higashi syndrome genes. *Nature* 382: 262–265
54 Vassalli JD, Granelli-Piperno A, Griscelli C, Reich E (1978) Specific protease deficiency in polymorphonuclear leukocytes of Chediak–Higashi syndrome and beige mice. *J Exp Med* 147: 1285–1290
55 Prigent D, Trancart MM, Seed MP, Willoughby DA (1996) Proteoglycan degrading activity in granulomatous inflammation: Comparison between the C57Bl/6 and C57bg/bg mouse. *Inflamm Res* 45: 494–498
56 Martorana PA, Cavarra E, Cortese S, Gambelli F, de Santi MM, Di Simplicio P, Lungarella G (1997) Neutrophil recruitment into the lungs of beige mice is followed by the onset of alveolar elastolytic lesions. *Am J Respir Crit Care Med* 155: A654

Molecular Biology of the Lung
Vol. 1: Emphysema and Infection
ed. by R. A. Stockley

CHAPTER 3
α_1-Antitrypsin Deficiency

Robert A. Stockley

Department of Medicine, Queen Elizabeth Hospital, Edgbaston, Birmingham, UK

1. Introduction

α_1-antitrypsin deficiency can be classified as a relatively modern disease. The first identification of the condition occurred in 1963, when Laurell and Eriksson [1] noticed several subjects with a deficient α_1-globulin band on paper electrophoresis. The authors subsequently showed that 90% of this band was caused by the presence of a single protein which was responsible for most of the plasma trypsin inhibitory activity. This observation led to the initial labelling of the protein as α_1-antitrypsin. Although subsequent information has indicated that the primary function of this protein may be to inhibit other serine proteinases, in particular neutrophil elastase, the original name of the protein still remains most commonly used. However, particularly in the USA, the term α_1-proteinase inhibitor has been accepted as an alternative.

Of the initial five subjects identified with this deficiency, it was noted that three had severe early onset emphysema. This led to an assumption that the deficiency in some way predisposed to the development of this condition.

Subsequent studies from the same group confirmed that α_1-antitrypsin deficiency was inherited and appeared to behave as an autosomal recessive condition [2]. The reason for the association with lung disease started to become clear when Gross and colleagues [3] demonstrated that proteolytic enzymes were capable of inducing pulmonary changes similar to human emphysema in experimental animals. Subsequently, a human enzyme (human neutrophil elastase) was shown to have the same effect [4]. It therefore became generally accepted that subjects with α_1-antitrypsin deficiency were unable to protect their lungs from proteolytic damage by human neutrophil elastase which therefore resulted in excess tissue degradation and the development of pathological changes typical of the condition.

Since these early studies much has been learnt about the evolution of the α_1-antitrypsin gene, its mutations, the structure – function relationships of α_1-antitrypsin and gradually more about the relationship of the deficiency to disease.

2. The Protein

The α_1-antitrypsin gene is found at q32.1 on chromosome 14. The mRNA for α_1-antitrypsin is 1.6 kilobases (kb) in length (in hepatocytes), and consists of four coding exons and three untranslated exons in the 5′-region. The 5′ sequences contain a variety of putative transcription regulatory sites and further controlling sequences have been identified 3′ (see Chapter 5). The α_1-antitrypsin molecule is a 52 kilodalton (52 kDa) glycoprotein of 394 residues with three asparagine-linked carbohydrate side chains. These side chains are either bi-antennary or tri-antennary complex carbohydrates.

The protein is polymorphic with many nucleotide substitutions, most of which are consistent with the protein functioning entirely normal. This polymorphism has, however, enabled the determination of the evolution of the gene and the phenotypic recognition of many of the polymorphims by isoelectric focusing.

In normal subjects the α_1-antitrypsin genes for both chromosomes 14 are transcribed equally. Thus, in true genetic terms, the α_1-antitrypsin gene is expressed in a co-dominant fashion, although phenotypically diseases associated with α_1-antitrypsin deficiency appear to follow a classic autosomal recessive mode of inheritance.

2.1. Protein Structure

α_1-antitrypsin is a member of the SERPIN family of proteinase inhibitors. As such it preferentially inhibits enzymes with serine at the active site. The molecular structure of the whole protein has yet to be studied, but its basic formation has been ascertained by analysis of the cleaved form of α_1-antitrypsin (where the active site of the carboxyl terminus has been disrupted) and comparison with the structure of other members of the SERPIN family. The protein consists of three β sheets (A–C) nine α helices (A–I) and six helical turns. In broad terms the lower three strands of β sheet B forms a highly conserved hydrophobic core, together with a vertically oriented helix B. Anterior to this is the planar β sheet A. The β sheet C is above β sheet B, with inferiorly and anteriorly positioned helices A, C, D and E, whereas helices G and H are found below and in front of β sheet B. The carboxyl terminus forms a taut extension which on cleavage is incorporated into the middle of sheet A. This structure has been based on the description by Priestle in 1988 [5] and is shown graphically in Figure 1.

The active site on the exposed carboxyl terminus has a critical amino acid at position 358. In native α_1-antitrypsin this is methionine which determines the specificity of the inhibitor towards serine proteinases. This specificity is demonstrated by a single substitution of the amino acid arginine at this site, changing the inhibitory function of α_1-antitrypsin from enzymes such as elastase to antithrombin [6].

Although α_1-antitrypsin inhibits many serine proteinases, including trypsin, chymotrypsin, cathepsin G and neutrophil elastase, it is the last that

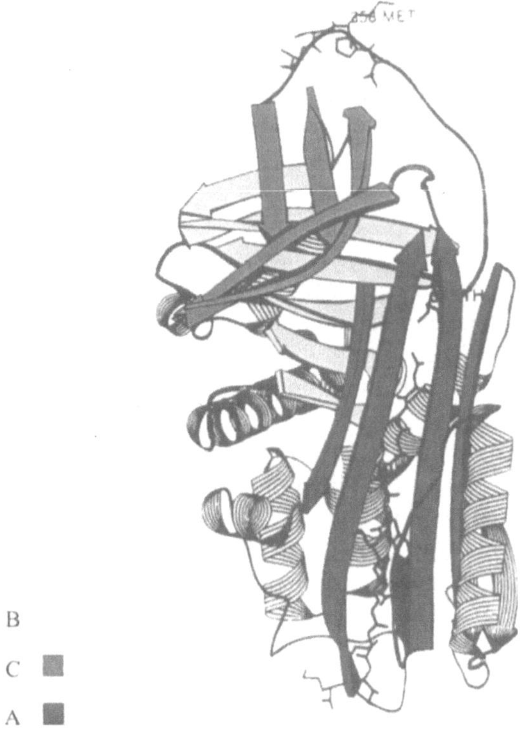

Figure 1. Ribbon-type stereo representation of the intact inhibitory form of α_1-antitrypsin. The reactive site methionine on the exposed reactive loop is shown. The β sheets A are indicated in dark shading, β sheets B in light shading, and β sheets C in intermediate shading.

is regarded as its major target enzyme. α_1-Antitrypsin has a high affinity for neutrophil elastase with an association constant (K_{ass}) of 9.6×10^6/mol s. The interaction results in cleavage of the Met/Ser bond at position 358/359, leading to burial of the carboxyl terminus within the central molecular structure of the α_1-antitrypsin (see above) and the formation of a stable complex that inactivates both proteins.

The protein is produced by a variety of cells, although most is believed to come from hepatocytes. About 34 mg α_1-antitrypsin/kg is produced per day with a half-life of 5–6 days. The half-life is rapidly reduced when α_1-antitrypsin is complexed with enzymes [7]. α_1-Antitrypsin is an acute phase protein which is able to show a two- to four-fold rise in concentration over 3–4 days from the onset of an inflammatory process (see later).

The normal α_1-antitrypsin alleles are heterogeneous. The archetypal sequence (20% of variants) in based on alanine at position 213 (M1) which resembles that in apes. There is a second version of the M1 variant with valine at position 213 (50%) and both these M1 version have arginine at position 101 and glutamic acid at position 376. The common Z and S variants are derived from M1 (Ala 213) and M1 (Val 213) respectively. The M2 variant (19%) has two replacements with histidine at position 101 and asparagine at 376, based on the Ala 213 variant. The M3 variant (10%) is similar but with arginine at position 101. Finally, the M4 variant (1%) is similar to the M1 (Val 213) with the exception of histidine at position 101 instead of arginine. Apart from these major variants of the M phenotype, 15 or so rarer variations have been described.

3. Deficiency

"Deficiency" of α_1-antitrypsin can occur for a variety of reasons. These range from variation of gene expression to the production of truncated protein, failure of secretion of the protein, increased intracellular degradation of the protein, failure of protein function and finally an inappropriate or absent acute phase response.

The α_1-antitrypsin gene is 12.2 kb in length and consists of seven exons, designated 1 a, 1 b, 1c, 2, 3, 4 and 5. The protein-coding region is contained within exons 2–5. Exons 1a and 1b are involved in the transcription start in macrophages, whereas exon 1c is involved in the transcription start in hepatocytes. The ATG site is at the start of exon 2 and is followed by a short lead peptide. Regulation of α_1-antitrypsin transcription is described in Chapter 5.

Among the mutations within the protein-coding regions, the mutations are relatively evenly dispersed, although two exceptions are the susceptibility of codons 51–53 and 361–363. The most likely explanation for the concentration of variants in these locations is that these regions represent mutational hotspots.

Studies have so far identified more than 30 genetic defects associated with decreased α_1-antitrypsin concentration or function. True gene deletion itself is rare, although the Q0 *isola di procida* [8] and the Q0 Reidenberg [9] variants are associated with major deletions from exon 2 to exon 5 of the protein.

3.1. Frameshift Mutations

A variety of nucleotide insertions and deletions have been associated with failure of α_1-antitrypsin secretion. Examples include Q0 granite falls in which tyrosine at position 160 (TAC) is changed by deletion of C. This results in a 5′-frameshift resulting in a stop codon TAG at position 160 [10].

Q0 Mattawa is based on an insertion at leucine position 353 (TTA), insert T and results in a 3′-frameshift mutation leading to a stop codon TGA at position 376 [11].

3.2. Nucleotide Change

Q0 Kowloon is associated with a change in a Tyr 38 (TAC) nucleotide change to TAA, resulting in the stop codon [12], whereas in Q0 Bellingham Lys 217 (AAG) is changed to TAG, resulting in a stop codon [13].

3.3. Impaired Translocation

The gene for α_1-antitrypsin contains a transit peptide of 21 residues at the amino terminus of the precursor α_1-antitrypsin. The role of the peptide was first reported by the discovery of a single point mutation (PiZ Wrexham) – Ser 19 being replaced by leucine within the peptide [14]. This mutation results in the replacement of a hydrophilic residue with a hydrophobic one, which leads either to abnormal processing, resulting in further impairment of secretion, or to a protein that is less stable than the normal Z protein. The net result is a loss of protein secretion and the failure to identify the Z band pattern on isoelectric focusing [14].

3.4. Deficiency States

Apart from the null variants, over 15 deficient or dysfunctional forms of α_1-antitrypsin have been described. More than 95% of these are related to the Z mutation which was the one originally described by Laurell and Eriksson [1]. The Z mutation is again the result of a single nucleotide change with glutamic acid (GAG) at position 342 being changed to AAG resulting in the production of lysine [15]. The gene itself is normally transcribed, resulting in α_1-antitrypsin production within hepatocytes. The normal transcription of the mRNA has been confirmed in cell-free translation systems [16]. Nevertheless, despite normal translation, the protein is not secreted from the cell in the normal way and this has also been confirmed in oocyte transfection studies of *Xenopus* [17].

The α_1-antitrypsin accumulates in the rough endoplasm reticulum resulting in the presence of inclusion bodies visible as periodic acid–Schiff (PAS)-positive globules on liver biopsy (Figure 2). Secretion of the α_1-antitrypsin is reduced to about 10–20% of normal and in plasma it shows only a slight acute phase response.

The mechanism for failure of secretion has been the subject of many studies. Initially it was felt that the critical change of glutamic acid at position 342 to lysine affected the tertiary structure of the protein. In the tertiary structure this amino acid lies opposite lysine at position 290. As glutamic acid and lysine are oppositely charged, it was felt that a salt bridge at this point was important in the correct conformation of the mature protein. Replacement of glutamic acid at position 342 with a further lysine resulted in the lysine at position 342 and that at position 290 repelling each

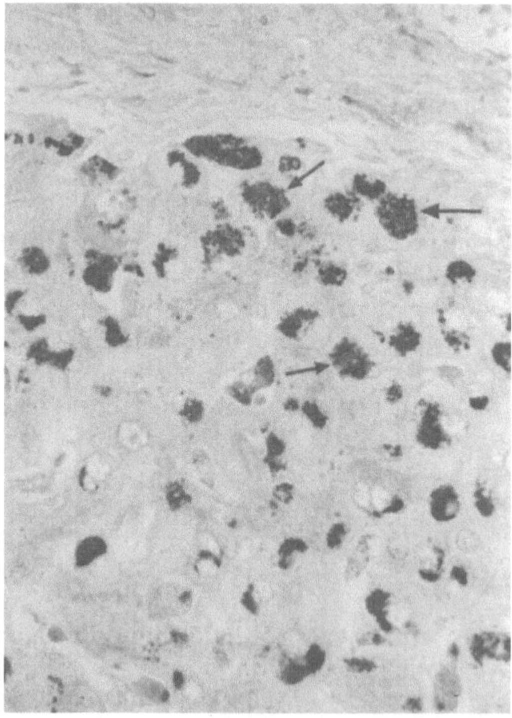

Figure 2. Liver biopsy from a patient with α_1-antitrypsin deficiency. PAS-positive globules are seen within hepatocytes (indicated by arrow).

other, disturbing the tertiary structure [18]. Nevertheless, subsequent studies have suggested that this may not be the cause and it is currently believed that the major reason for accumulation of α_1-antitrypsin in hepatocytes is the ability of the Z protein to undergo spontaneous polymerization as a result of the insertion of the carboxyl-terminal sequence of one protein into the A sheets of another [19]. The change of glutamic acid at the hinge region of the carboxyl terminus to lysine apparently facilitates this process. Polymerization itself is temperature and concentration dependent and can be prevented by insertion of an appropriate peptide into the space between the A sheets [19].

This mechanism of "loop-sheet polymerization" has also been suggested as an explanation of the deficiency associated with the Siiyami phenotype [20] and the M malton variant [21].

3.5. Dysfunctional α_1-antitrypsin

The very rapid association rate constant of α_1-antitrypsin and neutrophil elastase may be critical in the role of this inhibitor in protecting connective tissues (such as those in the lung) from damage. Not only is the concentration of the Z phenotype in plasma reduced, but its association rate constant for neutrophil elastase is also decreased about twofold [22]. This change results in a 20-fold delay in the association time between α_1-antitrypsin and neutrophil elastase. The importance of this delay has been demonstrated by Llewellyn-Jones et al. [23], indicating that when neutrophils are activated in close contact with connective tissue the Z variant of α_1-antitrypsin shows a reduced ability to prevent tissue degradation when compared with equimolar functional concentrations of the native M protein (Figure 3). This slight difference may prove critical in the development of chronic destructive lung disease because, with continued neutrophil migration into the lung over many years, a slight increase in the amount of connective tissue that is destroyed by the neutrophil would be cumulatively greater than in subjects with normal α_1-antitrypsin.

The F phenotype of α_1-antitrypsin has also been shown to have a decreased association rate constant for neutrophil elastase [24] and to be associated with the development of emphysema (see below). The F variant is based on the M1 (Val 213) base allele and shows a single point mutation in exon 3 with Arg 223 (CGT) being changed to Cys (TGT). Why this should affect the association rate constant is currently unknown. However, it is possible that the firm interaction between SERPINs and their inhibitors is dependent not only on the primary binding site in the exposed reactive loop but also on the presence of other binding sites elsewhere on the protein. Studies with the C1 esterase inhibitor have indicated that a secondary binding site is critical for the formation of stable enzyme inhibitor complexes. Elegant studies by He et al. have indicated a four amino acid

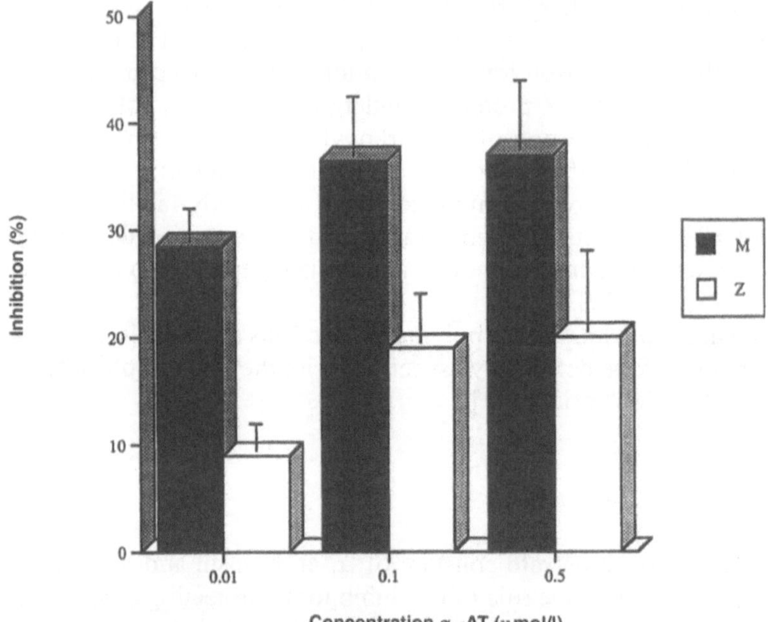

Figure 3. Inhibition of fibronectin degradation by neutrophils is shown for equimolar concentrations of α_1-antitrypsin purified from patients with M and Z α_1-antitrypsin as indicated. At all concentrations the Z α_1-antitrypsin (α1AT) was less inhibitory than the M α_1-antitrypsin (Adapted from [23]).

sequence in the distal hinge region of C1 inhibitor may be critical in the process of enzyme inhibition [25]. Whether the same is true of α_1-antitrypsin remains uncertain but the reduction in the association rate constant of the F variant may suggest that the area around amino acid 223 could also be critical in α_1-antitrypsin function.

4. Secondary Deficiency

The interaction of α_1-antitrypsin with oxidants derived from cigarette smoke or inflammatory cells results in a change of the methionine at position 358 to methionine sulphoxide. This changes the molecular shape at the active site resulting in a 2000-fold reduction in the association rate constant for neutrophil elastase [26]. This large change in association is likely to be of major importance in the control of the enzyme by α_1-antitrypsin. At present there is considerable debate about whether the oxidized variant of α_1-antitrypsin can be found within lung tissues and whether it plays a role in predisposing to the development of connective tissue destruction, leading to emphysema [27].

4.1. Failure of Acute Phase Response

Studies by Kalsheker et al. have indicated that a significant number of patients with lung disease have a polymorphism in the 3′-region of the α_1-antitrypsin gene [28]. This polymorphism at a Taq 1 restriction site is thought to occur in the middle of a sequence with potential enhancer function [29]. The proposed effect of this mutation is to in some way restrict the normal acute phase response of α_1-antitrypsin, leading to a selective partial deficiency when inflammatory processes occur. The nature and function of this mutation is described in Chapter 5.

5. Association of α_1-Antitrypsin Deficiency With Disease

5.1. Lung Disease

Of the first five subjects to be identified with α_1-antitrypsin deficiency, three had extensive emphysema at an early age [1]. Subsequent familial studies confirmed not only that the deficiency was inherited in what appeared to be an autosomal recessive pattern, but also that this was associated with a very high incidence of emphysema (about 80%). Larger epidemiological studies confirm that subjects with α_1-antitrypsin deficiency have a decreased life expectancy and that this decrease was accelerated in subjects who smoked [30]. As smoking has been a well-recognized cause of the development of emphysema, it was believed that, in subjects with α_1-antitrypsin deficiency, the additional risk factor of cigarette smoking accelerated the development of lung pathology.

The earlier studies had identified α_1-antitrypsin deficiency in young patients with severe emphysema and it became generally accepted, that this was the major lung problem associated with the condition. In view of this, the guidelines of both the American Thoracic Society and the European Thoracic Society suggested that the most appropriate group to test for α_1-antitrypsin deficiency was young subjects with severe emphysema. Over the years this has led to relatively limited testing for α_1-antitrypsin deficiency and this has been highlighted in the results of the extensive registry at the National Institutes of Health (NIH) in Bethesda, USA [31].

The results of this registry confirmed that the average age of subjects with α_1-antitrypsin deficiency and lung disease was about 46 years and that the peak onset of symptoms was between the ages of 25 and 40. The registry confirmed that over one-third of the patients also had evidence of airway disease as indicated by a history of chronic bronchitis. About 20% of the subjects had some reactive airway disease indicative of an asthmatic tendency and most subjects (93%) were smokers or ex-smokers. The disease was found to be exclusively confined to white subjects and the average degree of lung function impairment indicated approximately a 66% loss of forced expiratory volume in 1 second (FEV_1).

The mechanism for development of lung diseases was initially thought to be relatively simple. It was believed that the low α_1-antitrypsin concentration was itself the major problem. In view of the ability of this inhibitor to complex with and inactivate neutrophil elastase, it was believed that the development of the lung disease was a direct consequence of poorly controlled neutrophil elastase activity. Early studies of lung secretions obtained from the lower airways by bronchoalveolar lavage indicated that these secretions were devoid of elastase inhibitors, indicating that α_1-antitrypsin was the main inhibitor of this enzyme within the airways [32] and hence, by implication, in the interstitium of the lung. The importance of the latter site is that emphysema develops only when lung elastin is destroyed, and as this is one of the major connective tissues of the interstitial areas of the lung, it was believed that free elastase activity at this site was the major cause of the disease. In subjects with normal serum α_1-antitrypsin, diffusion of the protein from the plasma into the interstitium would provide a sufficient degree of protection to prevent the development of emphysema. However, in deficiency states, the concentrations of α_1-antitrypsin in the interstitium would be much lower and this is reflected in the even lower concentrations found in bronchoalveolar lavage fluid [33].

Currently, it is accepted that the scenario is much more complex than has been outlined above. First, where major studies have been carried out in patients with lung disease, it becomes apparent that most subjects with α_1-antitrypsin deficiency have not been identified. In most countries less than 10% of the predicted number of patients have been identified through patient or familial screening. This suggests two main possibilities: first that most subjects with α_1-antitrypsin deficiency remain well and, second, that our concepts of the way in which it affects individuals is incorrect, resulting in testing of the wrong group. There is evidence to suggest that both misconceptions play a role.

Routine screening at birth indicates that between 1 in 2000 and 1 in 3000 individuals from northern Europe (in particular Scandinavia) have severe α_1-antitrypsin deficiency [34]. When a similar screening programme was undertaken in the USA involving healthy blood donors, it was noted that the expected number of subjects was identified but that many of them remained well [35]. Indeed the study indicated that there may even be a familial component in addition to the α_1-antitrypsin deficiency which influences the development of lung disease. This finding was in agreement with that published previously by Cullen and workers [36] and is highlighted by the family tree outlined in Figure 4.

Studies have also suggested that confining α_1-antitrypsin testing to young subjects with established emphysema may also result in failure to identify many subjects. In the protein reference laboratory in Sheffield, in the UK, the age distribution of subjects identified with α_1-antitrypsin de-

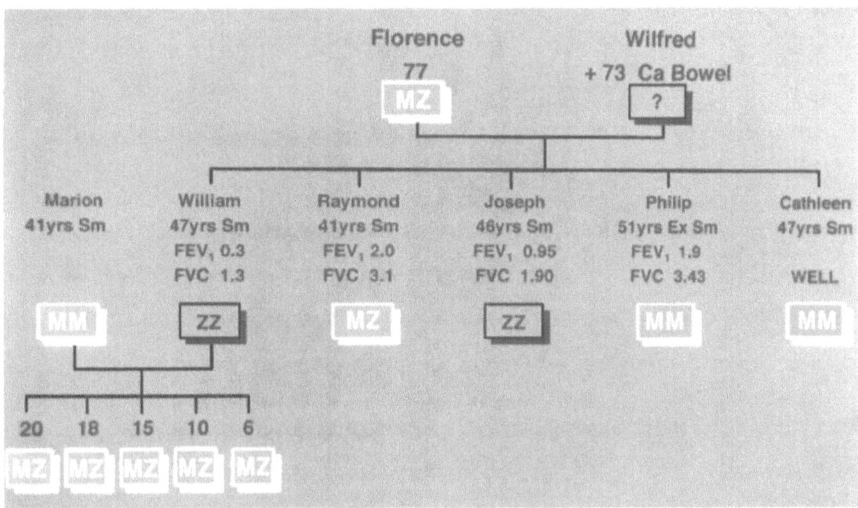

Figure 4. Familial emphysema highlighted by α_1-antitrypsin deficiency. Of the five siblings, the homozygote Z individuals have severely impaired lung function, whereas the heterozygote and the subject with normal α_1-antitrypsin have much less severely impaired lung function. FEV_1, forced expiratory volume in 1 second; FVC, forced vital capacity.

ficiency is much wider than was previously thought. Most subjects identified were between the ages of 50 and 60 (see Figure 5), giving an average age in excess of that identified by the NIH registry (see above). Finally, it may be that patients with other diseases are not being screened appropriately. α_1-antitrypsin deficiency has been recognized in subjects with bronchiectasis [37] and recent studies from Sweden have suggested that a history of wheezing with relatively normal lung function may be common in subjects with deficiency [38]. In view of these discrepancies, recent recommendations of the World Health Organization (WHO) are for screening of all subjects with chronic lung disease, including those with adult-onset asthma and bronchiectasis.

5.2. Mechanism of Lung Destruction

As indicated above, the pathogenesis of emphysema is thought to result from the release of neutrophil elastase into the interstitium of the lung by migrating neutrophils. These inflammatory cells are recruited to the lung in response to the release of chemoattractants and early studies suggested that even before significant disease develops α_1-antitrypsin-deficient subjects have an increase in concentrations of leukotriene B_4 (LTB_4) within the lung which is responsible for neutrophil recruitment [39].

As neutrophils migrate from the vascular space into the airways in response to chemoattractants, they must pass through a compact interstitium

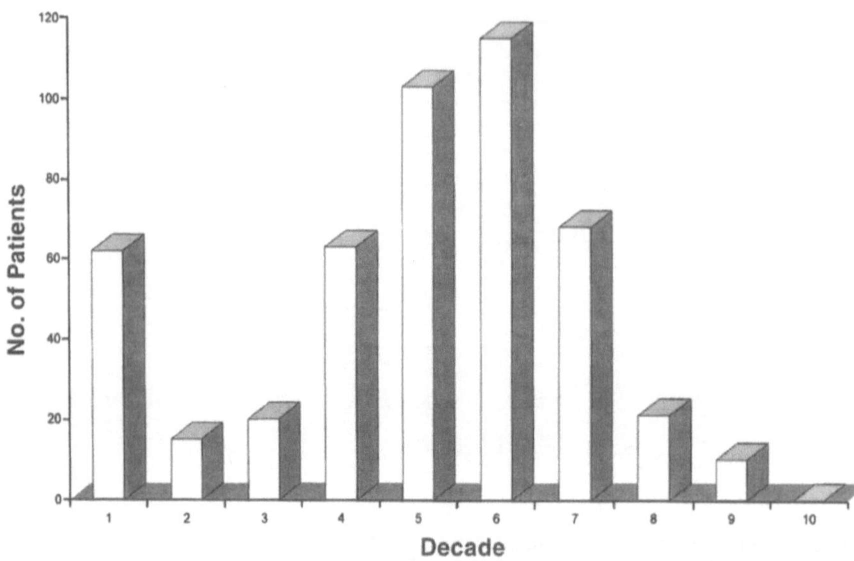

Figure 5. Age range of subjects identified with α_1-antitrypsin deficiency (Z) over the period 1995–1997, in the Protein Reference Laboratory, Sheffield, UK. (Data kindly supplied by A. Milford Ward).

of connective tissue. To do this it is believed that the cells need to digest a path, creating a natural hole through the matrix. Recent elegant studies using eosinophils have demonstrated this most graphically [40]. Studies by Campbell and colleagues have shown that, when neutrophils are in close contact with connective tissue, they are able to digest matrix proteins even in the presence of supranormal concentrations of proteinase inhibitors [41]. This clearly underlines the importance of the ability of these cells to digest connective tissue in order to migrate. It is believed that α_1-antitrypsin acts as an inhibitor that prevents destruction of connective tissue beyond the limits of the cell and its close contact with the substrate.

Studies with α_1-antitrypsin isolated from deficient subjects (PiZ) have shown that activated neutrophils are able to destroy more connective tissue in the presence of deficient protein, irrespective of its concentration when compared with the normal M protein [23]. This may reflect the slight difference in association rate constant and provide one reason why excessive connective tissue might be destroyed by migrating neutrophils in subjects with α_1-antitrypsin deficiency. However, more recent studies by Liou and Campbell, both on a theoretical [42] and a practical basis [43], have suggested that this might be a relatively minor component of the pathogenic process. It was demonstrated by these workers that the azurophil granule contains high concentrations of neutrophil elastase. As these granules are exocytosed when the cell is activated, supranormal concentrations of elastase would start to diffuse away from the granule. As the protein diffuses greater distances away from the granule, the concentration gradually falls until it equals that of the physiological inhibitors surrounding them. At this point connective tissue degradation ceases. Studies showed that the area of enzyme activity was quite well restricted until the concentration of α_1-antitrypsin fell below 10 μmol/l. At this point there was an exponential rise in the area of persistent activity of neutrophil elastase. The implications of this observation are that for subjects with α_1-antitrypsin deficiency where the concentration is less than 10 μmol/l (on average, about 5 μmol/l), for each neutrophil that enters the interstitium of the lung the degree of connective tissue degradation would be excessive as a result of the inability to prevent elastase activity for a wider area around the activated neutrophil.

Understanding this process is clearly critical in the development of therapeutic strategies for patients with α_1-antitrypsin deficiency. Whether treatment is given by α_1-antitrypsin replacement therapy or substitution with other forms of proteinase inhibitors, it will clearly be of importance to obtain concentrations of inhibitors in excess of 10 μmol/l in the interstitium of the lung in order to return to normal the area of surrounding connective tissue degradation produced by migrating neutrophils.

The above explanation clearly provides a mechanism to understand how emphysema will develop in subjects with α_1-antitrypsin deficiency. In addition it explains why cigarette smoking is likely to enhance this process because the lungs of smokers are known to contain more neutrophils than those of non-smokers [44]. Nevertheless, it is highly likely that there is some other familial component or risk factor involved in the development of lung disease. Indeed Silverman and colleagues had indicated that lower respiratory tract infections may be a critical factor and certainly a history of Chronic Obstructive Pulmonary Disease (COPD) or asthma in a parent appears to play a role [35].

The relationship of α_1-antitrypsin deficiency to other lung conditions, including asthma, bronchitis and bronchiectasis, is even less well understood. This is particularly true of airway disease because the major airways contain large quantities of Secretory Leukocyte Protease Inhibitor (SLPI) which is an effective inhibitor of neutrophil elastase at this site and predominates over α_1-antitrypsin.

Clearly further studies will be indicated to determine these more subtle relationship and the interplay of other genetic factors.

6. Liver Disease

The association between α_1-antitrypsin deficiency and liver disease was first reported by Sharpe and colleagues in 1969 [45]. Initially it was identified as a problem in children, but subsequently it was also shown to affect adults [46]. In 1976 Sveger reported that liver disease in some form or other affected about 10% of all neonates with Z α_1-antitrypsin deficiency [47].

The incidence in adults is, however, relatively unknown and probably not a direct consequence of neonatal problems. In 1987 Eriksson studied 35000 *post mortem* examinations and found 17 subjects with α_1-antitrypsin deficiency; of these eight had cirrhosis and five hepatocellular carcinoma [48]. This represents an overall incidence of deficient subjects *post mortem* of 1 in 2000, which is similar to the national prevalence.

In children the usual form of presentation is with neonatal jaundice. This is associated with cholestasis that may occur between 4 days and 2 months after birth, and may last for up to 8 months [49]. Longitudinal studies of subjects with α_1-antitrypsin deficiency identified at birth have indicated that abnormal lung function tests can be present in as many as 70% of neonates 6 months after birth, and this falls to less than 10% by the age of 18 [49]. The overall pattern is therefore for the liver problem to regress, although occasionally it may progress to cirrhosis and liver failure.

Again there is a suggestion that a further genetic influence may play a role because the likelihood of a sibling with α_1-antitrypsin deficiency developing neonatal jaundice is greatly increased when it has occurred in a first individual [50].

In adults there is a wide spectrum of abnormality. At its simplest it may involve only histopathological changes with α_1-antitrypsin inclusion bodies in hepatocytes. In some individuals there may be slightly abnormal liver function tests and in others evidence of hepatitis and fibrosis. The spectrum extends to those with end-stage cirrhosis and liver failure, and this process may lead to rapid progression of the liver disease. There is an increase in hepatocellular carcinoma in individuals with α_1-antitrypsin deficiency and liver problems seem to occur with more frequency in male subjects [48].

Although the liver disease is conventionally associated with the Z form of deficiency, it has also been described in other α_1-antitrypsin-deficient phenotypes in which failure to excrete protein also occurs. The M malton variant is also associated with liver inclusion bodies of α_1-antitrypsin and cirrhosis [51].

The pathogenesis of liver disease is not clearly understood, but is likely to relate to the accumulation of α_1-antitrypsin in hepatocytes. Early studies were uncertain about whether the serum deficiency of α_1-antitrypsin in some way failed to protect hepatocytes from damage. However, elegant studies using transgenic mice show that the animals transfected with the normal human α_1-antitrypsin gene retained normal liver histology whereas those transfected with the Z gene developed the histological changes of liver damage [52].

Clinical studies generally seemed to indicate that subjects who develop lung disease as a result of α_1-antitrypsin deficiency are unlikely to have significant liver damage and vice versa. The role of other genetic factors in determining the phenotype in patients with α_1-antitrypsin deficiency has been explored by several workers. Evidence has suggested that there is a relationship of the liver disease to HLA-DR3 haplotype and also an association with HLA-DW25 [53]. Death as a result of liver disease seems to be decreased in PiZ subjects who have been breast-fed [54], which may reflect a true association or be a reflection of social class. This concept of a subgroup susceptibility was discussed in detail by Teckman and colleagues in 1996 [55], indicating that factors involved in protein degradation may play a intracellular role.

Treatment for the liver disease is relatively unsatisfactory. Although replacement therapy may have a role to play in protecting distant organs such as the lung from proteolytic degradation, as a result of low levels of α_1-antitrypsin, the same cannot be true of the liver. The liver damage is thought to be a direct consequence of the build-up of α_1-antitrypsin in hepatocytes and, unless methodology can be developed to prevent gene transcription at this site and/or enhance protein degradation, it is unlikely that a realistic therapeutic strategy can be developed. Most subjects with severe liver disease therefore show gradual progression and transplantation is the only realistic treatment. This in itself not only restores a normal liver function but in addition corrects the α_1-antitrypsin defect.

The identification of α_1-antitrypsin deficiency has led to a major increase in our understanding of the genetic template and coding for this protein as well as its biological role. At present many questions remain to be answered. However, understanding of the molecular biology should lead to the development of successful strategies to counteract the clinical manifestations.

References

1 Laurell C-B, Eriksson S (1963) The electrophoretic α-1-globulin pattern of serum in α_1-antitrypsin deficiency. *Scand J Clin Lab Invest* 15: 132–140
2 Eriksson S (1965) Studies in α_1-antitrypsin deficiency. *Acta Med Scand* 432 (suppl): 1–85
3 Gross P, Pfitzer EA, Tolker E, Babyak MA, Kaschak M (1974) Experimental emphysema. Its production with papain in normal and silicotic rats. *Arch Environ* Health 11: 50–58
4 Janoff A, Sloane B, Weinbaum G, Damiano V, Sandhaus RA, Elias J, Kimbel P (1977) Experimental emphysema induced with purified human neutrophil elastase: tissue localisation of the instilled protease. *Am Rev Respir Dis* 115: 461–478
5 Priestle JP (1988) Ribbon: a stereocartoon drawing programme for proteins. *J Aplied Crystall* 21: 572–576
6 Owen MC, O'Brennan S, Lewis JH, Carrell RW (1983) Mutation of antitrypsin to antithrombin: antitrypsin Pittsburgh (358 Met to Arg), a fatal bleeding disorder. *N Engl J Med* 309: 694–698
7 Ohlsson K, Laurell C-B (1976) The disappearance of enzyme-inhibitor complexes from the circulation in man. *Clin Sci Mol Med* 51: 87–92
8 Takahashi H, Crystal RG (1990) α_1-antitrypsin $\text{null}_{\text{isola di procida}}$: an α_1-antitrypsin deficiency allele caused by deletion of all α_1-antitrypsin coding exons. *Am J Hum Genet* 47: 403–413
9 Poller W, Faber JP, Fiedinger S, Olek K (1991) DNA polymorphisms associated with a new α_1-antitrypsin PI Q0 variant (PI Q0 Reidenburg). *Hum Genet* 86: 522–524
10 Nukiwa T, Takahashi H, Brantly M, Courtney M, Crystal RG (1987) α_1-antitrypsin $\text{null}_{\text{granite falls}}$, a non expressing α_1-antitrypsin gene associated with a frameshift to stop mutation in a coding exon. *J Biol Chem* 262: 11999–12004
11 Curiel D, Brantly M, Curiel E, Steir L, Crystal RG (1989) α_1-antitrypsin deficiency caused by the α_1-antitrypsin $\text{null}_{\text{mattawa}}$ gene. *J Clin Invest* 83: 1144–1152

12 Brantly MA (1996) α_1-antitrypsin genotypes and phenotypes. In: RG Crystal (ed): *Lung biology in health and disease. α_1-antitrypsin deficiency*, Vol. 88. Marcel Dekker, New York, 45–59
13 Satoh K, Nukiwa T, Brantly M, Garvier RI, Hofker M, Courtney M, Crystal RG (1988) Emphysema associated with complete absence of α_1-antitrypsin of a stop codon in an α_1-antitrypsin coding exon. *Am J Hum Genet* 42: 77–83
14 Graham A, Kalsheker NA, Bamforth FJ, Newton CR, Markham AF (1990) Molecular characterisation of two α_1-antitrypsin deficiency variants: proteinase inhibitor (PI) $Null_{newport}$ (GLy 115-Ser) and (PI) $Z_{wrexham}$ (Ser 19-Leu). *Hum Genet* 85: 537–540
15 Nukiwa T, Sato K, Brantly ML, Ogushi F, Fells GA, Courtney M, Crystal RG (1986) Identification of a second mutation in the protein coding sequence of the Z type α_1-antitrypsin gene. *J Biol Chem* 261: 15989–15994
16 Verbanac KM, Heath EC (1986) Biosynthesis processing and secretion of M and Z variant human α_1-antitrypsin. *J Biol Chem* 261: 9979–9989
17 Foreman RC, Judah JD, Coleman A (1984) Xenopus oocytes synthesise but do not secrete Z variant of human α_1-antitrypsin. *FEBS Lett* 168: 84–88
18 Brantly ML, Courtney M, Crystal RG (1988) Repair of the secretion defect of the Z form of α_1-antitrypsin by addition of a second mutation. *Science* 242: 1700–1702
19 Lomas DA, Evans DL, Finch JT, Carrell RW (1992) The mechanism of Z α_1-antitrypsin accumulation in the liver. *Nature* 357: 605–607
20 Lomas DA, Finch JT, Seyama K, Nukiwa T, Carrell RW (1993) α_1-antitrypsin S_{iiyama} (Ser 53-Phe): further evidence for intracellular-sheet polymerisation. *J Biol Chem* 268: 15333–15335
21 Lomas DA, Elliott PR, Sidhar SK, Foreman RC, Finch JT, Cox DW, Whisstock JC, Carrell RW (1995) α_1-antitrypsin M malton (^{52}Phe deleted) forms loop-sheet polymers *in vivo*: evidence for the C-sheet mechanism of polymerisation. *J Biol Chem* 270: 16864–16870
22 Ogushi F, Fells GA, Hubbard RC, Straus SD, Crystal RG (1987) Z-type α_1-antitrypsin is less competent than M1 type α_1-antitrypsin as an inhibitor of neutrophil elastase. *J Clin Invest* 80: 1366–1374
23 Llewellyn-Jones CG, Lomas DA, Carrell RW, Stockley RA (1994) The effect of the Z mutation on the ability of α_1-antitrypsin to prevent neutrophil mediated tissue damage. *Biochim Biophys Acta* 1227: 155–160
24 Cook L, Burdon JDW, Brenton S, Knight KR, Janus ED (1996) Kinetic characterisation of α_1-antitrypsin F as an inhibitor of human neutrophil elastase. *Pathology* 28: 242–247
25 He S, Sim RB, Whaley K (1997) A secondary C1s interaction site on C1-inhibitor is essential for formation of an SDS-stable enzyme-inhibitor complex. *FEBS Lett* 405: 42–46
26 Beattie K, Bieth J, Travis J (1980) Kinetics of association of serine proteinases with native and oxidised α_1-proteinase inhibitor and α_1-antichymotrypsin. *J Biol Chem* 255: 3931–3934
27 Stockley RA (1992) Biochemical and cellular mechanisms: In: P Calverley, N Pride (eds): *Chronic obstructive pulmonary disease*. Chapman & Hall, London, 93–133
28 Kalsheker NA, Hodgson I, Watkins GL, White JP, Morrison HM, Stockley RA (1987) Deoxyribonuclei acid (DNA) polymorphism of the α_1-antitrypsin (AAT) gene in chronic lung disease. *BMJ* 294: 1511–1514
29 Morgan K, Scoby G, Kalsheker N (1992) The characterisation of a mutation of the 3′ flanking sequence of the α_1-antitrypsin gene commonly associated with chronic obstructive airways disease. *Eur J Clin Invest* 22: 134–137
30 Larsson C (1978) Natural history and life expectancy in severe α_1-antitrypsin deficiency, PiZ. *Acta Med Scand* 204: 345–351
31 Brantly ML, Paul LD, Miller BH, Falk RT, Wu M, Crystal RG (1988) Clinical features and history of the destructive lung disease associated with α_1-antitrypsin deficiency of adults with pulmonary symptoms. *Am Rev Respir Dis* 138: 327–336
32 Gadek JE, Felles GA, Zimmerman RL, Rennard SI, Crystal RG (1981) Antielastases of the human alveolar structures. Implications for the protease/antiprotease theory of emphysema. *J Clin Invest* 68: 889–898
33 Stockley RA (1988) Proteases/Antiproteases: Pathogenesis and role in therapy. *Clinical pulmonary medicine* 5: 203–210
34 Sveger T (1978) α_1-antitrypsin deficiency in early childhood. *Pediatrics* 62: 22–25

35 Silverman EK, Miletich JP, Pierce JA, Sherman LA, Broze GJ, Campbell EJ (1989) α_1-antitrypsin deficiency. High prevalence in the St. Louis area determined by direct population screening. *Am Rev Respir Dis* 140: 961–966
36 Cullen BH, Ball WC, Bias WB et al. (1975) A genetic-epidemiologic study of chronic obstructive pulmonary disease. *John Hopkins Med J* 137: 95–104
37 Jones DK, Godden D, Kavanagh P (1985) α_1-antitrypsin deficiency presenting as bronchiectasis. *Br J Dis Chest* 79: 301–304
38 Piitulainen E, Tornling G, Eriksson S (1997) Effect of age and occupational exposure to airway irritants on lung function in non-smoking individuals with α_1-antitrypsin deficiency (PiZZ). *Thorax* 52: 244–248
39 Hubbard RC, Fells G, Gadek J et al. (1991) Neutrophil accumulation in the lung in α_1-antitrypsin deficiency: spontaneous release of leukotriene B_4 by alveolar macrophages. *J Clin Invest* 88: 891–897
40 Okada S, Kita H, George TJ, Gleich TJ, Leiferman KM (1997) Migration of eosinophils through basement membrane components *in vitro*: role of matrix metalloproteinase-9. *Am J Respir Cell Mol Biol* 17: 519–528
41 Campbell EJ, Senior RM, McDonald JA, Cox DW (1982) Proteolysis by neutrophils. Relative importance of cell-substrate contact and oxidative inactivation of proteinase inhibitors *in vitro*. *J Clin Invest* 70: 745–852
42 Liou TG, Campbell EJ (1995) Non-isotropic enzyme-inhibitor interactions: a novel non-oxidative mechanism for quantum proteolysis by human neutrophils. *Biochemistry* 34: 16171–16177
43 Liou TG, Campbell EJ (1996) Quantum proteolysis resulting from release single granules by human neutrophils. *J Immunol* 157: 2624–2631
44 Reynolds HY, Newball HH (1974) Analysis of proteins in respiratory cells from human lungs by bronchial lavage. *J Lab Clin Med* 84: 559–573
45 Sharpe HL, Bridges RA, Krivit W, Freier EF (1969) Cirrhosis associated with α_1-antitrypsin deficiency: a previously unrecognised inherited disorder. *J Lab Clin Med* 73: 934–939
46 Berg NO, Eriksson S (1972) Liver disease in adults with α_1-antitrypsin deficiency. *N Engl J Med* 287: 1264–1267
47 Sveger T (1976) Liver disease in α_1-antitrypsin deficiency detected by screening of 200000 infants. *N Engl J Med* 294: 1316–1321
48 Eriksson S, Ohlsson J, Wellers R (1986) Risks of cirrhosis and primary liver cancer in α_1-antitrypsin deficiency. *N Engl J Med* 314: 736–773
49 Sveger T, Eriksson S (1995) The liver in adolescents with α_1-antitrypsin deficiency. *Hepatology* 22: 514–517
50 Cox DW, Mansfield T (1987) Prenatal diagnosis of α_1-antitrypsin deficiency and estimates of foetal risk for disease. *J Med Genet* 24: 52–59
51 Curiel DT, Holmes MD, Okayama H, Brantly ML, Vogelmeier C, Travis WD, Stier LE, Perks WH, Crystal RG (1989) Molecular basis of the liver and lung disease associated with the α_1-antitrypsin deficiency allele M malton. *J Biol Chem* 264: 13938–13945
52 Carlsen JA, Rogers BB, Sifers RN, Finegold MJ, Clift SM, DeMayo FJ, Bullock DW, Woo SLC (1989) Accumulation of PiZ α_1-antitrypsin causes liver damage in transgenic mice. *J Clin Invest* 83: 1183–1190
53 Doherty DG, Donaldson PT, Whitehouse DB, Mieli-Vergami G, Duthie A, Hopkinson DA, Mowat AP (1990) HLA phenotypes and gene polymorphism in juvenile liver disease associated with α_1-antitrypsin deficiency. *Hepatology* 12: 218–223
54 Udall JN, Dixon M, Newman AP, Wright JA, James B, Bloch KJ (1985) Liver disease in α_1-antitrypsin deficiency. *JAMA* 253: 267–282
55 Teckman JH, Qu D, Perlmutter DH (1996) Molecular pathogenesis of liver disease in α_1-antitrypsin deficiency. *Hepatology* 24: 1504–1516

Molecular Biology of the Lung
Vol. 1: Emphysema and Infection
ed. by R. A. Stockley

CHAPTER 4
Recombinant SLPI: Emphysema and Asthma

Jan Stolk and Pieter S. Hiemstra

Leiden University Medical Centre, Department of Pulmonology (C3-P), Leiden, The Netherlands

1. Introduction

Secretory leukocyte protease inhibitor (SLPI), also known as antileukoprotease (ALP) or mucus protease inhibitor, is a low-molecular-weight serine protease inhibitor of 11.7 kDa. In addition to neutrophil elastase, SLPI inhibits cathepsin G, trypsin, chymotrypsin, mast cell chymase and tryptase, but not proteinase 3. Besides acting as an antiprotease, SLPI also has other important biological properties. For example, SLPI increases glutathione levels in the lung, supports colony growth of human haemopoietic cells, shows antimicrobial activity and could have anti-HIV-1 activities.

2. Production in the Lung

In the airways, SLPI has been localized in serous cells of nasal and bronchial submucosal glands, in a non-ciliated epithelial cell population of bronchus and terminal bronchioles (Clara cells and goblet cells), and in cuboidal cells of the alveolar duct [1]. An immunoelectron microscopic study revealed that intracellular SLPI is localized in secretory granules. After fixation of these tissues with paraformaldehyde lysine periodate, four types of secretory granules with distinct SLPI-specific labelling patterns could be recognized in serous cells of bronchial glands. It may be that these types designate a state of maturation within a single population. Using light microscopy, the distribution of SLPI has also been studied in the developing lung from fetuses of 9–40 weeks of gestation [2]. SLPI was detected from 16 weeks in submucosal glands and in collecting ducts in the trachea and main bronchi, whereas SLPI in bronchiolar epithelium could only be detected after 36 weeks of gestation. In addition to detection in the airways, SLPI was also found in association with elastin fibres in the subepithelial connective tissue of the bronchial wall and in the parenchymal matrix of the alveolar septa [3]. This observation suggests that SLPI is a modulating factor in destructive pulmonary diseases such as emphysema.

The neutrophil is a key player in many inflammatory lung diseases. Two reports in the literature showed that SLPI is also produced in the neutrophil, where it is present in the cytoplasm as an active elastase inhibitor with a molecular mass of 14 kDa [4, 5]. However, when the cells were stimulated with phorbol myristate acetate (PMA), SLPI was secreted in an inactive form. PMA-stimulated neutrophils were shown to secrete 3 µg SLPI/10^6 cells per 24 h, about 100-fold more than secreted by stimulated epithelial cells derived from tumour cell lines such H322 and A549 [5]. The physiological importance of this finding remains to be established. It was speculated that the cytosolic SLPI is involved in the tight regulation of proteinases during maturation of neutrophils in the bone marrow. The reason why SLPI is excreted in an inactive form by neutrophils is unclear.

3. Genes and Gene Regulation

In 1986, the human SLPI gene was characterized by Stetler et al. and shown to include four exons, spanning 2.6 kb [6]. The cDNA encodes a predicted translation product of 14 kDa. As the N-terminus of the secreted protein starts at residue 26, residues 1–25 probably constitute a signal peptide. The predicted size of the mature secretion protein is approximately 12 kDa. In the 5′-flanking region close to exon 1, there are four potential binding sites for transcription factor activator protein-1 (AP-1), three for AP-2 and one for the CCAAT enhancer binding protein (C/EPB) [7]. Recently, a lung cell-specific regulatory region in the SLPI promoter was identified and shown to contain a recognition sequence for two nuclear proteins [8]. No polymorphisms in the major SLPI-coding exons have been noted, which is in contrast to the α_1-antitrypsin gene [7]. Even in individuals with chronic obstructive pulmonary disease (COPD) disease, who did not have α_1-antitrypsin deficiency or cystic fibrosis, no polymorphisms were detected at an early age in the SLPI coding exons 2–4.

The SLPI gene is constitutively expressed, but various stimuli have been shown to modulate SLPI expression in cultures of primary lung epithelial cells and cell lines *in vitro* (Figure 1). Whereas the mRNA for SLPI was

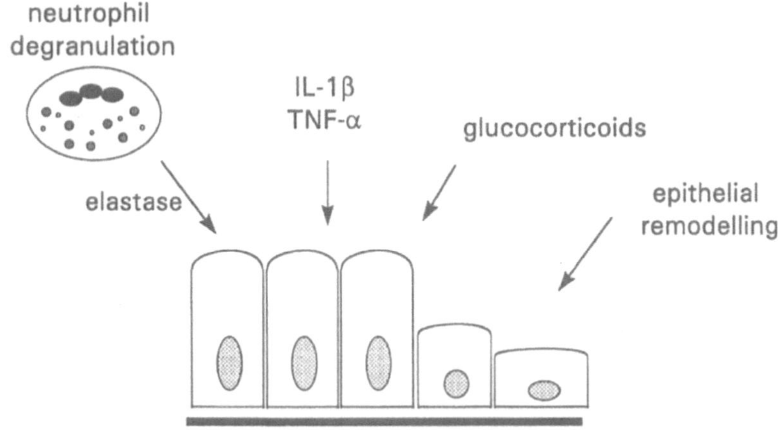

Figure 1. Regulation of SLPI production by epithelial cells (see text for details).

found to be relatively stable, its stability was further increased by treatment of an epithelial cell line with PMA [9]. Sallenave and co-workers reported increased SLPI production in airway epithelial cell lines upon stimulation with the proinflammatory cytokines interleukin 1β (IL-1β) and tumor necrosis factor α (TNF-α) [10]. This implies that epithelial cells may respond to cytokines from macrophages secreted during the onset of inflammation by increasing their antiprotease shield. Proinflammatory agents such as lipopolysaccharide (LPS), IL-6, IL-8 and substance P had no effect on SLPI production by cell lines. Both Sallenave et al. [10] and Abbinante-Nissen et al. [11] reported increased SLPI mRNA levels in epithelial cells treated with neutrophil elastase, but it was interesting that this was accompanied by a decrease in SLPI protein release [10]. Similar results were obtained using primary epithelial cell cultures derived from nasal polyps by Marchand et al. [12], who also noted an increase in the number of SLPI-containing cells in elastase-treated cultures. It was suggested that elastase may stimulate secretion of SLPI to the basal side of the cell, and thus protect the underlying tissue from proteolytic injury. In addition to proinflammatory mediators, glucocorticoids also increase SLPI production by epithelial cell lines, at both the mRNA and protein level [13]. So far these *in vitro* findings have not been confirmed by *in vivo* studies, because treatment of patients with chronic bronchitis and emphysema with inhaled steroids did not result in significant increases in sputum SLPI levels [14].

Although these data on the synthesis of SLPI in cell cultures suggest that the production of SLPI is regulated by various mediators, at present there is also evidence for dynamic regulation of SLPI production *in vivo*. *In vivo*, SLPI-containing cells in respiratory bronchioli are associated with parenchymal destruction in smokers [15]. In pneumonia, SLPI-containing cells in the bronchial/bronchiolar epithelium correlate with goblet cell hyperplasia, and with acute inflammatory infiltration in the adjacent alveolar area [16]. Further support for dynamic regulation of SLPI production *in vivo* was obtained by Marchand et al. in a study using nasal polyps [17], who demonstrated an association between the number of SLPI-containing cells and epithelial remodelling, but no such association with the local degree of inflammation. These data indicate that changes in local SLPI production may play a role in the regulation of the local defence against tissue destruction, inflammation and infection in the lung.

4. Proteinase Inhibitory Activities

4.1. Inhibitory Activities in the Lung

Although α_1-antitrypsin is considered as the major inhibitor of neutrophil elastase (NE) in the peripheral lung, SLPI is the major inhibitor of NE in the central airways [18]. However, SLPI could also protect the peripheral lung against proteolytic destruction. Indeed, SLPI has been found in bronchoalveolar lavage (BAL) fluid from healthy volunteers or patients, at lower, similar or slightly higher concentrations than α_1-antitrypsin [19–21]. In contrast to α_1-antitrypsin, SLPI is not considered to be an acute phase reactant. Different mechanisms may inactivate SLPI, including oxidation of critical methionine residues and inactivation by lipid peroxidation products [22]. The pathophysiological importance of these phenomena is not clear.

SLPI is able to inhibit tryptase Clara [23], a novel serine protease that is produced by bronchiolar epithelial Clara cells. The enzyme is able to cleave the haemagglutinin of the influenza virus, leading to enhancement of the infectivity of influenza A virus in a dose-dependent way. Similar results were obtained in an animal model of viral pneumonitis induced by the Sendai virus [24]. These results imply that therapy with recombinant SLPI (rSLPI) may reduce the pathogenicity of pneumonitis-inducing viruses.

4.2. SLPI Binding to Mucins and Heparin

SLPI is incompletely released in a free form by the extraction procedure used to isolate this inhibitor from human sputum. This is the result of the tight binding of SLPI to mucins, probably through ionic interactions between basic amino acid residues of SLPI and acidic residues of the carbohydrate chains of mucins [25]. These interactions protect bronchial mucins against proteolysis by neutrophil elastase, allowing them to retain their rheological properties. In addition to mucins, SLPI also forms a tight complex with heparin which involves seven ionic interactions [26]. This property is not restricted to SLPI, because heparin also interacts with members of the SERPIN family of proteinase inhibitors, including antithrombin III and the protease nexin. The binding strongly enhances the rate of association with NE (k_{ass}) [26]. This *in vitro* observation may have important pathophysiological implications which can be determined by using the k_{ass}. SLPI and α_1-antitrypsin are the physiological inhibitors that protect the lungs against tissue destruction by accidentally liberated NE. Earlier studies showed that heparin strongly decreased the rate of inhibition of NE by α_1-antitrypsin by a factor of 40 [27] but increased the k_{ass} of SLPI by a factor of 27 [26]. Heparin is abundantly present in the lung [28], because this organ has many heparin-containing mast cells present in the alveolar walls, the site where elastase attacks the lung matrix proteins to induce emphysematous lesions.

5. Antimicrobial and Anti-Inflammatory Properties

In addition to its proteinase inhibitory properties, which may serve to protect against proteolytic injury, it was recently shown that SLPI also displays antimicrobial and anti-inflammatory activities which appear to be independent of its ability to inhibit neutrophil serine proteinases (Figure 2). Studies by McNeely and co-workers identified SLPI as a major anti-HIV-1 component in human saliva, and suggested that this activity of SLPI was medi-

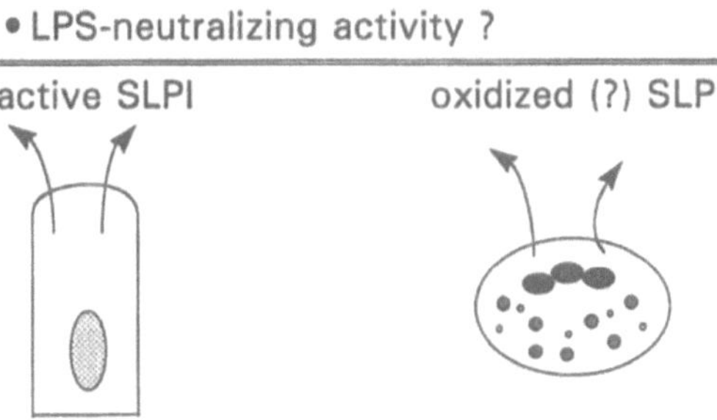

Figure 2. Multiple functions of SLPI in inflammation and infection. Several activities have been described for SLPI, and not all of these may be dependent on the proteinase inhibitory activity of SLPI (see text for details). This is important because the proteinase inhibitory activity of SLPI is sensitive to oxidative inactivation, and neutrophils, in contrast to epithelial cells, appear to secrete SLPI that lacks this activity.

ated by interaction with a target cell-associated protein [29]. In a follow-up study, a SLPI-binding protein on the surface of monocytes was identified as a protein with a molecular weight of 55 kDa [30]. SLPI was found to inhibit the HIV-1 infection process by interfering with it at a stage after virus binding to the cell and before reverse transcription. These studies still await confirmation, because others have reported that SLPI does not display any anti-HIV-1 activity [31].

Based on the identification of an equine antimicrobial protein that has some of the characteristics of SLPI [32], the antimicrobial activity of rSLPI against both Gram-negative (*Escherichia coli*) and Gram-positive (*Staphylococcus aureus*) bacteria [33], and towards the human fungal pathogens *Aspergillus fumigatus* and *Candida albicans* [34], was investigated. SLPI was found to display marked antibacterial and antiviral activity at concentrations in which SLPI is present in mucosal secretions, including those of the lung. Using purified domains obtained by cleavage of intact rSLPI, it was shown that, whereas the antiproteinase activity of SLPI is localized in its carboxyl-terminal domain, the antibacterial and antifungal activities are localized in the amino-terminal domain. The antibacterial and antifungal activities of SLPI, like those of other cationic antimicrobial peptides, are inhibited at increased ionic strength [33, 34]. This is of importance, because recently epithelial-derived, salt-sensitive, antimicrobial peptides, including human β-defensin-1 (hBD-1), have been implicated in the recurrent pulmonary infections of cystic fibrosis; these peptides may not function optimally in the epithelial lining fluid of cystic fibrosis patients as a result of the increased salt concentrations in this fluid [35, 36]. These results suggest that SLPI, in addition to other epithelial antimicrobial peptides including hBD-1 [36, 37], may contribute to host defence against infection at the mucosal surface.

Two recent studies demonstrate that SLPI inhibits monocyte/macrophage pro-inflammatory activities. Lipopolysaccharide (LPS) is a potent stimulator of gene expression in various cell types, including mononuclear phagocytes, and differences in LPS responsivenes have been noted between various strains of mice. Using differential display to analyse gene expression in the LPS-responsive and LPS-hyporesponsive strains of mice, the murine homologue of human SLPI was cloned and shown to be overexpressed in a macrophage cell line derived from LPS-hyporesponsive mice [38]. In contrast, cells from a macrophage cell line derived from LPS-responsive mice expressed little SLPI. Further support for an association between SLPI expression and LPS responsiveness was obtained by transfection of cells from LPS-responsive mice with the SLPI gene, resulting in a marked decrease in LPS-induced nuclear factor κB (NF-κB) activation and production of nitric oxide and TNF-α. In murine macrophages, SLPI expression was found to be induced by LPS and suppressed by interferon-γ. SLPI also inhibits other functions of cells from the mononuclear phagocyte lineage, because it was recently demonstrated that SLPI blocks the production of matrix metalloproteinases (MMPs) in human monocytes, suggesting that SLPI may also restrict MMP-mediated connective tissue destruction [39]. Inhibition of monocyte MMP production was mediated in part by interference with signal transduction, because SLPI inhibited LPS- and concanavalin A-stimulated production of monocyte prostaglandin H synthase-2, which is a critical enzyme in the prostaglandin E_2-cAMP-dependent pathway of monocyte MMP production. Using SLPI mutants that lack antiproteinase activity, it was demonstrated that these inhibitory activities of SLPI are not mediated by proteinase inhibitory activity. Furthermore, SLPI did not affect TNF-α or IL-10 production by monocytes stimulated with high concentrations (1 µg/ml) of LPS. Taken together, these data indicate that SLPI not only displays anti-inflammatory activity by regulating the activity of released serine proteinases, but also contributes to the anti-inflammatory screen by regulating selected proinflammatory activities of monocytes and macrophages.

6. Aerosol Inhalation of Recombinant SLPI in Animals and Humans

The therapeutic potential of rSLPI is underlined by the fact that at least three pharmaceutical companies are able to produce this protein by recombinant DNA technology. Although several elastase inhibitors have been available for clinical studies during the past 3 years, few or no clinical effects in humans have been reported to date. This is largely related to the fact that these compounds are tested in chronic inflammatory diseases such as cystic fibrosis or pulmonary emphysema, which can only show benefits in long-term clinical trials. To date, short-term interventions in cystic fibrosis with aerosolized rSLPI have not shown complete reduction of elastase activity (the presumed target) in epithelial lung lining fluid [40]. Thus the results do not indicate the clinical outcome of long-term studies in cystic fibrosis (CF). Moreover, the potential therapeutic effect of rSLPI in CF may be restricted by the fact that aerosolized rSLPI will only deposit in well-ventilated but only modestly inflamed areas [41]. It is not possible to administer rSLPI effectively either orally or intravenously because the compound is rapidly excreted by the kidneys, as demonstrated in rats [42]. Aerosol administration of rSLPI to sheep resulted in a marked increase in SLPI levels and anti-elastase activity in the epithelial lining fluid of sheep, but it also appeared to increase glutathione levels in epithelial lining fluid [43]. These results suggest that SLPI not only contributes to the formation of an antiproteinase screen, but also may increase antioxidant defences.

We studied the distribution and disappearance of aerosolized rSLPI in humans [41]. Recombinant SLPI was coupled to technetium-99m (^{99m}Tc) and inhaled by normal volunteers, as well as by patients with emphysema and cystic fibrosis. We found that only 10% of the aerosol was deposited in the lungs by using a Pariboy jet nebulizer. The remaining aerosol was deposited in the mouth and stomach (20%) and the outflow filter (70%). The inhaled portion of the aerosol deposited only in well-ventilated areas in the lung. In each of the three groups of volunteers, the SLPI aerosol disappeared biexponentially, with an initial rapid phase of about 2 h and a slow phase of more than 24 h. The results suggest that SLPI aerosol therapy is likely to be of more value in emphysema to protect normal lung tissue against elastase, than in a bronchial disease such as cystic fibrosis where the aerosol is rapidly cleared from bronchi.

7. SLPI in Models of Emphysema

In our laboratory we used two models for induction of emphysema in experimental animals. We induced emphysema in hamsters by a single intratracheal instillation of purified human NE [44]. After 21 days the animals were sacrificed and the emphysema was quantified by measuring mean linear intercepts in tissue sections of the lungs. We found that the development of emphysema was inhibited by SLPI in a dose-dependent way. Molar ratios of rSLPI over NE of 0.86, 1.3 or 1.74 inhibited elastase-induced emphysema by 45, 51 or 65%, respectively, which was similar to the results obtained by Lucey et al. [45]. When the interval of time between a single dose of rSLPI and elastase (in a molar ratio of 1.74) was increased from 1 to 20 h, the development of emphysema was inhibited by 79% [46]. This improvement may be explained by a more efficient and relevant distribution of rSLPI in the lungs before the instillation of elastase.

In a second model we induced emphysema by repeated intratracheal instillations of *E. coli* LPS [47]. In this way we recruited hamster neutrophils into the lungs, mediated by macrophage-derived inflammatory stimuli. The neutrophils released elastase that caused emphysema and bronchial cell metaplasia. Intratracheal instillation of 0.5 mg LPS twice a week for 4 weeks resulted in marked emphysema, which was inhibited by 54% when 1 mg rSLPI was instilled either several minutes before LPS or even 7 and 31 h after LPS. The recruitment of neutrophils into the lungs was not inhibited by rSLPI so the result suggests that endogenous hamster neutrophil elastase activity was inhibited, thereby preventing the development of emphysema. We postulated that this model resembles the situation in smokers-related emphysema in humans, where neutrophils are recruited into the lungs directly by cigarette smoke and by proinflammatory mediators from macrophages such as TNF-α', to release their elastase into the interstitium and bronchoalveolar airspaces. The results described above suggest that rSLPI would be of therapeutic value in a similar situation in humans.

8. SLPI in Models of Asthma

The participation of neutrophils and neutrophil-derived elastase in allergen-induced airway inflammation in human asthma has yet to be fully resolved. A possible role for elastase inhibitors in antigen-induced airway hyperresponsiveness (AHR) was demonstrated by a study in sheep [48]. Continuous administration of an elastase inhibitor before antigen challenge of the lungs of sheep significantly inhibited the late bronchoconstriction reaction, neutrophil recruitment in the airways and chemotactic activity of BAL. AHR had a tendency to be attenuated, but this did not reach statistical significance.

Recently, Abraham and collagues showed, in a sheep model, that the enzyme tryptase plays an important role in *Ascaris suum*-induced asthma [49]. The early and late bronchoconstrictor response, as well as the non-specific bronchoconstriction following 24 h after allergen challenge, could be significantly inhibited by rSLPI [50]. The authors postulated that rSLPI had antiallergic and anti-inflammatory properties, with tryptase as an important target in this model. The inhibitor α_1-antitrypsin had no effect in this model, suggesting that neutrophil elastase is of minor importance.

We recently evaluated the effect of rSLPI on ozone-induced airway hyperresponsivenes in humans. It has been shown that ozone inhalation causes acute, predominantly neutrophil-mediated, inflammatory changes in the lung [51, 52]. Acute exposure to ozone in healthy and asthmatic subjects causes dose-dependent (but transient) decrements in lung volumes and flow rates [51]. Ozone inhalation causes methacholine-inducible AHR in healthy subjects and asthmatic patients [53]. Animal and human studies have shown ozone-induced airway inflammation and neutrophil influx after a single exposure to 0.2–0.6 ppm over 2 h [51], with up to an eight-fold increase in percentage neutrophils in BAL [52]. Immunoreactive neutrophil elastase was elevated fourfold after exposure [51]. It was observed some time ago that the bronchial responses to inhaled methacholine and to histamine increase after acute exposure to ozone and return to control values by the following day [54]. The data suggested a correlation between elastase activity in the airways after ozone inhalation and induction of AHR. In our laboratory, we examined the effect of rSLPI treatment on ozone-induced AHR in people with mild asthma [55]. Sixteen hours after exposure to ozone in the laboratory, AHR to methacholine was increased after both placebo and rSLPI treatment. These results therefore indicated that neutrophil-derived serine proteinases do not play an important role in mediating ozone-induced hyperresponsiveness.

9. Concluding Remarks

In recent years, new information has been obtained concerning the *in vitro* properties of SLPI. Although SLPI was originally identified as a proteinase inhibitor involved in the protection against proteinase-mediated tissue destruction, it has more recently been shown also to act as an antimicrobial protein and to inhibit monocyte/macrophage proinflammatory activities. Furthermore, *in vitro* SLPI supports colony growth of human haemopoietic progenitor cells by neutralizing proteinases that are produced by accessory cells [56]. Studies in experimental animals support the therapeutic potential of rSLPI treatment in both pulmonary emphysema and asthma, but at present no data are available for the contribution of SLPI to host defence against infection *in vivo*. Although rSLPI has been used in short-term intervention studies in humans, the therapeutic efficacy of rSLPI in human disease remains to be demonstrated, and may require long-term intervention studies. The new information obtained recently on the *in vitro* and *in vivo* properties of SLPI may stimulate the development of new research programmes aimed to evaluate the therapeutic potential of SLPI in human lung disease.

Acknowledgements

The studies in our laboratory cited in this review were supported in part by grants from the Dutch Asthma Foundation (grant no. 87.13), the Dutch Ministry of Housing, Physical Planning and the Environment, and the European Union (EU Biomed 2 programme, grant no. BMH4 CT96-0152).

References

1 de Water R, Willems LNA, van Muijen GNP, Franken C, Fransen JAM, Dijkman JH, Kramps JA (1986) Ultrastructural localization of bronchial antileukoprotease in central and peripheral human airways by a gold-labelling technique using monoclonal antibodies. *Am Rev Respir Dis* 133: 883–890
2 Willems LNA, Kramps JA, Jeffery PK, Dijkman JH (1988) Antileukoprotease in the developing fetal lung. *Thorax* 43: 784–786
3 Kramps JA, te Boekhorst AHT, Fransen JAM, Ginsel LA, Dijkman JH (1989) Antileukoprotease is associated with elastin fibers in the extracellular matrix of the human lung. An immunoelectron microscopic study. *Am Rev Respir Dis* 140: 471–476
4 Bohm B, Aignet T, Kinne R, Burkhardt H (1991) The serine-protease inhibitor of cartilage matrix is not a chondrocytic gene product. *Eur J Biochem* 207: 773–779
5 Sallenave J-M, Si-Ta har M, Cox G, Chignard M, Gauldie J (1997) Secretory leukocyte proteinase inhibitor is a major leukocyte elastase inhibitor in human neutrophils. *J Leukocyte Biol* 61: 695–702
6 Stetler G, Brewer MT, Thomspon RC (1986) Isolation and sequence of a human gene encoding a potent inhibitor of leukocyte proteases. *Nucleic Acids Res* 14: 7883–7896
7 Abe T, Kobayashi N, Yoshimura K, Trapnell BC, Kim H, Hubbard RC, Brewer MT, Thompson RC, Crystal RG (1991) Expression of the secretory leukoprotease inhibitor gene in epithelial cells. *J Clin Invest* 87: 2207–2215
8 Kikuchi T, Abe T, Satoh K, Narumi K, Sakai T, Abe S, Shindoh S, Matsushima K, Nukiwa T (1997) *cis*-Acting region associated with lung cell-specific expression of the secretory leukoprotease inhibitor gene. *Am J Respir Cell Mol Biol* 17: 361–367
9 Maruyama M, Hay JG, Yoshimura K, Chu C-S, Crystal RG (1994) Modulation of secretory leukoprotease inhibitor gene expression in human bronchial epithelial cells by phorbol ester. *J Clin Invest* 94: 368–375

10 Sallenave J-M, Shulmann J, Crossley J, Jordana M, Gauldie J (1994) Regulation of secretory leukocyte proteinase inhibitor and elastase-specific inhibitor in human airway epithelial cells by cytokines and neutrophilic enzymes. *Am J Respir Cell Mol Biol* 11: 733–741

11 Abbinante-Nissen JM, Simpson LG, Leikauf GD (1993) Neutrophil elastase increases secretory leukocyte protease inhibitor transcript levels in airway epithelial cells. *Am J Physiol Lung Cell Mol Physiol* 265: L286–292

12 Marchand V, Tournier JM, Polette M, Nawrocki B, Fuchey C, Pierrot D, Burlet H, Puchelle E (1997) The elastase-induced expression of secretory leukocyte protease inhibitor is decreased in remodelled airway epithelium. *Eur J Pharmacol* 336: 187–196

13 Abbinante-Nissen JM, Simpson LG, Leikauf GD (1995) Corticosteroids increase secretory leukocyte protease inhibitor transcript levels in airway epithelial cells. *Am J Physiol Lung Cell Mol Physiol* 268: L601–606

14 Llewellyn-Jones CG, Harris TAJ, Stockley RA, Harris TA (1996) Effect of fluticasone proprionate on sputum of patients with chronic bronchitis and emphysema. *Am J Respir Crit Care Med* 153: 616–621

15 Willems LNA, Kramps JA, Stijnen T, Sterk PJ, Weening JJ, Dijkman JH (1989) Antileukoprotease-containing bronchiolar cells. Relationship with morphological disease of small airways and parenchyma. *Am Rev Respir Dis* 139: 1244–1250

16 Asano S, Kida K, Koyama T, Wada H, Izawa Y, Hosoda K, Masuda K, Suzuki Y (1995) A morphologic study of lung secretory leukoprotease inhibitor in pneumonia. *Am J Respir Crit Care Med* 151: 1576–1581

17 Marchand V, Tournier JM, Chevillard M, Polette M, Beorchia A, Klossek JM, Puchelle E (1995) Identification of antileucoprotease in remodelled human adult nasal surface epithelium. *Eur Respir J* 8: 15–21

18 Morrison HM, Kramps JA, Burnett D, Stockley RA (1987) Lung lavage fluid from patients with α_1-proteinase inhibitor deficiency or chronic obstructive bronchitis: anti-elastase function and cell profile. *Clin Sci* 72: 373–381

19 Gast A, Dietemann-Molard A, Pelletier A, Pauli G, Bieth JG (1990) The anti-elastase screen of the lower respiratory tract of α_1-antiproteinase inhibitor-sufficient patients with emphysema or pneumothorax. *Am Rev Respir Dis* 141: 880 – 883

20 Vogelmeier C, Hubbard RC, Fells GA, Schnebli H, Thompson RC, Fritz H, Crystal RC (1991) Anti-neutrophil elastase defense of the normal human respiratory epithelial surface provided by the secretory leukoprotease inhibitor. *J Clin Invest* 87: 482–487

21 Fujita J, Nelson NL, Daughton DM, Dobry CA, Spurzem JR, Irino S, Rennard SI (1990) Evaluation of elastase and antielastase balance in patients with chronic bronchitis and pulmonary emphysema. *Am Rev Respir Dis* 142: 57–62

22 Kramps JA, van Twisk C, Klasen EC, Dijkman JH (1988) Interactions among stimulated human polymorphonuclear leukocytes, released elastase and bronchial antileukoprotease. *Clin Sci* 75: 53–62

23 Kido H, Yokogoshi Y, Sakai K, Tashiro M, Kashino Y, Fukutomi A, Katunuma N (1992) Isolation and characterization of a novel trypsin-like protease found in rat bronchiolar epithelial Clara cells. *J Biol Chem* 267: 13573–13579

24 Tashiro M, Yokogoshi Y, Tobita K, Seto JT, Rott R, Kido H (1992) Tryptase Clara, an activating protease for Sendai virus in rat lungs, is involved in pneumopathogenicity. *J Virol* 66: 7211–7216

25 Fritz H (1988) Human mucus proteinase inhibitor. *Biol Chem Hoppe Seyler* 369: 79–82

26 Faller B, Mely Y, Gerard D, Bieth JG (1992) Heparin-induced conformational change and activation of mucus proteinase inhibitor. *Biochemistry* 31: 8285–8290

27 Frommherz KJ, Faller B, Bieth JG (1991) Heparin strongly decreases the rate of inhibition of neutrophil elastase by α_1-proteinase inhibitor. *J Biol Chem* 266: 15356–15362

28 Clark JG, Kuhn C, McDonald JA, Mecham RP (1983) Proteoglycans in the lung. *Int Rev Connect Tissue Res* 10: 249–331

29 McNeely TB, Dealy M, Dripps DJ, Orenstein JM, Eisenberg SP, Wahl SM (1995) Secretory leukocyte protease inhibitor: a human saliva protein exhibiting anti-human immunodeficiency virus type-1 activity *in vitro*. *J Clin Invest* 96: 456–464

30 McNeely TB, Shugars DC, Rosendahl M, Tucker C, Eisenberg SP, Wahl SM (1997) Inhibition of human immunodeficiency virus type 1 infectivity by secretory leukocyte protease inhibitor occurs prior to viral reverse transcription. *Blood* 90: 1141–1149

31 Turpin JA, Schaeffer CA, Bu M, Graham L, Buckheit RW Jr, Clanton D, Rice WG (1996) Human immunodeficiency virus type-1 (HIV-1) replication is unaffected by human secretory leukocyte protease inhibitor. *Antiviral Res* 29: 269–278
32 Couto MA, Harwig SSL, Cullor JS, Hughes JP, Lehrer RI (1992) eNAP-2, a novel cysteine-rich bactericidal peptide from equine leukocytes. *Infect Immun* 64: 5042–5047
33 Hiemstra PS, Maassen RJ, Stolk J, Heinzel-Wieland R, Steffens GJ, Dijkman JH (1996) Antibacterial activity of antileukoprotease. *Infect Immun* 64: 4520–4524
34 Tomee JFC, Hiemstra PS, Heinzel-Wieland R, Kauffman HF (1997) Antileukoprotease: an endogenous protein in the innate mucosal defense against fungi. *J Infect Dis* 176: 740–747
35 Smith JJ, Travis SM, Greenberg EP, Welsh MJ (1996) Cystic fibrosis airway epithelia fail to kill bacteria because of abnormal airway surface fluid. *Cell* 85: 229–236
36 Goldman MJ, Anderson GM, Stolzenberg ED, Kari UP, Zasloff M, Wilson JM (1997) Human β-defensin-1 is a salt-sensitive antibiotic in the lung that is inactivated in cystic fibrosis. *Cell* 88: 553–560
37 Zhao R, Wang I, Lehrer RI (1996) Widespread expression of β-defensin hBD-1 in human secretory glands and epithelial cells. *FEBS Lett* 396: 319–322
38 Jin FY, Nathan C, Radzioch D, Ding A (1997) Secretory leukocyte protease inhibitor: a macrophage product induced by and antagonistic to bacterial lipopolysaccharide. *Cell* 88: 417–426
39 Zjang Y, DeWitt DL, McNeely TB, Wahl SM, Wahl LM (1997) Secretory leukocyte protease inhibitor suppresses the production of monocyte prostaglandin H synthase-2, prostaglandin E_2, and matrix metalloproteinases. *J Clin Invest* 99: 894–900
40 McElvaney NG, Nakamura H, Birrer P, Hubert A, Wong WL, Alphonso M, Baker JB, Catalano MA, Crystal RG (1992) Modulation of airway inflammation in cystic fibrosis. *In vivo* suppression of interleukin-8 levels on the respiratory epithelial surface by aerosolization of recombinant secretory leukoprotease inhibitor. *J Clin Invest* 90: 1296–1301
41 Stolk J, Camps J, Feitsma HIJ, Hermans J, Dijkman JH, Pauwels EKJ (1995) Pulmonary deposition and disappearance of aerosolized secretory leukocyte protease inhibitor. *Thorax* 50: 645–650
42 Gast A, Anderson W, Probst A, Nick H-P, Thompson RC, Eisenberg SP, Schnebli H-P (1990) Pharmacokinetics and distribution of recombinant secretory leukocyte proteinase inhibitor in rats. *Am Rev Respir Dis* 141: 889–894
43 Gillissen A, Birrer P, McElvaney NG, Buhl R, Vogelmeier C, Hoyt RF, Hubbard RC, Crystal RG (1993) Recombinant secretory leukoprotease inhibitor augments glutathione levels in lung epithelial lining fluid. *J Appl Physiol* 75: 825–832
44 Rudolphus A, Kramps JA, Dijkman JH (1991) Effect of human antileukoprotease on experimental emphysema. *Eur Respir J* 4: 31–39
45 Lucey EC, Stone PJ, Coccolella DE, Breuer R, Christensen TG, Thompson RC, Snider GL (1990) Recombinant human secretory leukocyte-protease inhibitor: *in vitro* properties, and amelioration of human neutrophil elastase-induced emphysema and secretory cell metaplasia in the hamster. *J Lab Clin Med* 115: 224–232
46 Rudolphus A, Kramps JA, Mauve I, Dijkman JH (1994) Intratracheally-instilled antileukoprotease and α_1-proteinase inhibitor: effect on human neutrophil elastase-induced experimental emphysema and pulmonary localization. *Histochem J* 26: 817–824
47 Stolk J, Rudolphus A, Davies P, Osinga D, Dijkman JH, Agarwal L, Keenan KP, Fletcher D, Kramps JA (1992) Induction of emphysema and bronchial mucous cell hyperplasia by intractracheal instillations of lipopolysaccharide in the hamster. *J Pathol* 167: 349–356
48 Fujimoto K, Kubo K, Shinozaki S, Okada K, Matsuzawa Y, Kobayashi T, Sugane K (1995) Neutrophil elastase inhibitor reduces asthmatic responses in allergic sheep. *Respir Physiol* 100: 91–100
49 Clark JM, Abraham WM, Fishman CE, Forteza R, Ahmed A, Cortes A, Warne RL, Moore WR, Tanaka RD (1995) Tryptase inhibitors block allergen-induced airway and inflammatory responses in allergic sheep. *Am J Respir Crit Care Med* 152: 2076–2083
50 Forteza RM, Ahmed A, Lee T, Abraham WM (1997) Secretory leukocyte proteinase inhibitor, but not α_1-proteinase inhibitor blocks tryptase-induced bronchoconstriction. *Am J Respir Crit Care Med* 155: A654 (abstract)
51 Koren HS, Devlin RB, Graham DE, Mann R, McGee MP, Horstman DH, Kozumbo WJ, Becker S, House DE, McDonnell WF et al. (1989) Ozone-induced inflammation in the lower airways of human subjects. *Am Rev Respir Dis* 139: 407–415

52 Schelegle ES, Siefkin AD, McDonald RJ (1991) Time course of ozone-induced neutrophilia in normal humans. *Am Rev Respir Dis* 143: 1353–1358
53 Seltzer J, Bigby BG, Stulbarg M (1986) Ozone-induced change in bronchial reactivity to metacholine and airway inflammation in humans. *J Appl Physiol* 60: 1321–1326
54 Dimeo MJ, Glenn MG, Holtzman MJ (1981) Threshold concentration of ozone causing an increase in bronchial reactivity in humans and adaptation with repeated exposures. *Am Rev Respir Dis* 124: 245–248
55 Hilterman TJN, Peters EA, Alberts B, Kwikkers K, Borggreven PA, Hiemstra PS, Dijkman JH, van Bree LA, Stolk J (1998) Ozone-induced airway hyperresponsiveness in patients with asthma: role of neutrophil-derived serine proteinases. *Free Rad Biol Med* 24: 952–958
56 Goselink HM, Van Damme J, Hiemstra PS, Wuyts A, Stolk J, Fibbe WE, Willemze R, Falkenburg JHF (1996) Colony growth of human hematopoietic progenitor cells in the absence of serum is supported by a proteinase inhibitor identified as antileukoprotease. *J Exp Med* 184: 1305–1312

Molecular Biology of the Lung
Vol. 1: Emphysema and Infection
ed. by R. A. Stockley

CHAPTER 5
Elastase Inhibitors in the Lung: Expression and Functional Relationships

Jean-Michel Sallenave[1], Kevin Morgan[2], Jack Gauldie[3] and Noor Kalsheker[2]

[1] *Rayne Laboratory, Department of Medicine, Edinburgh Medical School, Edinburgh, Scotland, UK*
[2] *Division of Clinical Chemistry, School of Clinical Laboratory Sciences, Faculty of Medicine, Queen Medical Centre, Nottingham, UK*
[3] *Department of Pathology, McMaster University, Hamilton, Ontario, Canada*

1. Introduction

The acute-phase response (APR) is thought to be the response of the body to initiation and development of inflammation. This is a beneficial response, aimed at limiting damage and restoring normal haemostasis. A well-orchestrated sequence of events starts at the site of injury, leading to the systemic release of biological mediators, principally via the liver. The major hepatic acute-phase reactants are composed of serum amyloid A, C-reactive protein (CRP), serum amyloid P component, metal-binding proteins such as haptoglobin and ceruloplasmin and proteinase inhibitors such as α_1-proteinase inhibitor (also known as α_1-antitrypsin) and α_1-antichymotrypsin [1]. Proteinase inhibitors have been extensively studied, because of their ability to inhibit the deleterious effects of proteases, secreted either by foreign bodies such as bacteria, or by endogenous cells such as tissue macrophages, blood monocytes and polymorphonuclear cells.

The APR is a very tightly regulated process which is thought to be initiated locally by these inflammatory cells. Cytokines represent one of the major classes of chemical mediators responsible for initiating, regulating and terminating the APR. Their synthesis, switch-on and switch-off mechanisms, as well as their mode of action, are tightly regulated in what is now classically entitled a cytokine network. Indeed, early cytokines, such as interleukin 1 (IL-1) and tumour necrosis factor (TNF), are synthesized very quickly within one hour of the onset of inflammation, stimulated, for example, by bacterial products such as lipopolysaccharides. These cytokines seem to be necessary for the induction of secondary cytokines, such as members of the IL-6 family, which are extremely important for the initiation of the systemic acute-phase response [2].

"Secondary cytokines", such as IL-4, IL-6 and IL-10, are also important in the process by which the APR is limited and resolution of inflammation achieved. IL-4 is primarily released by T-helper 2 (Th2) lymphocytes and appears to have a significant role in modulating acute inflammation. In monocytes and macrophages, it causes the down-regulation of cytokines such as TNF, IL-1 and IL-8. IL-4 also up-regulates the expression of the IL-1 receptor antagonist (IL-1RA) thereby reducing further the IL-1 effects [3].

IL-6 has direct anti-inflammatory effects on cytokines, down-regulating IL-1 and TNF synthesis [3]. IL-10 has a broader origin because it is produced by Th2 lymphocytes, monocytes, macrophages and B cells. It was originally described as an inhibitory factor of cytokine synthesis because it inhibits monocyte/macrophage synthesis of IL-1, TNF, IL-6, IL-8 and colony-stimulating factors (CSFs), and up-regulates IL-1RA [3].

In a lipopolysaccharide (LPS) model of pulmonary neutrophilia, inflammation is more sustained in IL-6 knock-out mice than in wild-type mice [4]. Similarly, IL-10 can protect mice from the lethal effects of endotoxic shock [5, 6].

In parallel to the cytokine network, data are emerging which suggest the existence of an antiproteinase network; this involves sequential secretion of antiproteinases. Indeed, there is a close relationship between proteolysis and the acute-phase response to inflammation. Proteinases come from the infectious agents and the inflammatory host cells (neutrophils, macrophages, mast cells) [7]. To protect itself against these potentially harmful agents, the host secretes high amounts of antiproteinases [7].

Particularly relevant to this chapter is the protection provided by antiproteinases against the proteinases secreted by macrophages and neutrophils such as metalloproteases and serine proteases (for example, human neutrophil elastase (HNE) and proteinase 3).

It is not our objective to review exhaustively all the antiproteinases described to date (for a recent review, see Twining [8]). Seven inhibitor superfamilies have been described so far: the kunins, kazals, antileukoproteases (ALPs), SERPINs, α-macroglobulin, cystatins and tissue inhibitors of metalloproteinases (TIMPs) [9]. We propose classifying the antiproteases relevant to the lung in three groups: the first comprises early or alarm inhibitors, the second secondary or acute-phase inhibitors, and the third inhibitors of remodelling and repair processes such as the TIMPs and the plasminogen activator inhibitors (PAIs) [10]. We wish to focus on the first two groups ("alarm" and "acute-phase" inhibitors) in this chapter.

Alarm inhibitors include the two-low-molecular-weight proteinase inhibitors of the ALP family: antileukoprotease itself, also known as secretory leukocyte proteinase inhibitor (SLPI) [11], mucus proteinase inhibitor (MPI) or bronchial inhibitor (BrI) (this inhibitor will henceforth be referred to as SLPI) and elastase-specific inhibitor (ESI), also known as elafin or skin-derived antileukoprotease (SKALP) [12]. These molecules are synthesized and secreted locally at the site of injury. Interestingly, these molecules are produced in response to primary cytokines such as IL-1 and TNF and might therefore be part of a first wave of local, inducible defence in the antiproteinase network [13]. The concentration of these inhibitors is very low in the circulation, of the order of a few nanograms per millilitre (J.-M. Sallenave et al., unpublished data) [14] and they are not expressed in liver cells [15–17]. In addition, it was found that the serum concentration of SLPI rises very little during an acute-phase response [18], arguing against a prominent systemic anti-inflammatory role.

In contrast to these "alarm" inhibitors, the "secondary" antiproteinases such as α_1-antichymotrypsin or α_1-antitrypsin are produced in abundance by the liver and secreted in high concentration in the circulation as acute-phase reactants.

The liver produces these antiproteinases in response to secondary cytokines such as members of the IL-6 family, including IL-6 itself, leukaemia inhibitory factor (LIF) and oncostatin-M [3] (see below). Interestingly, "secondary" cytokines also up-regulate local synthesis of proteinase inhibitors, in inflammatory [19] and structural cells [20–22]. The existence of an integrated network between "alarm" and "acute-phase" inhibitors *in vivo* is inferred by *in vitro* data [23] showing that HNE can be transferred from SLPI to an α_1-antitrypsin inhibitor. If the existence of such a network is confirmed, this transfer makes sense both physiologically and thermodynamically, in that the binding of SLPI to HNE is not as tight as that of α_1-antitrypsin to HNE. It is therefore conceivable that SLPI (and possibly elafin) is present first at the scene of the crime and is able to bind HNE loosely and present it subsequently to α_1-antitrypsin, which is a very tight

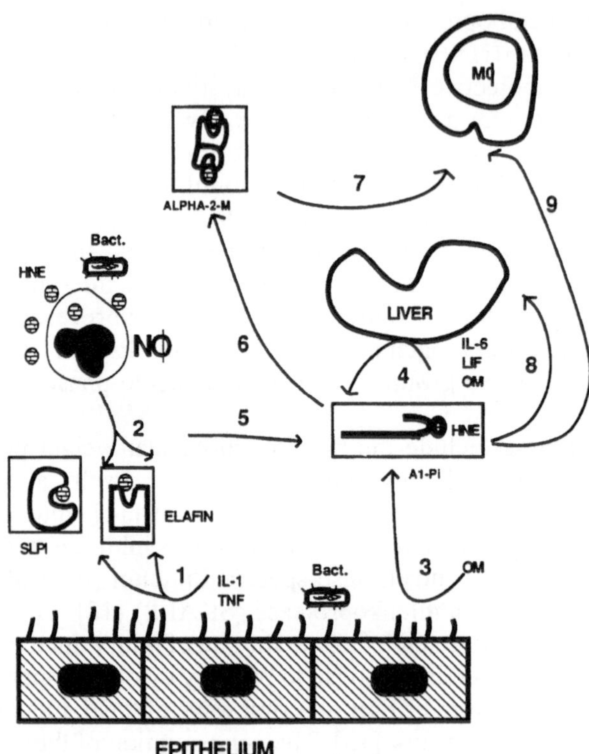

Figure 1. Regulation of synthesis of "alarm" and acute-phase elastase inhibitors by cytokines. (1) After an initial insult (bacterial infection for example), early cytokines (IL-1, TNF) up-regulate alarm elastase inhibitors (SLPI, elafin). (2) These inhibitors can bind human neutrophil elastase (HNE) when released in excess by neutrophils (NO). A second wave of cytokines, such as IL-6, LIF and OM up-regulate both (3) locally and (4) systemically acute-phase proteinase inhibitors such as α_1-antitrypsin and α_1-antichymotrypsin. (5) α_1-antitrypsin can then displace HNE from SLPI and transfer it to (6) α_2-macroglobulin (A2-M) or (7–9) the complexes HNE-α_1-antitrypsin and human NE – α_2-macroglobulin can be cleared by monocytes and hepatocytes after binding to a SERPIN – enzyme complex receptor.

inhibitor of HNE. The enzyme-inhibitor complex can then be cleared by monocytes and hepatocytes, through a SERPIN receptor-mediated pathway [24] (Figure 1). Interestingly, Dabbagh et al. [25] showed that α_1-antitrypsin might subsequently have a role in initiating repair processes by stimulating fibroblast proliferation and collagen deposition and could therefore be an intermediate between the early phase of the inflammatory response and the later phase involving repair and proliferation.

2. Alarm Antiproteinases

2.1. *Secretory Leukocyte Proteinase Inhibitor*

2.1.1. Protein, gene structure and antiproteinase activity: Secretary leukocyte protease inhibitor (SLPI) is one of the two members of the ALP superfamily of proteinase inhibitors (the other being elastase-specific inhibitor/elafin, see below). SLPI has been purified from different sources, including parotid, cervical, seminal and lung secretions [11]. It is a 11.7-kDa protein, consisting of 107 amino acids [26], and comprising two domains assembled in a boomerang-like shape. It contains 16 cysteines and these form eight disulphide bridges [27]. This makes the molecule very compact and presumably very resistant to proteolytic cleavage. Indeed, protocols for SLPI purification often include treatments with strong acids such as perchloric acid. The gene, approximately 2.65 kilobases (kb) in length [28, 29] is composed of four exons and three introns and contains typical 5′ TATAA and CAAT boxes as well as regulatory sequences (activator proteins AP-1, AP-2 and the CCAAT/enhancer binding protein C/EBP) [30]. The SLPI gene appears to be a relatively non-polymorphic, stable gene which can be modulated at both the transcriptional and the translational levels [30]. DNAse I hypersensitivity sites have been found in epithelial cells and not in fibroblasts, consistent with its synthesis in epithelial cells but not fibroblasts. Transfection studies using fusion elements composed of fragments of up to 1.2 kb of the 5′-flanking region of the SLPI gene demonstrated a high promoter activity in a 131-bp fragment (– 115 to + 16) relative to the transcription start site [30]. Recently Kikuchi et al. [31] have delineated within this region a proximal 41-base-pair (bp) region which confers lung specificity for SLPI expression. Two nuclear factors that bind to a 11-bp sequence within this region are being investigated (SLPI-B1 and SLPI-B2) and the authors propose that they could be members of the hepatocyte nuclear factor-3 (HNF-3) family.

The N-terminal moiety of SLPI is responsible for stabilizing the molecule by binding proteoglycan components such as heparan sulphates [32–34], whereas the C-terminal domain of the molecule contains the antiproteinase site [35–38]. SLPI has been shown to inhibit HNE, cathepsin G, trypsin, chymotrypsin and chymase [39, 40]. Its major target is thought to be HNE in view of its high affinity and kinetic constants (K_i in the nanomoles/litre range and K_{ass} in the micromoles/litre range) [41–43].

2.1.2. Synthesis and regulation: The mouse counterpart has recently been cloned [44] and was shown, like human SLPI, to be up-regulated at the transcriptional level by the early cytokines IL-1 and TNF [45]. In addition, Abbinante-Niessen et al. [46] and our own group [13] showed that HNE can up-regulate the gene for SLPI. SLPI is produced by epithelial cells and has been found mainly at mucosal sites (hence its pseudonym mucosal proteinase inhibitor) [11, 47]. In the case of the lung, it has been shown to be produced *in vitro* by tracheal, bronchial, bronchiolar and type II alveolar cells [15, 48–50]. It has also been produced *in vivo* by tracheal serous glands and bronchiolar Clara cells, and is closely associated with elastin fibres in the alveolar interstitium [51, 52].

However, SLPI can also be produced at other sites: Jin et al. [53] showed that mouse monocytes and neutrophils can produce SLPI, in agreement with studies in human neutrophils [54, 55]. Indeed, we have shown that these cells could potentially be a very significant contributor of SLPI in bronchial secretions [54]. Its role in inflammatory cells such as monocytes or neutrophils is uncertain but anti-bacterial or anti-inflammatory actions have been proposed. Hiemstra et al. [56] recently showed that SLPI was an effective antimicrobial against both *Escherichia coli* and *Staphylococcus aureus*, and they demonstrated that this activity depended upon the N-terminal domain of the molecule and not upon its C-terminal antiproteinase site [56]. The highly cationic nature of SLPI probably contributes at least partly to this activity; indeed, other antibiotic molecules such as lactoferrin and elastase are all cationic.

2.3.1. SLPI as an anti-inflammatory agent: Whether SLPI acts as an anti-inflammatory agent solely through its antiproteinase activity is unclear at present, but a recent report by Zhang et al. [57] showed that SLPI down-regulates LPS activity in monocytes independently of its antiproteinase activity. The authors also showed that treatment of human monocytes with human SLPI prevented production of pro-inflammatory reagents such as TNF and nitric oxide, and metalloproteinases upon stimulation with LPS. Similarly, Jin et al. [53] showed that a macrophage cell line derived from a mouse line naturally resistant to LPS (C3H/HeJ) consistently expressed SLPI, as opposed to C3H/HeN, a strain sensitive to LPS. However, surprisingly, this difference was not maintained when primary macrophages were examined in culture. If these findings were confirmed, this would be evidence for the concept that SLPI acts through a feedback mechanism and is protective in murine models of endotoxic shock involving LPS and downstream cytokines such as IL-1 and TNF (precisely the cytokines that up-regulate SLPI both in humans [13] and in mice [45]).

However, these models might be misleading and caution is necessary when extrapolating the results of these studies to interpretation of endotoxic shock in humans. For example, although inhibition of IL-1 or TNF results in reduced mortality in mice [58], inhibition of TNF in humans may actually worsen the outcome. In humans, it is possible that the amount and/or the timing of SLPI secretion may be important in the outcome of sepsis. Indeed, whereas groups have shown that SLPI administered as a recombinant protein is protective in elastase-T and LPS-induced models of emphysema in hamsters [59, 60] and allergic alveolitis in rats [61], we have shown that increased levels of SLPI in bronchoalveolar lavage (BAL) fluid correlates with a poor prognosis in the setting of overwhelming sepsis progressing to the acute respiratory distress syndrome (ARDS) [62]. One potential explanation for this association stems from work by Docke et al. [63], which showed that monocytes from patients with sepsis and a poor prognosis were hyporesponsive to LPS, leading to a profound immunodeficiency that the authors called immunoparalysis (which was shown to be reversible by interferon-γ), a state probably caused by an initial exposure to LPS inducing relative refractoriness to a subsequent exposure. Clinical studies designed to inhibit IL-1 or TNF-α have failed to improve outcome and in some cases have shown worsening of symptoms [64].

LPS hyporesponsiveness has been atributed to SLPI in murine models [53] but requires confirmation in human monocytes.

These data raise the intriguing possibility that SLPI is critically involved in regulating release of inflammatory mediators, but that excessive, dysregulated secretion of SLPI might equally be detrimental. These hypotheses are currently under investigation in our laboratory in murine models of inflammation where transient (using adenovirus, for example [65]) or constitutive (murine transgenic models) overexpression of elastase inhibitors is achieved.

2.2. Elastase-Specific Inhibitor (ESI)/Elafin/Skin-Derived Antileukoprotease (SKALP)

2.2.1. Protein structure and antiproteinase activity: The neutrophil elastase inhibitor elafin (the other member of the ALP superfamily of proteinase inhibitors) was first described by Hochstrasser et al. [66] and Kramps and Klasen [67] in bronchial secretions under the name elastase-specific inhibitor. In the early 1990s, both Wiedow et al. [68] and our group [69] sequenced part of the protein, derived from skin and lung secretions, respectively. The molecule is composed of 117 amino acids, including a hydrophobic signal peptide of 22 amino acids. It can be divided into two domains: the C-terminal domain containing the antiproteinase active site and the N-terminal domain containing characteristic VKGQ sequences, which have been called cementoin [16]. These sequences allow the elafin molecule to glue itself into polymers and bind other interstitial molecules, through transglutamination [70–72]. This mode of binding has also been described in seminal vesicle protein 1 from guinea-pigs. Although this binding has been demonstrated *in vitro* and *ex vivo*, it still remains to be formally demonstrated *in vivo*. This particular binding characteristic may allow a close association of the inhibitor to the interstitium, conferring protection against degradation by neutrophilic enzymes at the site of inflammation. This feature could make elafin maximally effective as a tissue-bound inhibitor as opposed to α_1-antitrypsin which is present in high amounts in the circulation. Interestingly, SLPI has also been suggested to have a protective role locally, against neutrophilic damage, presumably because of its small size and negative charge [73–75]. The elafin molecule shows a 40% homology with the SLPI molecule and the active sites of both inhibitors are identical, except for the P1 residue (alanine for elafin and leucine for SLPI), which probably explains its specificity. Elafin has been shown to be very specific in its spectrum of inhibition: it inhibits porcine pancreatic elastase, human neutrophil elastase and proteinase-3 [68, 69, 76]. It is a fast acting inhibitor and association with the enzyme follows a bimolecular process, in the micromoles/litre range [68, 69, 77].

Like SLPI, elafin has a high content of cysteines (eight), which are arranged in four disulphide bonds in the C-terminal proteinase-inhibiting region and makes it, like SLPI, a very compact and proteolytically resistant molecule [78]. Small proteins such as SLPI and elafin are part of a "four-disulphide" core protein family which includes such different proteins as whey acidic protein and the Na^+/H^+ ATPase inhibitor 1 (SPAI-1) [79, 80]. The crystal structure of a portion of the elafin molecule (57 amino acids) has recently been determined in a complex with porcine pancreatic elastase [81]. The 57 amino acid polypeptide chain of elafin has a planar spiral shape with an exposed external part and an internal core part which is very similar to the crystal structure of SLPI and the solution structure of SPAI-1. Importantly, the "full picture" will be obtained only when the complete inhibitor (95 amino acids excluding the signal peptide) is crystallized. Indeed, the N-terminus (for which the crystal structure is not available yet) contain the VKGQ sequences mentioned above which are a major feature of the whole molecule.

2.2.2. Gene sequence, synthesis and regulation: We and others subsequently sequenced the elastase-specific gene [71, 82], showing that it is approximately 2300 bp, and is composed of three exons and two introns and contains typical 5′-TATA and CAAT boxes, as well as 5′-regulatory sequences such as AP1 and NF-κB sites [71, 83]. It is a member of the recently described REST family of genes, which are expressed principally in seminal vesicles [84, 85]. Zhang et al. [83] demonstrated that a positive regulatory *cis*-element present in the region between –505 to –368 bp is responsible for up-regulation of the elafin gene in normal breast epithelial cells. Whether this region is tissue specific or is also important for expression in lung cells is currently under investigation in our laboratory. Consistent with the presence of putative NF-κB sites, we found that IL-1-β and TNF-α are potent inducers of the elafin gene [13]. In 1993, Molhuizen et al. [70] showed that SKALP, initially thought to be SLPI, was in fact the same molecule as ESI/elafin. They further demonstrated that the ESI-elafin/SKALP gene is localized in the q12 and q13 region of chromosome 20 [86].

As mentioned above, elafin was first demonstrated in the skin and in lung secretions [66–69]. Its purification from sputum [66, 67, 69], its presence in tracheal biopsies [16] and in BAL from normal subjects as well as patients [72], in addition to its synthesis by Clara cell and type II cells [13, 50], indicates a tracheobronchioalveolar origin. It is not, however, restricted to these tissues; interestingly, northern blot analysis and RNAse protection assays have shown that it is produced mainly in the trachea, stomach, tongue, pharynx and, to a lesser degree in lung, small intestine and duodenum, all tissues characterized by their richness in elastic fibres [16, 17]. We have recently investigated its presence in the peripheral lung and have shown by immunohistochemistry that macrophages are strongly positive (J.-M. Sallenave et al., unpublished data).

Interestingly, several forms of the ESI/elafin molecule have been demonstrated in lung secretions, including the native 10-kDa molecule [66, 71], a 45-kDa species probably consisting of ESI bound to an as yet uncharacterized molecule [72], and 2.5- and 6-kDa proteolytic fragments of the molecule [67, 69, 71]. Whether these fragments represent products of physiological activation of the molecule or merely artefactual products after purification is unknown at present, but it is conceivable that they could represent a portion of the physiological ESI.

2.3. *SLPI and ESI/Elafin* In Vivo

Although a genetic deficiency such as the one for α_1-antitrypsin has not yet been described for the low-molecular-weight elastase inhibitors, the presence and role of SLPI in the lung has been assessed in chronic obstructive pulmonary disease (COPD) (see Chapter 4) and recently in ARDS [62]. Comparatively less information is available concerning the physiological role of ESI/elafin in the lung. We have found that it is increased in the acute-phase of hypersensitivity pneumonitis [72]. In chronic conditions, such as COPD and cystic fibrosis, we found that SLPI and elafin were regulated in a different fashion; SLPI levels were augmented whereas elafin levels were down-regulated (Figure 2).

Although the mechanism for this is unclear, this suggests that SLPI and elafin are regulated differently in acute and chronic inflammation.

3. Acute Phase Antiproteinases

3.1. *α_1-Antitrypsin in Lung Disease*

α_1-Antitrypsin deficiency is one of the most common hereditary disorders in white Europeans [87]. The physiological role of α_1-antitrypsin was first observed when it was noted that, in patients with pulmonary emphysema, there was a deficiency of α_1-globulin [88]. Subsequently, the major component α_1-globulin was found to be α_1-antitrypsin. The major physiologi-

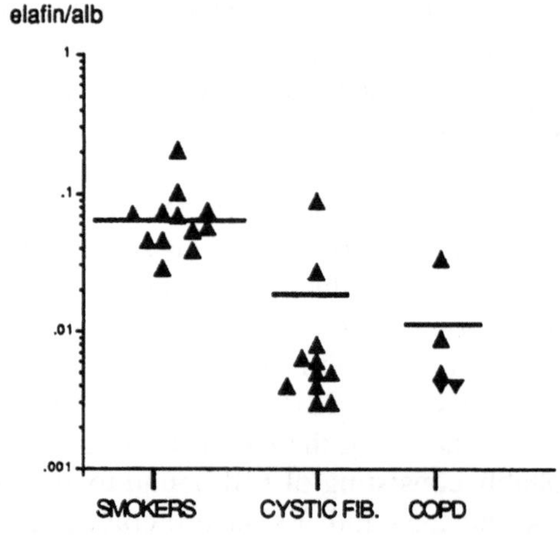

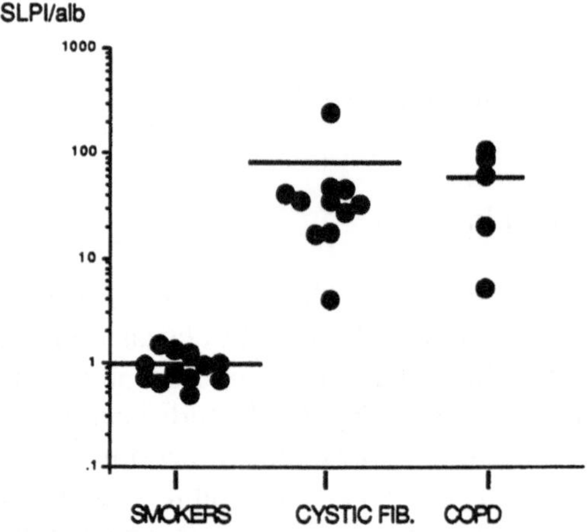

Figure 2. Secretory leukocyte proteinase inhibitor (SLPI) and elafin levels (as assessed by enzyme-linked immunosorbent assay in sputa from normal smokers, patients with COPD and cystic fibrosis. Results are expressed as a molar ratio to albumin.

cal function of α_1-antitrypsin is to inhibit neutrophil elastase, which is released by neutrophils recruited to the lung during inflammation, and thus prevent excessive damage to lung tissue [89]. α_1-Antitrypsin is the archetypal member of the serine protease inhibitor (SERPIN) supergene family which includes a number of other proteins that inactivate serine proteinases by forming stable covalent complexes [90]. Severe deficiency of α_1-antitrypsin is also associated with chronic liver disease in early childhood [91, 92]. Chronic obstructive airway disease (COAD), which includes diseases such as pulmonary emphysema, affects about 3% of the population in Western countries [93], and as more people live longer it is expected that its associated morbidity will increase. Around 20% of patients with COAD have a familial component which is predominantly genetic in origin [94].

Genetic deficiency of α_1-antitrypsin leads to progressive lung damage in early adult life for cigarette smokers [91] and accounts for about 2% of all patients with COAD [92]. The deficiency states are caused by mutations in the α_1-antitrypsin gene with the two most common forms being the S and Z variants. Clinical manifestations (increased susceptibility to emphysema) occur when the mean serum concentration of α_1-antitrypsin is less than 35% of normal [95]. The Z variant arises from a glutamic acid to lysine substitution at amino acid position 342 in the mature protein [96]. The Z protein is synthesized at a normal rate but it accumulates in the rough endoplasmic reticulum of hepatocytes; the clinical consequence of this is that around 10% of patients develop severe cirrhosis and liver failure. MZ heterozygotes have a relatively low risk of developing COAD compared with ZZ homozygotes. The other common cause of deficiency is the result of valine at position 264 being replaced by glutamic acid giving rise to the S variant [97]. In addition, over 75 rare molecular variants have been described; some of these are the null alleles.

Other studies [98, 99] have identified a mutation in the 3′-flanking sequence of the α_1-antitrypsin gene which is associated with COAD and occurs in around 15–18% of patients. This mutation occurs in a motif that demonstrates weak intrinsic enhancer activity with the wild-type sequence, which is abolished by the mutant sequence [100]. However, after IL-6 stimulation, the 3′ enhancer assumes a major role in conjunction with the 5′ enhancer [101]. The mutation results in a markedly diminished IL-6-induced acute-phase response [101] and may therefore contribute to disease at a time when α_1-antitrypsin is most needed, i.e. during an inflammatory response such as occurs during a lung infection. The 3′ enhancer mutation does not segregate with a specific protein type and it occurs only very rarely with the Z allele [102]. In fact these patients have normal basal circulating levels of α_1-antitrypsin. It appears therefore that this mutation is an independent risk factor for COAD. Heterozygotes with the enhancer mutation appear to be predisposed to disease with a higher risk than that associated with the MZ heterozygotes. The reason for this is not completely clear but it may be that a diminished acute-phase response in individuals who harbour the mutation results in lower α_1-antitrypsin concentrations during inflammation in comparison with MZ patients (where the M allele is regulated normally), particularly at local sites.

Genetic deficiencies of another closely related SERPIN α_1-antichymotrypsin, have also been found to be associated with lung function abnormalities in some rare instances [103]. Individual family studies have revealed that a leucine to proline substitution at position 55 causes a defective α_1-antichymotrypsin allele as does a proline to alanine at position 229 [104]. The target for α_1-antichymotrypsin is cathepsin G which like neutrophil elastase is capable of damaging lung tissue [105]. It is evident that protease/antiprotease (SERPIN) imbalance has a central role to play in the pathogenesis of lung disease.

3.2. α_1-Antitrypsin and the Acute-Phase Response

α_1-Antitrypsin is a positive acute-phase reactant, its serum concentration rises three- to fourfold during inflammation [106] and a major function is to protect the lower respiratory tract from damage by neutrophil elastase [91]. α_1-Antitrypsin is synthesized in human liver cells, blood monocytes and bronchoalveolar macrophages [107–109]. α_1-Antitrypsin synthesis in human hepatoma cells (HepG2/Hep3B) is modulated by IL-6 [19, 110] whereas in monocytes it is modulated by LPS and IL-6 [19, 111].

3.3. Organization of the Human α_1-Antitrypsin Gene

The α_1-antitrypsin gene (Figure 3) is located on the long arm of chromosome 14 at position q31–31.2 [112]. The gene is within 12.2 kilobases (kb) of genomic sequence [113] and the full length liver cDNA is 1.6-kb. The gene consists of five exons with the first exon being split into three segments: A, B and C. The translational start site is at the beginning of exon 2 and the active site of the molecule is in exon 5. Two promoter regions are utilized: one specific for hepatocytes and the other over 3.7-kb upstream (unpublished observation) which is specific for monocytes and other tissues

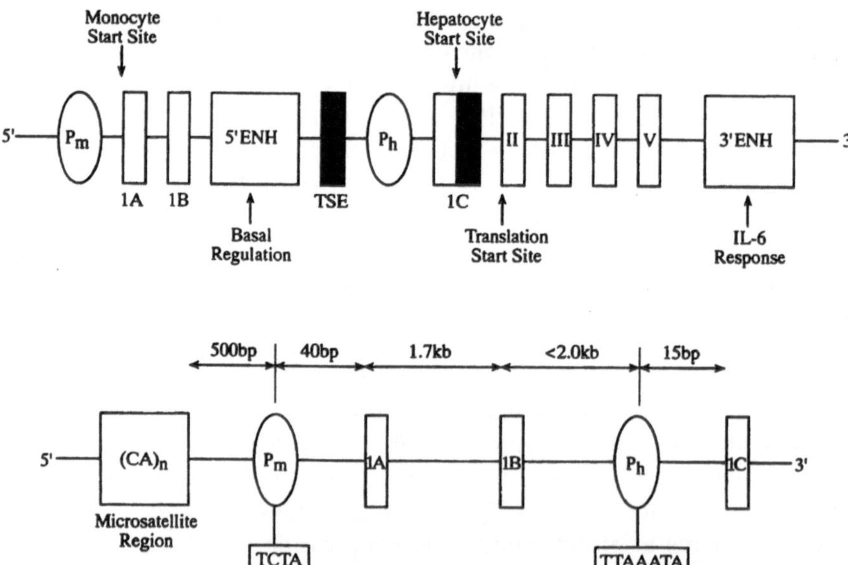

Figure 3. Organization of the α_1-antitrypsin gene. Pm and Ph represent the monocyte and hepatocyte promoters, respectively and the exons are shown as numbered boxes. The locations of the tissue-specific element (TSE), 5′ enhancer (5′ENH) and 3′ enhancer (3′ENH) are also shown. The lower portion of the figure indicates the spatial arrangement and organization of exon 1 (A, B and C) in relation to the monocyte and hepatocyte promoters.

[114]. Two transcription initiation start sites have been mapped. The hepatocyte-specific start site is located within exon 1C and the macrophage-specific start site is in exon 1A. Monocyte AAT has been reported to be expressed as four alternatively spliced transcripts with lengths of 1.8-kb, 1.9 kb, 1.95 kb and 2.0 kb [114, 115]. Monocyte transcripts contain four mRNA species which include all of exon 1A, 1B and 1C, exon 1A – 50 bp, 1B and 1C, and the transcripts in which all of exon 1A or all of exon 1B is missing (Figure 4). IL-6 stimulation of U937 cells (leukaemic monocyte cell line) results in the preferential exclusion of exon 1B from monocyte transcripts [116].

3.4. *Basal Regulation of α_1-Antitrypsin by the 5′ Enhancer*

The region 500-bp upstream of the liver-specific start site contains three regulatory elements including a minimal promoter element within 261 nucleotides of the transcription initiation site [117–119]. The hepatocyte promoter TATA box (actual sequence TTAAATA) is 15 bp upstream, i.e. at nucleotide positions –15 to –21, of the hepatocyte transcription start site in exon 1C (numbering starts at the first base in exon 1C). Tissue-specific expression is predominantly modulated by the 100 bp tissue-specific ele-

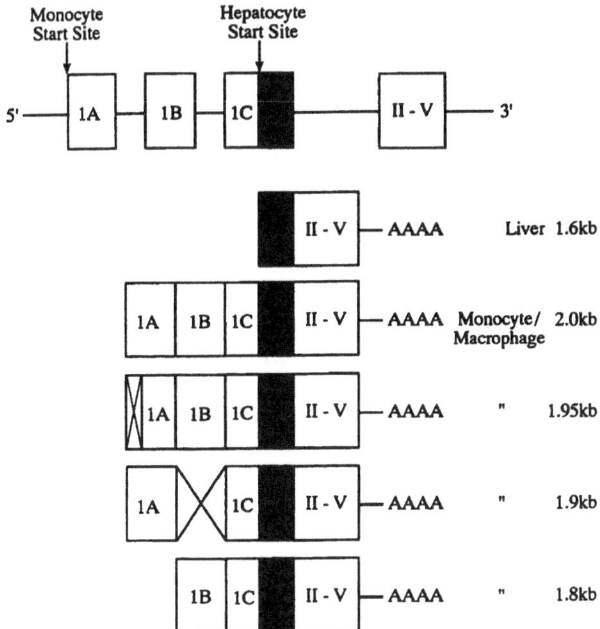

Figure 4. α_1-antitrypsin transcripts generated by alternative processing of the α_1-antitrypsin gene in the liver and monocyte/macrophage cells. Sizes for each transcript are given in kilobases (kb).

ment (TSE) located between nucleotidees –37 to –137. The presence of this element is sufficient to activate a heterologous promoter in hepatoma cells [114]. The TSE has a two-domain structure, both of which are necessary for efficient transcription [120]. The distal domain, located at –110 to –137, also acts as a tissue-specific repressor in non-hepatic cells [121]. Deletion of this region with the remainder of the element intact results in increased transcriptional efficiency when placed upstream of the SV40 (simian virus 40) promoter in a reporter gene system with near equivalent expression in both hepatic and HeLa cells [120]. A second element, which has the characteristics of an enhancer, is located between nucleotides –210 to –261 and can increase transcription four- to fivefold but not in a tissue-specific manner [117]. This sequence is of a modular nature and has binding sites for the transcription factors AP-1, hepatocyte nuclear factor-3 (HNF-3) and those in the C/EBP family [122]. The region increases transcriptional activity indepenent of distance and orientation which are two of the characteristic features of eukaryotic enhancers [117]. It has recently been demonstrated that, under basal conditions, this enhancer is dominant [101]. The third regulatory element, also an enhancer, is located between nucleotides –356 to –488 and is capable of increasing transcriptional activity three- or fourfold [122].

3.5. IL-6 Stimulation of α_1-Antitrypsin by the 3′ Enhancer

The 3′-enhancer is located 1.2–1.3 kb from the end of exon 5 and within these 100 bp are binding sites for AP-1, octamer-1 protein (Oct-1) and C/EBP isoforms [100]. We have recently shown that this region modulates the expression of the CAT reporter gene when transfected into HepG2 cells which have been treated with IL-6; under basal conditions the 3′ enhancer has a minimal effect on expression whereas the 5′ enhancer is dominant [101]. However, the up-regulation by IL-6 relies on the presence of both the 5′ and 3′ enhancers; this suggests a synergistic interaction between these two regions, one possibility being via looping out of the intervening DNA between the 5′ and 3′ enhancers, thereby making the gene more accessible to the transcription machinery.

To elucidate the molecular mechanism for the IL-6 stimulation of the α_1-antitrypsin gene, the interaction of transcription factors with the 3′ enhancer has been explored in some detail. Using electrophoretic mobility shift assays (EMSA) and antibody supershift assays we have demonstrated that the ubiquitous transcription factor Oct-1 and the tissue-specific factor NF-IL-6, one of the key mediators of the effects of IL-6, bind to neighboring sites in the 3′ enhancer. There appears to be a cooperative interaction between these two transcription factors such that binding at the Oct-1 site assists the binding of NF-IL-6. Interestingly, this cooperation is lost when the previously described COAD-associated mutation [98, 99] at the

Oct site is present [101]. It is not known at this stage if the interaction between Oct-1 and NF-IL-6 is direct or if the cooperation is assisted by an additional integrator molecule which bridges these two factors. Recently [123, 124], a B-cell co-activator, termed Bob 1/OBF-1, which interacts with Oct factors has been identified so it is possible that such a moiety exists in other cell types.

3.6. Functional Consequence of Oct-1 Binding to the 3′ α_1-Antitrypsin Enhancer

The interaction of a ubiquitous factor and a factor that regulates tissue-specific expression is intriguing and similar mechanisms may exist for regulation of other members of the SERPIN family/acute-phase genes. Oct-1 is capable of regulating genes in both a positive and a negative manner. As is seen with the α_1-antitrypsin gene the predominant effect of binding of Oct-1 transcription factor is to promote transcription [125]; however, there are instances where negative regulation of transcription has been described. Oct-1 negatively modulates mouse μ-opioid receptor (MOR) gene expression by binding to an element in the promoter region of the gene [126]. The 5′ flanking region of the rat *CYP1A1* gene contains a negative response element that binds Oct-1 [127], and Oct-1 also binds to the negative response element of the rat 3α-hydroxysteroid/dihydrodiol dehydrogenase gene [128]. In the human insulin gene promoter Oct-1 possibly interacts with an adjacent positive element to form a silencer complex [129]. Several other studies have shown that Oct proteins have the ability to recruit factors into the pre-initiation complex and examples include the recruitment of Jun protein to the IL-2 promoter octamer site upon antigenic stimulation [130] and OBF-1 co-activator to the immunoglobulin octamer sites [131]. It has also been demonstrated that the binding of Oct-1/2 to the lipoprotein lipase gene promoter octamer site was stimulated by transonphon factor IIB (TFIIB) [132], raising the possibility that the octamer site in this gene replaces the TATA box. It is conceivable that Oct-1-induced conformational changes aid the recruitment of additional transcription factors and in this way play a major role in gene regulation [132]; this phenomenon has been described in the steroid hormone family of transcription factors [133, 134]. It appears that Oct-1 harbours a number of effects that are gene specific and hence explain its diverse regulatory potential.

3.7. LPS and the α_1-Antitrypsin Gene

Lipopolysaccharide stimulation results in an increase in the synthesis of α_1-antitrypsin in monocytes by around five- to tenfold but α_1-antitrypsin mRNA levels only increase by 1.5- to 2.5-fold [115], suggesting that both transcription and the efficiency of translation play a role in α_1-antitrypsin expression. The LPS effect on rabbit monocyte S2 α_1-antitrypsin levels is mediated by NF-κB [135]. We have identified two potential LPS elements/NF-κB-binding sites within the vicinity of the human monocyte promoter, but as yet it is not known if this region is functionally active. IL-1 does not induce the α_1-antitrypsin acute-phase response, either alone or in combination with other cytokines. However, like LPS it induces the acute-phase response of α_1-antichymotrypsin in astrocytes [136] and epithelial cells [137]. All of these data suggest a possible alternative pathway for the activation of NF-κB by LPS in the α_1-antitrypsin gene; the potential role, if any, of regulation of human monocyte α_1-antitrypsin by NF-κB needs to be explored.

3.8. *Cytokine Regulation of Acute-Phase Proteins*

The changes in concentrations of the secondary acute-phase proteins reflect changes in gene expression and it is clear that the cytokine network, especially IL-6 and IL-1, also plays a central role in the induction of these genes as was seen for the "alarm" antiproteinases elafin and SLPI. It is probable that, as well as regulation by cytokines, steroid hormones such as oestrogens play a role. An oestrogen response element has been identified in the angiotensinogen gene [138]. Levels of α_1-antitrypsin are reported to increase during pregnancy so it is feasible that this gene is capable of responding in a similar manner. Several other regulators, besides IL-1 and IL-6, have been shown to have an effect on expression of acute-phase genes. Leukaemia inhibitory factor (LIF, previously called hepatocyte-stimulating factor III) has major stimulatory activity on fibrinogen and haptoglobin [139] and appears to mediate this effect via the response element for IL-6 (IL-6-RE) [140]. Oncostatin M (OM) has a potent effect on α_1-antichymotrypsin, fibrinogen and haptoglobin in HepG2 cells and again this effect appears to be mediated by IL-6-RE [140]. Thus, although LIF and OM bind to different receptors they induce similar signal transduction pathways to that seen with IL-6. Recently, OM has been shown to be a potent cytokine for inducing α_1-antitrypsin expression in the alveolar epithelial cell line A549 [22]. IL-1 has also been shown to regulate the hepatic expression of the same plasma protein genes as IL-6 [141]. Our current understanding of the molecular mechanisms involved during the cytokine-induced acute-phase response are outlined below.

Acute-phase genes can be divided into two major classes: class 1 genes are regulated mainly by IL-1 or combinations of IL-1 and IL-6 [142] and class 2 genes are regulated mainly by IL-6 and include AAT [143].

3.8.1. Interleukin-1: IL-1 mediates its stimulatory effect via the transcription factor NF-κB [144] which binds to the AP-3/enhancer core DNA consensus sequence GGGRHTYYC, also termed the κB site. NF-κB sites have been identified in the serum amyloid A (SAA), CRP and angiotensinogen genes. In rabbit blood monocytes the S2 form of α_1-antitrypsin can be induced by LPS and a distal enhancer located 2000 bases upstream of the hepatocyte transcription start site accounts for this LPS-induced increase in rabbit α_1-antitrypsin [135]. LPS mediates its effect via NF-κB [135] as does TNF [145].

The typical form of NF-κB, which exists as a result of activation of extracellular signals, is a heterodimer consisting of two proteins, namely a p65 (Rel A) subunit and a p50 subunit [146]. The transcriptional activity of NF-κB resides with the p65 subunit [147, 148]; both subunits contribute to the DNA-binding capability. Other subunits include v-Rel, c-Rel, RelB and p52, and almost all combinations of homo- and heterodimer can exist [149]. In unstimulated cells NF-κB is found in the cytoplasm bound to the inhibitor IκBa/b which precludes its entry into the nucleus [150]. Upon stimulation IκB is phosphorylated thereby releasing NF-κB and allowing it to pass into the nucleus [151, 152]. Activation of gene expression by NF-κB is terminated as a result of a feedback loop whereby NF-κB induces synthesis of IκB that enters the nucleus, binds to activated NF-κB and carries it back to the cytoplasm [153].

3.8.2. Interleukin-6: Two types of DNA sequences mediate the IL-6 response: type I and type II, each via distinct mechanisms.

3.8.2.1. Type I IL-6 response. This response is mediated by members of the C/EBP family of transcription factors through type I IL-6-REs which have the DNA consensus sequence TKNNGNAAK. These elements have been found in several acute-phase genes including α_1-antitrypsin, CRP and haptoglobin. Several members of the C/EBP family have been cloned and expressed, namely C/EBPα, C/EBPβ (also more commonly known as NF-IL-6) and C/EBPγ (NF-IL-6β). All of these molecules share a high degree of homology and have a characteristic leucine zipper essential for dimerization and basic domains which bind to DNA [154]. IL-6 regulates the concentration and/or activity of each of these isoforms by signal transduction mechanisms routed through the IL-6 receptor. In some tissues, during the acute-phase response to IL-6, C/EBPα levels decrease, whereas C/EBPβ (NF-IL-6) and C/EBPγ (NF-IL-6β) levels increase [155, 156]. C/EBPβ undergoes a nuclear post-translational threonine specific phosphorylation by Mitogen-activated protein (MAP) kinases [157] which increases its binding capacity for the DNA consensus sequence. In contrast C/EBPγ increases by transcriptional induction and has transcription activation potential [158]. It has been suggested that, during IL-6 induction of acute-phase genes, C/EBPα may be displaced by the other isoforms thus switching on transcription [155].

3.8.2.2. Type II IL-6 response. Type II IL-6-REs, also known as acute-phase response elements (APRE), are involved in the JAK (Janus kinase)–STAT

Table 1. Pathway for SERPIN gene regulation

Transcription factor	*Stimulus*	*Gene*	*Mechanism*
NF-κB	IL-1 LPS TNF	SAA CRP Angiotensinogen α_1-Antichymotrypsin α_1-Antichymotrypsin	Binds to AP3/core enhancer site
C/EBP family C/EBPα C/EBPβ (NF-IL-6) C/EBPγ (NF-IL-6β)	IL-6 OM? LIF?	AAT CRP Haptoglobin	Type I IL-6-RE MAP kinase
STAT 3	IL-6 OM? LIF?	C3 complement α_2-Macroglobulin Fibrinogen α_1-Antichymotrypsin	Type II IL-6-RE JAK/STAT

(signal transducers and activators of transcription) pathway [159] and interact with the DNA consensus KTMYKGKAA. These elements have been identified in complement C3, α_2-macroglobulin, fibrinogen and α_1-antichymotrypsin genes [159–161]. IL-6 has been shown to up-regulate the transcription factor STAT-3 in liver cells [162] which has a role in acute-phase gene expression [163]. Type II IL-6 responses are also mediated by the IL-6 receptor. In the case of STAT-3, homodimerization of the IL-6-associated gp130 subunits results in activation of JAK kinases followed by tyrosine- and serine-specific phosphorylation of STAT-3 [164], with subsequent translocation into the nucleus.

Some acute-phase genes, e.g. α_1-antichymotrypsin, SAA and CRP, are capable of responding to both IL-1 and IL-6, and this suggests that, although each cytokine evokes a distinct pathway, there is also the possibility of some degree of overlap between the molecular mechanisms responsible for induction. In this regard there is evidence for cooperation between NF-κB and NF-IL-6 in the SAA gene [165] which results in the synergistic effect seen with IL-1 and IL-6. The pathways by which IL-1 and IL-6 induce acute-phase gene expression are summarized in Table 1.

Acknowledgements

We are indebted to Anabel Silva and Mark Marsden for their involvement in the characterization of the elastase-specific inhibitor. We are grateful to Drs G. Cunningham, P. Reid and John Simpson for reviewing the manuscript. We also wish to thank the Salvesen Emphysema Research Trust, the EU Biomed 2 programme (Eurolung consortium) and the Wellcome Trust (grant numbers 044161 and 035324) for support.

References

1 Mackiewicz I, Kushner I, Baumann H (eds) (1993) *Acute phase proteins. Molecular biology, biochemistry, and clinical applications*. Boca Raton, FL, CRC Press

2 Koy A, Gauldie J (1993) Biological perspectives of cytokine and hormone networks. In: I Mackiewicz, I Kushner, H Baumann (eds): *Acute phase proteins. Molecular biology, biochemistry, and clinical applications*. Boca Raton, FL, CRC Press, 275–287

3 Baumann H, Gauldie J (1994) The acute phase response. *Immunol* Today 15: 74–80

4 Xing Z, Achong M, Lei X-F, Cox G, Jordana M, Gauldie J (1997) Enhanced pulmonary inflammatory responses to local endotoxin challenge in interleukin-6-deficient mice. *Am J Respir Crit Care Med* 155: A500

5 Howard M, Muchamuel T, Andrade S, Menon S (1993) Interleukin-10 protects mice from lethal endotoxemia. *J Exp Med* 177: 1205–1208

6 Standiford TJ, Strieter RM, Lukacs NW, Kunkel SL (1995) Neutralization of IL-10 increases lethality in endotoxemia. Cooperative effects of macrophage inflammatory protein-2 and tumor necrosis factor. *J Immunol* 155: 2222–2229

7 Bode W, Huber R (1992) Natural protein proteinase inhibitors and their interaction with proteinases. *Eur J Biochem* 204: 433–451

8 Twining SS (1994) Regulation of proteolytic activity in tissues. *Crit Rev Biochem Mol Biol* 29: 315–383

9 Salvesen G, Enghild JJ (1993) Proteinase inhibitors: an overview of their structure and possible function in the acute phase. In: Mackiewicz I, Kushner I, Baumann H (eds): *Acute phase proteins. Molecular biology, biochemistry, and clinical applications*. Boca Raton, FL, CRC Press, 117–147

10 Booth NA (1994) The natural inhibitors of fibrinololysis. In: AL, Bloom, DP, Thomas, CD, Forbes, EGD, Tuddenham (eds): *Haemostasis and thrombosis*. London, Churchill Livingstone, 699–717

11 Fritz H (1988) Human mucus proteinase inhibitors (human MPI). *Biol Chem Hoppe Seyler* 369: 79–82

12 Molhuizen HOF, Schalkwijk J (1995) Structural, biochemical, and cell biological aspects of the serine proteinase inhibitor SKALP/elafin/ESI. *Biol Chem Hoppe Seyler* 376: 1–7

13 Sallenave JM, Shulmann J, Crosley J, Jordana M, Gauldie J (1994) Regulation of secretory leukocyte proteinase inhibitor (SLPI) and elastase-specific inhibitor (ESI/elafin) in human airway epithelial cells by cytokines and neutrophilic enzymes. *Am J Respir Cell Mol Biol* 11: 733–741

14 Kramps JA, Franken C, Dijkman JH (1984) ELISA for quantitative measurement of low molecular weight bronchial protease inhibitor in human sputum. *Am Rev Respir Dis* 129: 959–963

15 Abe T, Kobayashi N, Yoshimura K, Trapnell BC, Kim H, Hubbard RC, Brewer MT, Thompson RC, Crystal RG (1991) Expression of the secretory leukoprotease inhibitor gene in epithelial cells. *J Clin Invest* 87: 2207–2215

16 Nara K, Ito S, Ito T, Suzuki Y, Ghoneim MA, Tachibana S, Hirose S (1994) Elastase inhibitor elafin is a new type of proteinase inhibitor which has a transglutaminase-mediated anchoring sequence termed "cementoin". *J Biochem* 115: 441–448

17 Pfundt R, van Ruissen F, van Vlijmen-Willems IMJJ, Akemade HAC, Zeeuwen PLJM, Schalkwijk J (1996) Constitutive and inducible expression of SKALP/elafin provides anti-elastase defence in human epithelia. *J Clin Invest* 98: 1389–1399

18 Asano S, Kida K, Koyama T, Wada H, Isawa Y, Hosoda K, Masuda K, Suzuki Y (1995) A morphologic study of lung secretory leukoprotease inhibitor in pneumonia. *Am J Respir Crit Care Med* 151: 1576–1581

19 Perlmutter DH, May LT, Sehgal PB (1989) Interferon b2/interleukin 6 modulates synthesis of α_1-antitrypsin in human mononuclear phagocytes and in human hepatoma cells. *J Clin Invest* 84: 138–144

20 Molmenti EP, Ziambaras T, Perlmutter DH (1993) Evidence for an acute phase response in human intestinal epithelial cells. *J Biol Chem* 268: 14116–14124

21 Cichy J, Potempa J, Chawla RK, Travis J (1995) Stimulatory effect of inflammatory cytokines and α_1-antichymotrypsin expression in human lung-derived epithelial cells. *J Clin Invest* 95: 2729–2733

22 Sallenave J-M, Tremblay GM, Gauldie J, Richards CD (1997) Oncostatin M but not interleukin-6 or leukaemia inhibiting factor, stimulates expression of α_1-proteinase inhibitor in A549 human alveolar epithelial cells. *J Interferon Cytokine Res* 17: 337–346
23 Fryksmark U, Ohlsson K, Rosengren M, Tegner H (1983) Studies on the interaction between leukocyte elastase, antileukoproteinase and the plasma proteinase inhibitors α_1-proteinase inhibitor and α_2-macroglobulin. *Hoppe-Seyler's Z Physiol Chem* 364: 793–800
24 Perlmutter DH, Glover GI, Rivetna M, Schasteen CS, Fallon RJ (1990) Identification of a serpin-enzyme complex receptor on human hepatoma cells and human monocytes. *Proc Nat Acad Sci USA* 87: 3753–3757
25 Dabbagh GJ, Laurent GJ, Chambers RC (1997) α_1-antitrypsin stimulates proliferation and procollagen production by human lung fibroblasts. *Am J Respir Crit Care Med* 155: A185
26 Seemuller U, Arnhold M, Fritz H, Wiedenmann K, Machleidt, W, Heinzel R, Appelhans H, Gassen HG, Lottspeich F (1986) The acid-stable proteinase inhibitor of human mucous secretions (HUSI-I, antileukoprotease). Complete amino acid sequence as revealed by protein and cDNA sequencing and structural homology to whey proteins and red sea turtle proteinase inhibitor. *FEBS Lett* 199: 43–48
27 Grutter MG, Fendrich G, Huber R, Bode W (1988) The 2.5 Å X-ray crystal structure of the acid-stable proteinase inhibitor from human mucous secretions analysed in its complex with bovine α-chymotrypsin. *EMBO J* 7: 345–351
28 Stetler G, Brewer MT, Thompson RC (1986) Isolation and sequence of a human gene encoding a potent inhibitor of leukocyte proteases. *Nucleic Acids Res* 14: 7883–7886
29 Heinzel R, Appelhans H, Gassen G, Seemuller U, Machleidt W, Fritz H, Steffens G (1986) Molecular cloning and expression of cDNA for human antileukoprotease from cervix uterus. *Eur J Biochem* 160: 61–67
30 Maruyama M, Hay JG, Yoshimura K, Chu CS, Crystal RG (1994) Modulation of secretory leukoprotease inhibitor gene expression in human bronchial epithelial cells by phorbol ester. *J Clin Invest* 94: 368–375
31 Kikuchi T, Abe T, Satoh K, Narumi K, Sakai T, Abe S, Shindoh S, Matsushima K, Nukiwa T (1997) *cis*-Acting region associated with lung-cell-specific expression of the secretory leukoprotease inhibitor gene. *Am J Respir Cell Mol Biol* 17: 361–367
32 Faller B, Mely Y, Gerard D, Bieth JG (1992) Heparin-induced conformational change and activation of mucus proteinase inhibitor. *Biochemistry* 31: 8285–8290
33 Ying QL, Kemme M, Simon SR (1994) Functions of the N-terminal domain of secretory leukoprotease inhibitor. *Biochemistry* 33: 5445–5450
34 Mellet P, Ermolieff J, Bieth JG (1995) Mapping the heparin-binding site of mucus proteinase inhibitor. *Biochemistry* 34: 2645–2652
35 Kramps JA, van Twisk C, Appelhans H, Meckelein B, Nikiforov T, Dijkman JH (1990) Proteinase inhibitory activities of antileukoprotease are represented by its second COOH-terminal domain. *Biochim Biophys Acta* 1038: 178–185
36 Meckelein B, Nikoforov T, Clemen A, Appelhans H (1990) The location of inhibitory specificities in human mucus proteinase inhibitor (MPI): separate expression of the COOH-terminal doamin yields an active inhibitor of three different proteinases. *Protein Engineering* 3: 215–220
37 Eisenberg SP, Hale KK, Heimdal P, Thompson RC (1990) Location of the protease-inhibitory region of secretory leukocyte protease inhibitor. *J Biol Chem* 265: 7976–7981
38 Masuda KI, Kamimura T, Watanabe K, Suga T, Kanesaki M, Takeuchi A, Imaizumi A, Suzuki Y (1995) Pharmacological activity of the C-terminal and N-terminal domains of secretory leukoprotease inhibitor *in vitro*. *Br J Pharmacol* 115: 883–888
39 Ohlsson K, Tegner H (1976) Inhibition of elastase from granulocytes by the low molecular weight bronchial protease inhibitor. *Scand J Lab Clin Invest* 36: 437–445
40 Fink E, Nettelbeck R, Fritz H (1986) Inhibition of mast cell chymase by eglin C and antileukoprotease (HUSI-I). *Biol Chem Hoppe Seyler* 367: 567–571
41 Gauthier F, Fryksmark U, Ohlsson K, Bieth JG (1982) Kinetics of the inhibition of leukocyte elastase by the bronchial inhibitor. *Biochim Biophys Acta* 700: 178–183
42 Boudier C, Bieth JG (1989) Mucus proteinase inhibitor: a fast-acting inhibitor of leukocyte elastase. *Biochim Biophys Acta* 995: 36–41
43 Boudier C, Bieth JG (1992) The proteinase-mucos proteinase inhibitor binding stoichiometry. *J Biol Chem* 267: 4370–4375

44 Zitnik RJ, Zhang J, Kashem MA, Kohno T, Lyons DE, Wright CD, Rosen E, Goldberg I, Hayday AC (1997) The cloning and characterization of a murine secretory leukocyte protease inhibitor cDNA. *Biochem Biophys Res Commun* 232: 687–697

45 Zitnik R, Zhang J, Gao X (1997) Cloning and characterization of the murine secretory leukocyte protease inhibitor (SLPI) gene. *Am J Respir Crit Care Med* 155: A657

46 Abbinante-Niessen JM, Simpson LG, Leikauf GD (1993) Neutrophil elastase increases secretory leukocyte protease inhibitor transcript levels in airway epithelial cells. *Am J Physiol* 265: L286–292

47 Kramps JA, Willems LNA, Franken C, Dijkman JH (1988) Antileukoprotease, its role in the human lung. *Biol Chem Hoppe-Seyler* 369: 83–87

48 Jacquot J, Spilmont C, Burlet H, Fuchey C, Buisson AC, Tournier JM, Gaillard D, Puchelle E (1994) Glandular-like morphogenesis and secretory activity of human tracheal gland cells in a three-dimensional collagen gel matrix. *J Cell Physiol* 161: 407–418

49 Appelhans B, Sachse EG, Nikiforov T, Appelhans H, Ebert W (1987) Secretion of antileukoprotease from a human lung tumor cell line. *FEBS Lett* 224: 14–18

50 Sallenave JM, Silva A, Marsden ME, Ryle AP (1993) Secretion of mucus proteinase inhibitor and elafin by Clara cell and type II pneumocyte cell lines. *Am J Respir Cell Mol Biol* 8: 126–133

51 Kramps JA, Franken C, Meijer CJLM, Dijkman JH (1981) Localization of low molecular weight protease inhibitor in serous secretory cells of the respiratory tract. *J Histochem Cytochem* 29: 712–719

52 Kramps JA, Te Boekhorst AH, Fransen JA, Gensel LA, Dijkman JH (1989) Antileukoprotease is associated with elastin fibers in the extracellular matrix of the human lung. An immunoelectron microscopy study. *Am Rev Respir Dis* 140: 471–476

53 Jin FY, Nathan C, Radzioch D, Ding A (1997) Secretory leukocyte protease inhibitor: a macrophage product induced by and antagonistic to bacterial lipopolysaccharide. *Cell* 88: 417–426

54 Sallenave JM, Si-Tahar M, Cox G, Chignard M, Gauldie J (1997) Secretory leukocyte proteinase inhibitor is a major leukocyte elastase inhibitor in human neutrophils. *J Leuk Biol* 61: 695–702

55 Bohm B, Aigner T, Kinne R, Burkhardt H (1992) The serine-protease inhibitor of cartilage matrix is not a chondrocytic gene product. *Eur J Biochem* 207: 773–779

56 Hiemstra PS, Maassen RJ, Stolk J, Heinzel-Wieland R, Steffens GJ, Dijkman JH (1996) Antibacterial activity of antileukoprotease. *Infect Immun* 64: 4520–4524

57 Zhang Y, DeWitt DL, McNeely TB, Wahl SM, Wahl LM (1997) Secretory leukocyte protease inhibitor suppresses the production of monocyte prostaglandin H synthase-2, prostaglandin E_2, and matrix metalloproteinases. *J Clin Invest* 99: 894–900

58 Beutler B, Milsark IW, Cerami AC (1985) Passive immunization against cachectin/tumor necrosis factor protects mice from lethal effect of endotoxin. *Science*229: 869–871

59 Rudolphus A, Kramps JA, Dijkman JH (1991) Effect of human antileukoprotease on experimental emphysema. *Eur Respir J* 4: 31–39

60 Rudolphus A, Stolk J, Dijkman JH, Kramps JA (1993) Inhibition of lipopolysaccharide-induced pulmonary emphysema by intratracheally instilled recombinant secretory leukocyte proteinase inhibitor. *Am Rev Respir Dis* 147: 442–447

61 Mulligan MS, Desrochers PE, Chinnaiyan AM, Gibbs DF, Varani J, Johnson KJ, Weiss SJ (1993). *In vivo* suppression of immune complex-induced alveolitis by secretory leukoproteinase inhibitor and tissue inhibitor of metalloproteinases 2. *Proc Natl Acad Sci USA* 90: 11523–11527

62 Sallenave JM, Donnelly SC, Gauldie J, Haslett C (1997) Secretory leukocyte proteinase inhibitor (SLPI), α_1-proteinase inhibitor (Alpha-1Pi) and elafin levels are augmented in the adult respiratory distress syndrome (ARDS). *Am J Respir Crit Care Med* 155: A651

63 Docke WD, Randow F, Syrbe U, Krausch D, Asadullah K, Reinke P, Volk HD, Kox W (1997) Monocyte deactivaton in septic patients: restoration by IFN-gamma treatment. *Nature Med* 3: 678–681

64 Fisher CJ Jr, Dhainaut JF, Opal SM, Pribble JP, Balk RA, Slotman GJ, Iberti TJ, Rackow EC, Shapiro MJ, Greenman RL et al. (1994) Recombinant human interleukin 1 receptor antagonist in the treatment of patients with sepsis syndrome: results from a randomized, double-blind, placebo-controlled trial. *JAMA* 271: 1836–1843

65 Sallenave J-M, Xing Z, Simpson AJ, Graham FL, Gauldie J (1998) Adenovirus-mediated expression of an elastase-specific inhibitor (elafin): a comparison of different promoters. *Gene Therapy* 5: 352–360
66 Hochstrasser K, Albrecht GJ, Schonberger G, Rasche B, Lempart K (1981) An elastase-specific inhibitor from human bronchial mucus. Isolation and characterization. *Hoppe-Seyler's Z Physiol Chem* 362: 1369–1375
67 Kramps JA, Klasen EC (1985) Characterization of a low molecular weight anti-elastase isolated from human bronchial secretion. *Exp Lung Res* 9: 151–165
68 Wiedow O, Schroder J, Gregory H, Young JA, Christopers E (1990) Elafin: an elastase specific inhibitor of human skin. Purification, characterization, and complete amine acid sequence. *J Biol Chem* 265: 14791–14795
69 Sallenave JM, Ryle AP (1991) Purification and characterization of elastase-specific inhibitor. Sequence homology with mucus proteinase inhibitor. *Biol Chem Hoppe-Seyler* 372: 13–21
70 Molhuizen HOF, Alkemade HAC, Zeeuwen PLJM, de Jongh GJ, Wieringa B, Schalkwijk J (1993) SKALP/Elafin: an elastase inhibitor from cultured human keratinocytes. Purification, cDNA sequence, and evidence for transglutaminase cross-linking. *J Biol Chem* 268: 12028–12032
71 Sallenave JM, Silva A (1993) Characterization and gene sequence of the precursor of elafin, an elastase-specific inhibitor in bronchial secretions. *Am J Respir Cell Mol Biol* 8: 439–445
72 Tremblay GM, Sallenave JM, Israel-Assayag E, Cormier Y, Gauldie J (1996) Elafin/elastase-specific inhibitor in bronchoalveolar lavage of normal subjects and farmer's lung. *Am J Respir Crit Care Med* 154: 1092–1098
73 Campbell EJ, Campbell MA (1988) Pericellular proteolysis by neutrophils in the presence of proteinase inhibitors: effects of substrate opsonization. *J Cell Biol* 106: 667–676
74 Rice W, Weiss SJ (1990) Regulation of proteolysis at the neutrophil–substrate interface by secretory leukoprotease inhibitor. *Science* 249: 178–181
75 Llewellyn-Jones CG, Lomas DA, Stockley RA (1994) Potential role of recombinant secretory leucoprotease inhibitor in the prevention of neutrophil mediated matrix degradation. *Thorax* 49: 567–572
76 Wiedow O, Ludemann J, Utecht B (1991) Elafin is a potent inhibitor of proteinase 3. *Biochem Biophys Res Commun* 174: 6–10
77 Ying QL, Simon SR (1993) Kinetics of the inhibition of human leukocyte elastase by elafin, a 6 kilodalton elastase-specific inhibitor from human skin. *Biochemistry* 32: 1866–1874
78 Tsunemi M, Kato H, Nishiuchi Y, Kumagaye S, Sakakibara S (1992) Synthesis and structure-activity relationship of elafin, an elastase-specific inhibitor. *Biochem Biophys Res Commun* 185: 967–973
79 Henninghausen LG, Sippel AE, Hobbs AA, Rosen JM (1982) Comparative sequence analysis of the mRNAs coding for mouse and rat whey protein. *Nucleic Acid Res* 10: 3733–3744
80 Araki K, Kuwada M, Ito O, Kuroki J, Tachibana S (1990) Four disulfide bonds allocation of Na^+/H^+-ATPase inhibitor (SPaI). *Biochem Biophys Res Commun* 172: 42–46
81 Tsunemi M, Matsuura Y, Sakakibara S, Katsube Y (1996) Crystal structure of an elastase-specific inhibitor elafin complexed with procine pancreatic elastase determined at 1.9 A resolution. *Biochemistry* 35: 11570–11576
82 Saheki T, Ito F, Hagiwara H, Saito Y, Kuroki J, Tachibana S, Hirose S (1992) Primary structure of the human elafin precursor preproelafin deduced from the nucleotide sequence of its gene and the presence of unique repetitive sequences in the prosegment. *Biochem Biophys Res Commun* 185: 240–245
83 Zhang M, Zou Z, Maass N, Sager R (1995) Differential expression of elafin in human normal mammary epithelial cells and carcinomas is regulated at the transcriptional level. *Cancer Res* 55: 2537–2541
84 Lundwall A, Lazure C (1995) A novel gene family encoding proteins with highly differing structure because of a rapidly evolving exon. *FEBS Lett* 374: 53–56
85 Lundwall A, Ulvsback M (1996) The gene of the protease inhibitor SKALP/Elafin is a member of the Rest gene family. *Biochem Biophys Res Commun* 221: 323–327

86 Molhuizen HOF, Zeeuwen PLJM, Weghuis DO, Geurts van Kessel A, Schalkwijk J (1994) Assignment of the human gene encoding the epidermal serine proteinase inhibitor SKALP (P13) to chromosome region 20q12-q13. *Cytogenet Cell Genet* 66: 129–131

87 Crystal RG (1989) The α_1-antitrypsin gene and its deficiency states. *TIG* 5: 411–417

88 Laurell C-B, Eriksson S (1963) The electrophoretic α_1-globulin pattern of serum in α_1-antitrypsin deficiency. *Scand J Lab Invest* 15: 132–140

89 Carrell RW, Jeppsson J-O, Laurrel C-B, Brennan SO, Owen MC, Vaughn L, Boswell DR (1987) Structure and variation of human α_1-antitrypsin (Review). *Nature (Lond)* 298: (5872) 329–334

90 Travis J, Salvesen G (1983) Human plasma proteinase inhibitors. *Annu Rev Biochem* 52: 655–709

91 Crystal RG (1990) α_1-Antitrypsin deficiency, emphysema and liver disease. *J Clin Invest* 85: 1343–1352

92 Mittman C, Barbela T, Liebermann J (1973) α_1-Antitrypsin deficiency as an indicator of susceptibility to pulmonary disease. *J Occup Med* 15: 33–38

93 Hay JW, Robin ED (1991) Cost-effectiveness of α_1-antitrypsin replacement therapy in treatment of congenital chronic obstructive pulmonary disease. *Am J Public Health* 81: 427–433

94 Cohen BH, Ball WC, Bias WB (1975) A genetic epidemiologic study of chronic obstructive pulmonary disease I: study design and preliminary observation. *Johns Hopkins Med J* 137: 94–104

95 Brantly M, Nukiwa T, Crystal RG (1988) Molecular basis of α_1-antitrypsin deficiency. *Am J Med* 84: 13–31

96 Yoshida A, Lieberman J, Gaidulis I, Ewing C (1976) Molecular abnormality of human α_1-antitrypsin variant (Pi-ZZ) associated with plasma activity deficiency. *Proc Natl Acad Sci USA* 73: 1324–1328

97 Owen MC, Carrell RW (1976) α_1-Antitrypsin: molecular abnormality of S variant. *BMJ* 1: 130–131

98 Kalsheker N, Hodgson, Watkins GL, White JP, Morrison HM, Stockley RA (1987) DNA Polymorphism of the α_1-antitrypsin gene in chronic lung disease. *BMJ* 294: 1511–1514

99 Poller W, Meissen C, Olek K (1990) DNA polymorphims of the α_1-antitrypsin gene region in patients with chronic obstructive disease. *Eur J Clin Invest* 20: 1–7

100 Morgan K, Scobie G, Kalsheker N (1993) Point mutation in a 3′ flanking sequence of the α_1-antitrypsin gene associated with chronic respiratory disease occurs in a regulatory sequence. *Hum Mol Genet* 2: 253–257

101 Morgan K, Scobie G, Marsters P, Kalsheker NA (1997) Mutation in an α_1-antitrypsin enhancer results in an interleukin-6 deficient acute-phase response due to loss of co-operativity between transcription factors. *BBA* 1362: 67–76

102 Cox DW, Billingsley GD, Mansfield T (1987) DNA restriction-site polymorphisms associated with the a_1-antitrypsin gene. *Am J Hum Genet* 41: 891–906

103 Lindmark BE, Arborelius M, Erikksson S (1990) Pulmonary deficiency in middle-aged women with heterozygous deficiency of the serine proteinase inhibitor α_1-antichymotrypsin. *Am Rev Respir Dis* 141: 884–888

104 Poller W, Faber J-P, Weidinger S, Tief K, Scholz S, Fischer M, Olek K, Kirkgesser M, Heidtmann HH (1993) A Leucine-to-Proline substitution causes a defective α_1-antichymotrypsin allele associated with familial obstructive lung disease. *Genomics* 17: 740–743

105 Janoff A (1985) Elastases and emphysema. Current assessment of the protease–antiprotease hypothesis. *Am Rev Respir Dis* 132: 417–433

106 Dickson I, Apler CA (1974) Changes in serum proteinase levels following bons surgery. *Clin Chem Acta* 54: 381

107 Mornex JF, Chytil-Weir A, Martinet Y, Courtney M, LeCocq JP, Crystal RG (1986) Expression of the α_1-antitrypsin gene in mononuclear phagocytes of normal and α_1-antitrypsin deficient individuals. *J Clin Invest* 77: 1952–1961

108 Perlmutter DH, Cole FS, Kilbridge P, Rossing TH, Cotten HR (1985) Expression of the α_1-proteinase inhibitor gene in human monocytes and macrophages. *Proc Natl Acad Sci USA* 82: 795–799

109 Lodish HF, Kong N, Snider M, Strous GJAM (1983) Hepatoma secretory proteins migrate from rough endoplasmic reticulum to Golgi at characteristic rates. *Nature (Lond)* 304: 80–83

110 Castell JV, Gomez-Lechon MJ, David M, Hirano T, Kishimoto T, Heinrich PC (1986) Recombinant human interleukin-6 (IL-6/BSF-2/HSF) regulates the synthesis of acute phase proteins in human hepatocytes. *FEBS Lett* 232: 347–352

111 Barbey-Morel C, Pierce JA, Campbell EJ, Perlmutter DH (1987) Lipopolysaccharide modulates the expression of α_1-proteinase inhibitor and other serine proteinase inhibitors in human monocytes and macrophages. *J Exp Med* 166: 1041–1054

112 LaI EC, Kao FT, Law ML, Woo SLC (1983) Assignment of the α_1-antitrypsin gene and a sequence-related gene to human chromosome 14 by molecular hybridisation. *Am J Hum Genet* 35: 385–392

113 Long GL, Chandra T, Woo SLC, Davie EW, Kurachi K (1984) Complete sequence of the cDNA for human α_1-antitrypsin and the gene for the S variant. *Biochemistry* 23: 4828–4837

114 Perlino E, Cortese R, Ciliberto G (1987) The human α_1-antitrypsin gene is transcribed from two different promoters in macrophages and hepatocytes. *EMBO J* 6: 2767–2771

115 Hafeez W, Ciliberto G, Perlmutter DH (1992) Constitutive and modulated expression of the human α_1-antitrypsin gene: different transcriptional initiation sites used in three different cell types. *J Clin Invest* 89: 1214–1222

116 Kalsheker N, Swanson T (1990) Exclusion of an exon in monocyte α_1-antitrypsin mRNA after stimulation of U937 cells by interleukin-6. *Biochem Biophys Res Commun* 172: 1116–1121

117 Shen R-F, Li Y, Sifers RN, Wang H, Hardick C, Tsai SY, Woo SLC (1987) Tissue-specific expression of the human α_1-antitrypsin gene is controlled by multiple *cis*-regulatory elements. *Nucleic Acid Res* 15: 8399–8415

118 Ciliberto G, Dente L, Cortese R (1985) Cell-specific expression of a transfected human α_1-antitrypsin gene. *Cell* 41: 531–540

119 De Simone V, Ciliberto G, Hardon E, Paonessa G, Palla F, Lundberg L, Cortese P (1987) *Cis* and *trans*acting elements responsible for the cell-specific expression of the human α_1-antitrypsin gene. *EMBO J* 6: 2759–2766

120 Hardon EM, Fain M, Poonessa G, Cortese R (1987) Two distinct factors interact with the promoter regions of several liver-specific genes. *EMBO J* 7: 1711–1719

121 De Simone, Cortese R (1989) A negative regulatory element in the promoter of the human α_1-antitrypsin gene. *Nucleic Acid Res* 17: 9407–9415

122 Wu Y, Foreman RC (1991) The molecular genetics of α_1-antitrypsin deficiency. *Bioessays* 13: 163–169

123 Gstaiger M, Knoepfel L, Georgiev O, Schaffner W, Hovens CM (1995) A β-cell co-activator of octamer-binding transcription factors. *Nature* 373: 360–362

124 Schubart DB, Sauter P, Massa S, Friedl EM, Schwarzenbach H, Matthias P (1986) Gene structure and characterisation of the murine homologue of the cell-specific transcriptional co-activator OBF-1. *Nucleic Acid Res* 24: 1913–1920

125 Ruvkin G, Finney M (1991) Regulation of transcription and cell identity by POU domain proteins. *Cell* 64: 475–478

126 Liang Y, Carr LG (1996) Identification of an octamer-1 transcription factor binding site in the promoter of the mouse m-opioid receptor gene. *J Neurochem* 67: 1352–1359

127 Sterling K, Weaver J, Ho K-L, Xu LC, Bresruck E (1993) Rat CYP 1A1 negative regulatory element: biological activity and interaction with a protein from liver and hepatoma cells. *Mol Pharmacol* 44: 560–568

128 Lin HK, Penning TM (1995) Cloning, sequencing and functional analysis of the 5′ flanking region of the rat 3α-hydroxysteroid/dihydrodiol dehydrogenase gene. *Cancer Res* 55: 4105–4113

129 Clark AR, Wilson ME, Leibiger I, Scott V, Docherty K (1995) A silencer and an adjacent postive element interact to modulate the activity of the human insulin promoter. *Eur J Biochem* 232: 627–632

130 Ullman KS, Northrop JP, Admon A, Crabtree GR (1993) Jun family members are controlled by a calcium-regulated cyclosporin A-sensitive signalling pathway in activated T lymphocytes. *Genes Devel* 7: 188–196

131 Strubin M, Newell JW, Matthias P (1995) OBF-1, a novel B cell-specific co-activator that stimulates immunoglobulin promoter activity through association with octamer-binding proteins. *Cell* 80: 497–506

132 Nakshatri H, Nakshatri P, Currie RA (1995) Interaction of Oct-1 with TFIIB: implications for a novel response elicited through the proximal octamer site of the lipoprotein lipase promoter. *J Biol Chem* 270: 19613–19623
133 Saatcioglu F, Deng T, Karin M (1993) A novel *cis* element mediating ligand-independent activation by c-ErbA: implications for hormonal regulation. *Cell* 75: 1095–1105
134 Pearce D, Yamamoto KR (1993) Mineralocorticol and glucocorticoid receptor activities distinguished by non-receptor factors at a composite response element. *Science* 259: 1161–1165
135 Ray A, Goa X, Ray BK (1995) Role of a distal enhancer containing a functional NFκB binding site in lipopolysacchardie-induced expression of a novel α_1-antitrypsin gene. *J Biol Chem* 270: 29201–29208
136 Das S, Potter H (1995) Expression of the Alzheimer amyloid-promoting factor antichymotrypsin is induced in human astrocytes by IL-1. *Neuron* 14: 447–456
137 Cichy J, Potempa J, Chawla RK, Travis J (1995) Regulation of α_1-antichymotrypsin synthesis in cells of epithelial origin. *FEBS Lett* 359: 262–266
138 Gaillard I, Clauser E, Correl P (1989) Structure of the human angiotensinogen gene. *DNA* 8: 87–99
139 Gauldie JC, Richards C, Northemann W, Fey G, Baumann H (1989) IFN-β2/BSF2/IL-6 is the monocyte-derived HSF that regulates receptor-specific acute phase gene regulation in hepatocytes. *Ann NY Acad Sci* 557: 46
140 Richards CD, Brown TJ, Shoyab M, Baumann H, Gauldie J (1992) Recombinant oncostatin M stimulates the production of acute-phase proteins in Hep G2 and rat primary hepatocytes *in vitro*. *J Immunol* 148: 1731–1736
141 Baumann H, Schendel P (1991) Interleukin-11 regulates the hepatic expression of the same plasma protein genes as interleukin-6. *J Biol Chem* 266: 1
142 Baumann H, Gauldie J (1990) Regulation of hepatic acute-phase plasma protein genes by hepatocyte stimulating factors and other mediators of inflammation. *Mol Biol Med* 7: 147–160
143 Heinrich PC, Castell JV, Andus T (1990) Interleukin-6 and the acute-phase response. *Biochem J* 265: 621–636
144 Brasier AR, Ron D, Tate JE, Habener JF (1990) A family of constitutive C/EBP-like DNA binding proteins attenuate the IL-1 a induced NFκB mediated transactivation of the angiotensinogen gene acute-phase response element. *EMBO J* 9: 3933–3944
145 Adcock IM, Brown CR, Gelder CM, Shiraski H, Peters MJ, Barnes PJ (1995) Effects of glucocorticoids on transcription factor activation in human peripheral blood mononuclear cells. *Am J Physiol* 268: C331–C338
146 Barnes PJ, Larin M (1997) Nuclear factor-κB – a pivotal transcription factor in chronic inflammatory diseases. *N Engl J Med* 336: 1066–1071
147 Fujita T, Nolan GP, Ghosh S, Baltimore D (1992) Independent modes of transcriptional activation by the p50 and p65 sub-units of NFκB. *Genes Devel* 6: 775–787
148 Schmitz ML, Baeuerle PA (1991) The p65 sub-unit is responsible for the strong transcription activating potential of NFκB. *EMBO J* 10: 3805–3817
149 Roff M, Thompson J, Rodriquez MS, Jacques J-M, Baleux F, Arenzana-Seisdedos F, Hay RT (1996) Role of IκBα ubiquitination in signal-induced activation of NFκB *in vivo*. *J Biol Chem* 271: 7844–7850
150 Baldwin AS Jr (1996) The NFκB and IκB proteins: new discoveries and insights. *Annu Rev Immunol* 14: 649–683
151 DiDonato J, Merairio F, Rosette, Wuli J, Suyang H, Ghosh S, Karin M (1996) Mapping of the inducible IκB phosphorylation sites that signal its ubiquitination and degradation. *Mol Cell Biol* 16: 1295–1304
152 Chen ZI, Parent L, Maniatis T (1996) Site-specific phosphorylation of IκBa by a novel ubiquitination-dependent protein kinase activity. *Cell* 84: 853–862
153 Arenzana-Seisdedos F, Thompson J, Rodriquez MS, Bachelerie F, Thomas D, Hay RT (1995) Inducible nuclear expression of newly synthesised IκBα negatively DNA-binding and transcriptional activities of NFκB. *Mol Cell Biol* 15: 2689–2696
154 Hirano T, Akiva S, Taga T, Kishimoto T (1990) Biological and clinical aspects of interleukin-6. *Immunol Today* 11: 443–449
155 Akira S, Isshiki H, Sugita T, Tambe O, Kinoshita S, Nishio Y, Nakajima T, Hirano T, Kishimoto T (1990) A nuclear factor for IL-6 expression (NF-IL-6) is a member of a C/EBP family. *EMBO J* 9: 1897–1906

156 Isshiki H, Akira S, Sugita T, Nishio Y, Hashimoto S, Pawlowski T, Suematus S, Kishimoto T (1991) Recipricol expression of NF-IL-6 and C/EBP in hepatocytes: possible involvement of NF-IL-6 in acute phase protein gene expression. *New Biol* 3: 63–70
157 Nakajima T, Kinoshita S, Sasagawa T, Sasaki K, Naruto M, Kishimoto T, Akira S (1993) Phosphorylation at threonine-235 by a ras-dependent mitogen-activated protein kinase cascade is essential for transcription factor NF-IL-6. *Proc Natl Acad Sci USA* 90: 2207–2211
158 Ramji DP, Vitelli A, Tronche F, Cortese R, Ciliberto G (1993) The two isoforms IL-6DBP/NF-IL-6 and C/EBPγ/NFIL-6β, are induced by IL-6 to promote acute phase gene transcription via different mechanisms. *Nucleic Acid Res* 21: 289–294
159 Wegemka UM, Luttichen C, Bischman J, Yvan J, Lottspeich F, Muller-Esterl W, Schindler C, Roeb E, Heinrich PC, Horn F (1994) The interleukin-6 activated acute-phase response factor is antigenically and functionally related to members of the signal transduced and activator (STAT) family. *Mol Cell Biol* 14: 3186–3196
160 Wilson DR, Juan TS-C, Wilde MD, Fey GH, Darlington GJ (1990) A 58-base-pair region of the human C3 gene confers synergistic inducibility by interleukin-1 and interleukin-6. *Mol Cell Biol* 10: 6181–6191
161 Hocke GM, Barry D, Fey GH (1992) Synergistic action of interleukin-6 and glucocorticoids is mediated by the interleukin-6 response element of the rat α2 macroglobulin gene. *Mol Cell Biol* 12: 2282–2294
162 Kordula T, Bugno M, Goldstein J, Travis J (1995) Activation of signal transducer and activator of transcription-3 (STAT-3) expression by interferon γ and interleukin-6 in hepatoma cells. *Biochem Biophys Res Commun* 216: 999–1005
163 Kishimoto T, Akira S, Narazaki M, Taga T (1995) Interleukin-6 family of cytokines and gp 130. *Blood* 86: 1243–1254
164 Wen Z, Zhong Z, Darnell JE Jr (1995) Maximal activation of transcription by Stat 1 and Stat 3 requires both tyrosine and serine phosphorylation. *Cell* 82: 241–250
165 Betts JC, Cheshire JK, Akira S, Kishimoto T, Woo P (1993) The role of NFκB and NF-IL-6 transactivating factors in the synergistic activation of serum amyloid A gene expression by interleukin- 1 and interleukin-6. *J Biol Chem* 268: 25624–25631

Molecular Biology of the Lung
Vol. 1: Emphysema and Infection
ed. by R. A. Stockley

CHAPTER 6
Regulation of Neutrophil Proteinases

Anne B. Sturrock and John R. Hoidal

Division of Respiratory, Critical Care and Occupational Pulmonary Medicine, University of Utah School of Medicine, Salt Lake City, UT, USA

1. Introduction

Proteinases play a central role in the degradation of proteins by hydrolyzing peptide bonds. Originally thought to fulfill primarily digestive functions, it now is believed that these enzymes are the principal regulators of a multitude of crucial and diverse physiologic processes and have a central role in pathologic tissue destruction of many organs. Their role in tissue destruction has been investigated in the greatest detail in the lungs, especially in relationship to the pathogenesis of emphysema. Recent investigations suggest prominent roles for proteinases in growth and development and in intracellular signaling.

Proteolytic activity in tissues is controlled at multiple levels. Three principal regultory mechanisms have been devised by nature to control proteinase activity: (1) regulation of their gene expression; (2) activation of their inactive precursors (zymogens) by limited proteolysis; and (3) inactivation by complexing with inhibitors. The relative importance of these various mechanisms differs for different proteinases. In addition to the principal regulatory mechanisms, several factors may modify the activity of proteinases including phosphorylation and glycosylation, storage in vesicles, localization on membranes, pH, and the concentrations of calcium ions and ATP. This chapter addresses the regulation of gene expression and activation of neutrophil proteinases focusing, in particular, on the granule-associated neutral serine proteinases, proteinase-3 (PR-3), human leukocyte elastase (HLE), and cathepsin G (Cat G).

2. Transcriptional Regulation of Granule-Associated Neutral Serine Proteinases

A distinctive feature of granule-associated neutral serine proteinases is the striking cell and development specificity of their distribution and synthesis. The genes of these cells are expressed only in cells of myeloid lineage, and their expression is confined to the late myeloblast and promyelocytic stages of maturation. A single report of PR-3 expression in endothelial cells has not as yet been confirmed [1]. Regulation of gene transcription is primarily via transcriptional factors binding to specific 5′-regulatory elements and appears to be coordinated for the granule-associated neutral serine proteinases. Transcriptional factors often function together. For the PR-3, HLE and Cat G genes to be coordinately expressed they require common 5′-regulatory elements. In the following section, a descriptive overview of the organization of the 5′-regulatory elements of PR-3, HLE and Cat G is given, and common elements identified and discussed.

A schematic summary is given in Figure 1. A more detailed discussion of the properties of the 5′-regulatory elements and the transcriptional factors that are common to the genes of the azurophil serine proteinases follows.

3. Granule-Associated Neutral Serine Proteinase Promoters

3.1. Proteinase 3

Analysis of the first 680 base-pairs (bp) of the proximal promoter of PR-3 reveals several putative 5′-regulatory elements (Figure 1). A TATA [2] box is present at –44, although there is no CAAT box [3]. The core element of the *ets* family (GGAA [4]) occurs at –101 and on the complementary strand at –366 and –418. The sequence at –101 corresponds to a PU-1 regulatory element [5, 6]. The immediate 5′-region of the PR-3 promoter also contains a potential binding site for the CAAT/enhancer binding protein (C/EBP, –82 [7, 8]) and for c-Myb transcription factors [9]. Other recognized elements include a nuclear factor κB (NF-κB) element [10] at –606 on the antisense strand and five β-globin elements (–16, –361, –539, –565, and –622). Three of the β-globin elements (–361, –539, and –565) are preceded by a T forming the retinoic regulatory element, TCACC [11].

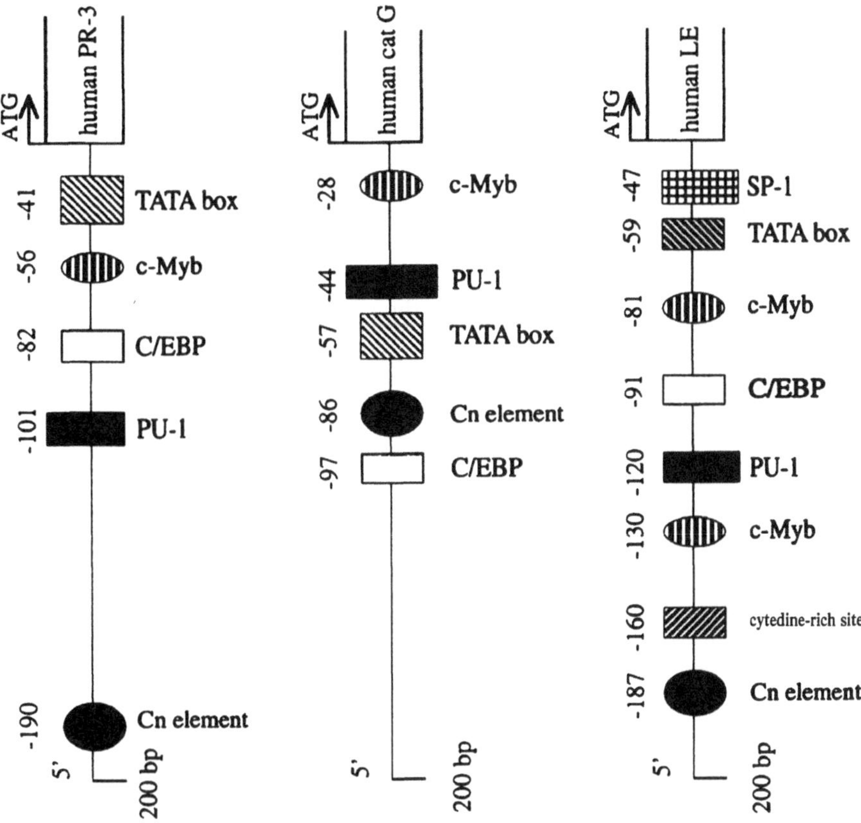

Figure 1. Putative transcriptional elements in the proximal promoters of granule-associated neutral serine proteinases.

The proximal 200 bp of the PR-3 promoter, the region that contains identifiable TATA, c-Myb, C/EBP and PU-1 regulatory elements, is sufficient to give maximal activity. However, an element upstream of PU-1 accounts for 75% of the PR-3 promoter activity when transiently transfected into myeloid cells as a pGL3-luciferase reporter construct. The regulatory element responsible for this increased activity has been identified as CCCCGCCC (–190) and was initially termed the CG element; it is now referred to as the C*n* element since replacing the central G nucleotide with an A or a T does not affect activity [12]. The PU-1 element (–101) accounts for 50% of the remaining activity. About 10% of maximal activity remains after step deletion of both the PU-1 and C*n* elements. This probably results from *trans*-activation of one or a combination of the C/EBP, c-Myb, and TATA elements present in the first 85 bp of the PR-3 promoter. The first 200-bp of the PR-3 promoter has no activity when transfected into HeLa cells, suggesting that this region is sufficient to confer myeloid specificity.

Some of the transcriptional factors binding to the putative 5′-regulatory elements of the PR-3 gene have been identified. The protein that binds to the PU-1 element at −101 has a molecular mass of about 45 kDa and is "supershifted" upon addition of PU-1 antibody in a gel retardation assay. The binding of the transcriptional factor can be blocked by addition of the CD11b PU-1 element [13] to the gel retardation assay suggesting that, in myeloid cells, PU-1 protein is the transcriptional factor binding to the site. The transcriptional factor binding to the C*n* element is unknown. Cross-linking studies indicate that the protein has a molecular mass of about 40 kDa and that it is present in cells of the myeloid lineage as well as non-myeloid cells such as HeLa. Differentiation of HL60 promyelocytic cells towards granulocytes with dimethyl sulfoxide (DMSO), or HL60 and U937 cells towards monocytes with phorbol myristate acetate (PMA), reduces the level of the protein that binds to the C*n* element, indicating a potential role for the protein in development-specific gene expression [12]. The minus strand sequence of the C*n* element is similar to the binding sequence for SP-1. However, neither SP-1 protein nor SP-1 binding sequence blocks the binding of the 40-kDa protein to the C*n* element [12]. The sequence of the minus strand is also similar to the sequence GGGTGGG that corresponds to a PuF/NM23 sequence [14], which is known to regulate c-*myc* transcription *in vitro* [15]. The factor binding to the PuF/NM23 site is a protein of 17 kDa and is therefore unlikely to be the 40-kDa factor described above [14].

Transcriptional factors may also act as suppressors. A reduction in luciferase activity occurs when the first 300 bp of the PR-3 promoter are transiently transfected into myeloid cells. This suggests that there is a suppressor region present within the sequence between −200 and −300 bp. The importance of this region in directing development- and cell type-specific expression of PR-3 is not currently known.

3.2. Leukocyte Elastase

The promoter of HLE contains several 5′-regulatory elements and maximal myeloid-specific activity also occurs within its first 200-bp [16]. Putative 5′-regulatory elements include: an SP-1 [17] site at −47, a TATA box at −59, a c-Myb-like element at −81, a C/EBP CAAT element at −91, a PU-1 element at −120, a c-Myb element at −138, a cytidine-rich element at −160, and a C*n* element at −187. Initial experiments indicate that the PU-1 regulatory element, but not the C*n* element, is important for expression of the HLE gene. A cytidine-rich site (CTCCCCC)) at −160 has also been identified as important for activation of the HLE gene [18] and our unpublished data.

In HLE, control of gene expression is not confined to the proximal promoter. Sequences further upstream of the gene can enhance the activity conferred by the proximal promoter. As one example, a 53 bp repetitive element located at −716 to −1032 confers a two- to threefold increase in HLE promoter activity in a reporter construct assay. Typical of an enhancer sequence, the increased activity occurs independently of the orientation of the sequence. Moreover, enhancement is not myeloid specific because a similar degree of enhancement occurs in HeLa cells as in myeloid K562 cells [19].

The murine LE (MLE) promoter has been studied extensively by Nuchprayoon and colleagues [20] and shows similarities to as well as differences from its human counterpart. Analysis of 1800 bp of MLE flanking sequence indicates that only the proximal 100 bp contains functional elements and that this region confers myeloid specific activity (activity of the proximal 100 bp is several hundred-fold greater in induced 32D c13 myeloid cells than in non-myeloid mouse L cells) [20]. A comparison of the MLE promoter region with the first 100 bp of the human promoter reveals conserved regulatory elements for PU-1, PEBP2/CBF (polyoma enhancer-binding protein/core-binding factors [21, 22]) C/EBP, c-Myb, and TATA. The PEBP2/CBF site is, however, disrupted in the HLE promoter.

Cooperative regulation of the MLE promoter is conferred by transcriptional factors that bind the c-Myb, C/EBP, and PU-1 elements. The promoter is activated via c-Myb and C/EBP in both non-myeloid (NIH3T3) and myeloid (32D c13) cells. These factors, together with PU-1, direct restricted expression of the MLE promoter to immature myeloid cells [23]. Deletion of the PU-1 site in the MLE promoter reduces promoter activity by 90%. However, recent studies show that the PU-1 regulatory element only moderately activates the MLE promoter. This element therefore should be considered a more general *ets* regulatory element. The *ets* factor GABPα from myeloid cells avidly binds the MLE *ets* element and increases transcription sevenfold in U937 cells. Again cooperation with c-Myb and C/EBP sites has been demonstrated [24].

3.3. Cathepsin G

The organization of the proximal promoter of the human Cat G gene shows interesting similarities and differences to PR-3 and HLE genes. The common 5′-regulatory elements TATA and CAAT are located within the first 100 bp of the promoter [25]. The putative myeloid-specific elements, PU-1 and a C*n* element are present within the first 200 bp of the Cat G promoter, indicating similarities to the promoters of PR-3 and HLE. However, the organization of these elements in the proximal promoter of Cat G differs from that of PR-3 and HLE. Most striking is the fact that the PU-1 site is downstream of the TATA box. Several 8-bp sequences within the first 300 bp of the Cat G promoter are homologous to regions within the HLE promoter. The relevance of these sequences for cell type- and development-specific regulation is not known because no transcriptional factors for these sequences have been identified. Unlike the PR-3 and HLE genes the Cat G proximal promoter does not contain the full C/EBP [T(T/G) NNGNAA(T/G)] consensus sequence. There is, however, a CAAT sequence in the Cat G promoter that can bind C/EBPα. The presence of PU-1, C*n*, C/EBPα and c-Myb regulatory elements in the proximal promoter of Cat G provides a possible basis for coordinate gene regulation of the granule-associated neutral serine proteinases of myeloid cells. To date, the functional importance of these elements and the proteins that bind them has not been characterized for the Cat G gene.

There is now information about the activity of the Cat G promoter *in vivo*. The human Cat G gene has been transgenically expressed in mice [26]. A 6-kb fragment comprising 2.7 kb of the coding sequence, about 2.5 kb of the 5′-flanking sequence and 0.8 kb of the 3′-flanking sequence contains regulatory elements sufficient to direct the cell type-specific expression of human Cat G. Furthermore, these elements target the expression of human Cat G exclusively to cells of the myeloid lineage. Expression is integration site dependent and relatively low compared with endogenous murine Cat G gene. This implies that the 6-kb human Cat G gene fragment lacks regulatory information (locus control) which insulates the gene from effects of the surrounding chromatin [27, 28].

4. Regulatory Elements Common to the Granule-Associated Neutral Serine Proteinase Promoters

From the above descriptions of the proteinase promoters several functional elements appear to be common and are probably central to the regulation of the genes for the granule-associated neutral serine proteinases of myeloid cells (Table 1). These regulatory elements include the C*n* element, a member of the *ets* family (probably PU-1), c-Myb, and C/EBP. TATA, although present in all three promoters in the expected position for forming a basal RNA polymerase II complex (within about 10 – 30 bp of the initiation site),

Table 1. Elements likely to be important in regulation of granule-associated neutral serine proteinases

Protein	DNA-binding domain	Consensus sequence
C*n* protein (40 kDa)	?	CCCC N CCC
Pu-1	*ets*	TGGGGAAGT AA
C/EBP	Basic leucine Zipper	TTNNCCAAC
c-Myb	Myb	CAACGG T T

is not myeloid specific; although important, it is not essential for regulation of the genes with respect to myeloid differentiation. In the following sections we address each regulatory element individually with respect to its role in the regulation of myeloid genes during differentiation.

4.1. *Cn*-element

The *Cn* element is within 200 bp of the initiation site in all three granule-associated neutral serine proteinase promoters and within 100 bp of a PU-1 (*ets*) element. In the PR-3 promoter the central nucleotide is a guanidine, whereas in HLE and Cat G it is an adenosine. Mutational studies show that interchange between a G or an A is irrelevant to the binding of the element of the 40-kDa protein in myeloid nuclear protein extracts [12]. Moreover, the core element and flanking sequence of the *Cn* elements in PR-3, HLE, and Cat G can compete with each other for the binding of the specific 40-kDa protein, suggesting that it is the same protein that binds to the *Cn* element in all three promoters.

Mutation of the cytidines on either side of the central guanidine or adenosine nucleotide abrogates binding of the factor to the specific 40-kDa protein in the *Cn* elements of PR-3, HLE, and Cat G. This leads to a significant loss of promoter function (close to 50% in the PR-3 promoter) [12]. The importance of the *Cn* element is also suggested by its presence in the promoters of other azurophil granule-associated proteins including myeloperoxidase (MPO). It accounts for 50% of the MPO promoter activity in transient transcription studies [29]. Thus, control of gene activity via a *Cn* element appears to be important in the regulation of the granule-associated neutral proteinase genes and perhaps azurophil granule constituents in general. Identification of the specific 40-kDa protein that binds this site will lead to greater understanding of the regulation of granule-associated neutral serine proteinase expression and azurophil granule formation.

4.2. Pu-1 (the *ets* Family)

PU-1 was first isolated as the *Spi-1* oncogene about a decade ago [5]. It was subsequently identified as a regulator of myelopoietic development and as a member of the *ets* family of regulatory elements [30]. Its central role in myelopoiesis is emphasized by its presence in the promoters of the M-CSF, GM-CSF and G-CSF receptors (M, macrophage; G, granulocyte; CSF, colony-stimulating factor), and it is involved in the maturation processes governed by these growth factors [31–33].

There is evidence that the consensus sequence for binding PU-1 in the proximal promoter of PR-3 [12] does indeed bind PU-1. Similar studies characterizing the proteins binding to the PU-1 elements in the HLE and Cat G promoters have yet to be done. However, it is known that the PU-1 element in the MLE promoter binds PU-1. A second *ets* protein GA-binding protein α (GABPα) also binds to the PU-1 element of the MLE promoter. GABPα and PU-1 compete with each other for the binding to this site, but the GABPα protein is a more powerful activator of MLE than PU-1 [24]. These results suggest that the PU-1 elements in the proteinase promoters can bind other members of the *ets* family of regulatory elements in addition to PU-1. Additional studies are needed to determine the relative importance of PU-1 compared with other members of the *ets* family of transcription factors in granule-associated neutral serine proteinase regulation.

PU-1 shows a specific pattern of hemopoietic expression. It is expressed in myeloid and B cells but not in T cells [5, 30]. Interesting from the perspective of expression of granule-associated neutral serine proteinase is the fact that PU-1 is specifically up-regulated with myeloid differentiation at a time that coincides with early myeloid maturation [34, 35]. There is no further increase in either PU-1 mRNA or its binding to DNA during the maturation of the promyelocyte to more mature stages [5, 36], but high levels of PU-1 mRNA remain in human monocytes and neutrophils [36]. Binding of PU-1 protein to specific DNA sequences has been found in mature neutrophils [36] and PU-1 mRNA has been detected in eosinophils [37]. Thus, the initial assertion that PU-1 expression is confined to B cells and monocytes is now in doubt.

One feature of the *ets* family members of transcriptional factors is the requirement to interact with other factors in order to stimulate transcription. A candidate for such interaction in the promoters of the granule-associated neutral serine proteinase is the C*n* element because it is always within 100 bp of the PU-1 (or *ets*) regulatory element, allowing physical interaction between the two factors. PU-1 also interacts with other regulatory elements. In B cells, for example, PU-1 is associated with a second B-cell-specific factor, NF-EM5 or Pip [38–40].

Increased specificity of PU-1 may occur via a mechanism other than interaction with additional regulatory elements. One hypothesis is that PU-1 interacts with TATA transcriptional factors *in vitro* to use the basal transcriptional machinery on myeloid promoters and replace the function of the TATA box which is often absent in myeloid genes [37, 41, 42]. This function of PU-1 is unlikely to be important in the regulation of the granule-associated neutral serine proteinases because they possess a TATA box, but it should be noted that PU-1 is downstream of the TATA box in the Cat G promoter. The importance of this is not known. Phosphorylation and dephosphorylation of PU-1 itself or a protein it interacts with are another level of control. PU-1 is unphosphorylated in both multipotential and granulocyte-committed cells but it is phosphorylated in B cells [43]. PU-1 can physically interact with the retinoblastoma protein, which in turn can negatively regulate another *ets* regulatory element, Elf-1, during T cell activation [44]. Moreover, retinoblastoma protein becomes hyperphosphorylated during myeloid differentiation and is therefore a possible regulator of PU-1 [45, 46].

The importance of PU-1 in myeloid differentiation has been examined in models of loss of function. Inhibition by the addition of competitor oligonucleotides to human CD34$^+$ cells blocks differentiation if added before the up-regulation of PU-1 [34]. Additional information on the role of PU-1 comes from inhibition of PU-1 function on murine development using targeted disruption of the PU-1 gene. In one knockout the –/– embryos died *in utero*. The animals had anemia, and did not produce leukocytes. The lack of monocytes, neutrophils, and B cells was predictable, but surprisingly the animals also lacked T cells. PU-1 is not known to be expressed in T cells [47]. A second knockout produced results that differ from the first. The –/– animals lived for 5 days, lacked monocytes and mature B cells, but produced B-cell progenitors. After birth T cells and cells similar to neutrophils were observed [48]. The basis for the difference in the two –/– models is not known.

4.3. C/EBP

C/EBPs are members of a family of leucine zipper *trans*-acting proteins that appear to promote differentiation. They bind as dimers (either homo- or heterodimers) and are differentially regulated during cell maturation [7, 49]. In the hemopoietic system they are specifically expressed in myeloid cells [50] which express at least four C/EBPs: α, β (NF-IL-6), δ and ε. C/EBPε expression appears to be confined to myeloid cells [51, 52].

The C/EBP transcriptional factors must play a role in myeloid differentiation as suggested from their pattern of expression in murine 32D cells, and human HL60 and U937 cells [50, 53]. In proliferating cells C/EBPα is highly expressed and its level is subsequently down-regulated with maturation, whereas C/EBPβ and C/EBPδ are up-regulated. More recent studies indicate that C/EBPα expression is maintained during granulocytic differentiation [37] and its level up-regulates as single CD34$^+$/CD38$^-$ cells differentiate into granulocytic colonies. In contrast, no up-regulation occurs during macrophage colony formation [35]. These studies imply that C/EBPα plays a role in granulocyte but not monocyte development.

A knockout of C/EBPα is lethal (–/–) within a few hours of birth and analysis of the hemopoietic system shows no mature neutrophils, although immature myeloid cells are present in blood. Eosinophils are also absent but peripheral blood monocytes, peritoneal macrophages, erythrocytes, platelets, and lymphoid cells are normal [54, 55]. In these mice the G-CSF receptor mRNA is selectively and significantly reduced [56]. This finding suggests that much of the phenotype may result from decreased or absent

G-CSF signaling. However, G-CSF receptor knockout animals produce mature granulocytes, implying that there must be important C/EBPα target genes in myeloid progenitors in addition to the G-CSF receptors. Disruption of the C/EBPβ gene does not adversely affect myelopoiesis, suggesting that C/EBPβ is not involved in myeloid development [57, 58].

C/EBP regulatory elements, such as PU-1, are critical for the activity of a number of myeloid CSF-receptor promoters, including the M-CSF receptor [31], the GM-CSF receptor α [32], and the G-CSF receptor [33].

In summary, the relevance of C/EBP regulatory element in gene regulation of granule-associated neutral serine proteinase is inferred because C/EBP proteins are differentially expressed and interact with other family members as well as other regulatory elements such as c-Myb and PU-1. At least one family member, C/EBPα, is intimately involved in granulocyte maturation and although this effect is exerted via the regulation of the G-CSF receptor it involves other unidentified myeloid genes.

4.4. c-Myb

Myb was first isolated as a retroviral oncogene and shown to transform chicken hemopoietic cells [59, 60]. The form c-Myb is expressed in proliferating immature hemopoietic cells and is down-regulated upon differentiation [61]. It is expressed in myeloid cells but not confined to myeloid lineages [62]. Down-regulation of c-Myb is required for differentiation of myeloid cells [63, 64]. Knockout of the c-*Myb* gene confirms its central role in hemopoiesis. The mice die *in utero* with a failure of hemopoiesis in the fetal liver [65].

A direct effect of c-Myb on expression of granule-associated neutral serine proteinase is suggested by studies demonstrating that c-Myb is synergistic with C/EBP in the MLE promoter [23]. The c-Myb regulatory element, has not, however, been identified as central to promoter activity in the HLE [16, 18] or the PR-3 promoter [12]. However, as it is present in the proximal promoter of all three of the granule-associated neutral serine proteinases, it is likely to be important in regulation of these genes. Further studies are required to delineate the role of c-Myb in expression of granule-associated neutral serine proteinase.

5. A Model for the Distribution of Granule-Associated Neutral Serine Proteinases Based on Gene Regulation

The granule-associated neutral serine proteinases are stored in the azurophil (primary) granules of neutrophils [66, 67]. These granules are heterogeneous and have been classified by size, morphology, electron density, and protein content [66–68]. Not all azurophil granules contain each proteinase and a spectrum of distribution is observed [69]. However, most azurophil granules do contain PR-3, HLE, and Cat G along with MPO [70]. Any model for regulation of granule-associated neutral serine proteinase has to account for their confinement to the azurophil granule as well as their heterogeneity of distribution within the population of azurophil granules.

Neutrophil granules are formed starting at the transition from the myeloblast to the promyelocyte [66, 67] and extending to the later stages of differentiation to the mature granulocyte [71]. Azurophil granules, the first granules to be formed, develop during the late myeloblast and the promyelocytic stages of development. All neutrophil granules are formed from the aggregation of small vesicles that bud from the *cis* or *trans*-networks in the Golgi apparatus [66, 67]. How granule contents are sorted to the "correct" granule population has been studied extensively by Borregaard and Berliner and recently reviewed [72, 73]. Borregaard has demonstrated that the destination of a neutrophil granule protein is dependent upon its time of expression and is not a result of the complex sorting information present on individual proteins [74]. This hypothesis is supported by the work of Sigurdsson and colleagues who demonstrated that the expression of secondary (specfic) granule protein genes is coordinately regulated at the level of mRNA transcription and occurs only during the transition to myelocytes concomitant with secondary granule formation [75].

Proteinase-3 [12, 76], HLE [77, 78], and Cat G [79] mRNA expression is largely confined to the promyelocytic stage of neutrophil development. Maturation to either a monocyte or granulocyte down-regulates their gene expression. The temporal pattern for this down-regulation, upon differentiation of U937 and HL60 cells towards either monocyte-type cells or a granulocyte, is similar for all three genes (A.B. Sturrock, unpublished observation). Thus, the granule-associated neutral serine proteinases, PR-3, HLE, and Cat G are also coordinately expressed at the level of mRNA transcription and this expression occurs at the same time as the development of azurophil granules. It is probable that this regulation at the transcriptional level is responsible for the coordinate stage-specific expression of granule-associated neutral serine proteinases and their packaging into azurophil granules. We have described the promoters of PR-3, HLE, and Cat G, and identified the common regulatory elements to be C*n*, PU-1, C/EBP, and c-Myb. These then are the putative regulatory elements responsible for this coordinate expression. We have discussed these regulatory elements in relation to myelogenesis and it is evident that none of the regulatory elements alone is sufficient for the temporal and myeloid-specific expression of granule-associated neutral serine proteinases. It is likely to be the interaction of these four relevant regulatory elements that is responsible for the coordinated and stage-specific expression of the granule-associated neutral serine proteinase genes. The precise interplay and relative importance of each regulatory element is not, however, known.

We have primarily limited our examination of granule-associated neutral serine proteinase genes to the proximal promoter regions. It is certain that the regulation of expression is more complex and involves distal enhancer and suppressor elements. A 6-kb genomic fragment containing the entire human Cat G gene and 2.5-kb fragment of the 5′-flanking sequence was used to direct cell type-specific expression of human Cat G in mice [26]; however, it is not known whether a smaller fragment would suffice. Distal locus control regions may control gene expression in both PR-3 and HLE because they reside within 3 kb of each other on chromosome 19 at p13.3 [76, 80]. A common locus that controls all three genes is unlikely because human Cat G resides on chromosome 14 at q11.2 [79].

If the hypothesis that C*n* PU-1, C/EBP, and c-Myb regulatory elements in the proximal promoters of PR-3, HLE, and Cat G are central to the expression of the genes, and if the timing of the expression of these genes determines their packaging into azurophil granules, it could be predicted that the same regulatory elements would occur in the proximal promoter of other proteins contained within the azurophil granules. An examination of the proximal promoter of MPO shows this to be the case. The proximal promoter of human MPO contains a C*n* and a PU-1 regulatory element and both sites are functional [29]. Moreover, the murine MPO proximal promoter contains two functional c-Myb regulatory elements [20, 81, 82].

Indirect support for the role of these common, proximal, promoter regulatory elements in controlling expression and distribution of granule-associated neutral serine proteinases comes from the observations that cooperative interaction of a different group of regulatory elements is responsible for the coordinate expression and distribution of specific granule proteins [75]. Although the putative regulatory elements for secondary granule protein expression include PU-1, it is the GATA element and a down-regulation of CAAT displacement protein that appear to be the partners of PU-1 in controlling gene expression of proteins contained in specific granules [83].

How does one account for the heterogeneous distribution of granule-associated neutral serine proteinases if expression of all three genes is tightly coordinated at the level of transcription? One suggestion is that this heterogeneity is possible because, although transcription is coordinate, there may be variations in the timing of translation of proteins [75]. All the regulatory elements that are involved in translational regulation of granule-associated neutral serine proteinases are unknown, and so the inference of translational control accounting for the distribution differences remains to be proved.

6. Post-Translational Processing of Granule-Associated Neutral Serine Proteinases

In addition to their tightly regulated development- and cell type-specific gene expression, a distinctive feature of the granule-associated neutral serine proteinases of leukocytes and mast cells is that they are stored fully active in secretory granules. In contrast, the more extensively characterized serine proteinases of non-hemopoietic origin, such as trypsin, chymotrypsin, or pancreatic elastase, are stored as inactive zymogens in secretory vesicles of cells and are activated only after secretion into the intestinal lumen. Nevertheless, based on their cDNA sequences, and studies of synthesis and processing, the immune/inflammatory cell proteinases are initially translated as zymogens. The processing of the granule-associated neutral serine proteinases requires three proteolytic cleavages: two on the amino-terminal side and one on the carboxyl-terminal side (Figure 2) [84–87]. The initial amino-terminal cleavage is produced by a signal peptidase and results in the removal of an endoplasmic reticulum-targeting of sequence 25 amino acids. An additional cleavage removes a carboxyl-terminal extension from the mature enzyme. The enzyme responsible for removal of the carboxyl-terminus has not been identified. The result of these two cleavage steps is that the mature enzymes are attached to two amino acid properties. The processing of the propeptides, which occurs in a post-Golgi compartment, is unusual in that it occurs at an acidic residue, in contrast to most proteinase zymogens which are processed at a basic or, rarely, an aromatic residue. We view this processing step as a potential central point for control of granule-associated neutral serine proteinases that is of both basic and clinical importance. Recent studies suggest that the enzyme responsible for removal of the activation dipeptide is a cysteine protease, most probably dipeptidyl-peptidase I. The hydrolytic action of dipeptidyl-peptidase I probably represents the final control point in the formation of the mature enzymes.

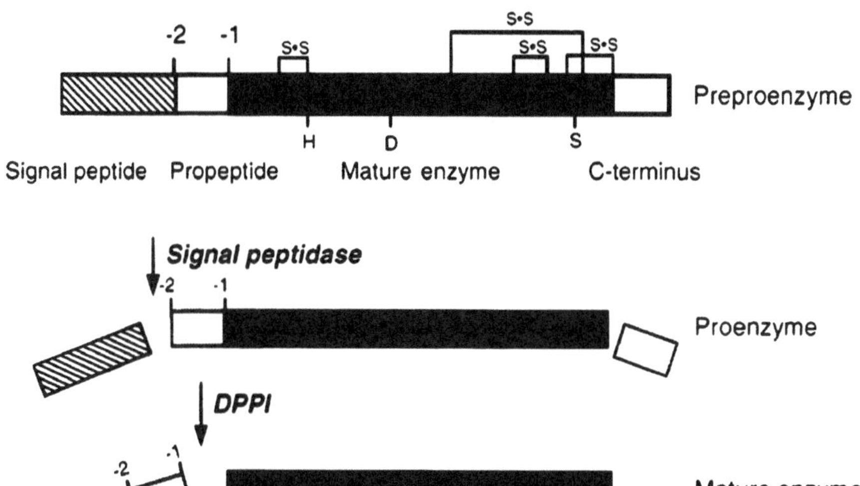

Figure 2. Biosynthesis and processing of granule-associated neutral serine proteinases.

In summary, the regulation of granule-associated neutral serine proteinases of myeloid cells is complex. There is coordinate expression at the transcriptional level. There may be discoordinate expression at the translational level which accounts for the heterogeneity of the distribution of PR-3, HLE, and Cat G proteins in azurophil granules, but this has not been proved. After translation, a number of proteolytic processing steps occur before the proteinases are stored in azurophil granules as active enzymes. Each of these steps offers a potential site to control the expression of the proteinases.

References

1 Mayet WJ, Csernok E, Szymkowiak C, Gross WL, Meyer-zum-Buschenfelde KH (1993) Human endothelial cells express proteinase 3, the target antigen of anticytoplasmic antibodies in Wegener's granulomatosis. *Blood* 382: 1221–1229
2 Corden J, Wasylyk B, Buchwalder A, Sassone-Corsi P, Kedinger C, Chambon P (1980) Promoter sequences of eukaryotic protein-coding genes. *Science* 209: 1406–1414
3 Myers RM, Tilly K, Maniatis T (1986) Fine structure genetic analysis of a beta-globin promoter. *Science* 232: 613–618
4 Mitchell PJ, Wang C, Tjian R (1987) Positive and negative regulation of transcription *in vitro*: enhancer-binding protine AP-2 is inhibited by SV40 T antigen. *Cell* 50: 847–861
5 Moreau-Gachelin F, Tavitian A, Tambourin P (1988) Spi-1 is a putative oncogene in virally induced murine erythroleukaemias. *Nature* 331: 277–280
6 Paul R, Schuetze S, Kozak SL, Kozak CA, Kabat D (1991) The Sfpi-1 proviral integration site of Friend erythroleukemia encodes the *ets*-related transcription factor PU-1. *J Virol* 65: 464–467
7 Johnson PF, Landschulz WH, Graves BJ, McKnight SL (1987) Identification of a rat liver nuclear protein that binds to the enhancer core element of three animal viruses. *Genes Dev* 1: 133–146
8 Landschulz WH, Johnson PF, Adashi EY, Graves BJ (1988) Isolation of a recombinant copy of the gene encoding C/EBP. *Genes Dev* 2: 786–800
9 Biedenkapp H, Borgmeyer U, Sippel AE, Klempnauer KH (1988) Viral myb oncogene encodes a sequence-specific DNA-binding activity. *Nature* 335: 835–837
10 Parry GC, Mackman N (1994) A set of inducible genes expressed by activated human monocytic and endothelial cells contain κB-like sites that specifically bind c-Rel-p65 heterodimers. *J Biol Chem* 269: 20823–20825
11 Vasios GW, Gold JD, Petkovich M, Chambon P, Gudas LJ (1989) A retinoic acid-responsive element is present in the 5′ flanking region of the laminin B1 gene. *Proc Natl Acad Sci USA* 86: 9099–9103
12 Sturrock AB, Franklin KF, Hoidal JR (1996) Human proteinase-3 expression is regulated by PU-1 in conjunction with a cytidine-rich element. *J Biol Chem* 271: 32392–32402
13 Pahl HL, Rosmarin AG, Tenen DG (1992) Characterization of the myeloid-specific CD11b promoter. *Blood* 79: 865–870
14 Postel EH, Berberich SJ, Flint SJ, Ferrone CA (1993) Human c-myc transcription factor PuF identified as nm23-H2 nucleoside diphosphate kinase, a candidate suppressor of tumor metastasis. *Science* 261: 478–480
15 Spencer CA, Groudine M (1991) Control of the c-myc regulation in normal and neiplastic cells. *Adv Cancer Res* 56: 1–48
16 Han J, Unlap T, Rado TA (1991) Expression of the human neutrophil elastase gene: positive and negative transcriptional elements in the 5′ flanking region. *Biochem Biophys Res Commun* 181: 1462–1468
17 Dynan WS, Tjian R (1983) The promoter-specific transcription factor Sp1 binds to upstream sequences in the SV40 early promoter. *Cell* 35: 79–87
18 Srikanth S, Rado TA (1994) A 30-base pair element is responsible for the myeloid-specific activity of the human neutrophil elastase promoter. *J Biol Chem* 269: 32626–32633

19 Yoshimura K, Chu C-S, Crystal RG (1994) Enhancer function of a 53-BP repetitive element in the 5′ flanking region of the human neutrophil elastase gene. *Biochem Biophys Res Commun* 204: 38–42
20 Nuchprayoon I, Meyers S, Scott LM, Suzow J, Hiebert S, Friedman AD (1994) PEBP2/CBF, the murine homolog of the human myeloid AML1 and PEBP2β/CBFβ proto-oncoproteins, regulates the murine myeloperoxidase and neutrophil elastase genes in immature myeloid cells. *Mol Cell Biol* 14: 5558–5568
21 Kamachi Y, Ogawa E, Asano M, Ishida S, Murakami Y, Satake M, Ito Y, Shigesada K (1990) Purification of a mouse nuclear factor that binds to both the A and B cores of the polyomavirus enhancer. *J Virol* 64: 4808–4819
22 Wang SW, Speck NA (1992) Purification of core-binding factor, a protein that binds the conserved core site in murine leukemia virus enhancers. *Mol Cell Biol* 12: 89–102
23 Oelgeschlager M, Nuchprayoon I, Luscher B, Friedman AD (1996) C/EBP, c-Myb, and PU-1 cooperate to regulate the neutrophil elastase promoter. *Mol Cell Biol* 16: 4717–4725
24 Nuchprayoon I, Simkevich CP, Luo M, Friedman AD, Rosmarin AG (1997) GABP cooperates with c-Myb and C/EBP to activate the neutrophil elastase promoter. *Blood* 89: 4546–4554
25 Hohn PA, Popescu NC, Hanson RD, Salvesen G, Ley TJ (1989) Genomic organization and chromosomal localization of the human cathepsin G gene. *J Biol Chem* 264: 13412–13419
26 Grisolano JL, Sclar GM, Ley TJ (1994) Early myeloid cell-specific expression of the human cathepsin G gene in transgenic mice. *Proc Natl Acad Sci USA* 91: 8989–8993
27 Grosveld E, van Assendelft GB, Greaves DR, Kollias G (1987) Position-independent, high-level expression of the human β-globin gene in transgenic mice. *Cell* 51: 975–985
28 Ley TJ (1991) The pharmacology of hemoglobin switching: of mice and men. *Blood* 77: 1146–1152
29 Zhao W-G, Lu JP, Regmi A, Austin GE (1997) Identification and functional analysis of multiple murine myeloperoxidase (MPO) promoters and comparison with human MPO promoter region. *Leukemia* 11: 97–105
30 Klemsz MJ, McKercher SR, Celada A, Van-Beveren C, Maki RA (1990) The marophage and B cell-specific transcription factor PU-1 is related to the *ets* oncogene. *Cell* 61: 113–124
31 Zhang DE, Hetherington CJ, Chen HM, Tenen DG (1994) The macrophage transcription factor PU-1 directs tissue-specific expression of the macrophage colony-stimulating factor receptor. *Mol Cell Biol* 14: 373–381
32 Hohaus S, Petrovick MS, Voso MT, Sun Z, Zhang DE, Tenen DG (1995) PU-1 (Spi-1) and C/EBP α regulate expression of the granulocyte-macrophage colony-stimulating factor receptor α gene. *Mol Cell Biol* 15: 5830–5845
33 Smith LT, Hohaus S, Gonzalez DA, Dziennis SE, Tenen DG (1996) PU-1 (Spi-1) and C/EBP-α regulate the granulocyte colony-stimulating factor receptor promoter in myeloid cells. *Blood* 88: 1234–1247
34 Voso MT, Burn TC, Wulf G, Lim B, Leone G, Tenen DG (1994) Inhibition of hematopoiesis by competitive binding of transcription factor PU-1. *Proc Natl Acad Sci USA* 91: 7932–7936
35 Cheng T, Shen H, Goikas D, Gere J, Tenen DG, Scadden DT (1996) Temporal mapping of gene expression levels during the differentiation of individual primary hematopoietic cells. *Proc Natl Acad Sci USA* 93: 13158–13163
36 Zhang D-E, Hohaus S, Voso MT, Chen H-M, Smith LT, Hetherington CJ, Tenen DG (1996) Function of PU-1 (Spi-1), C/EBP, and AML1 in early myelopoiesis: regulation of multiple myeloid CSF receptor promoters. *Curr Topics Microbiol Immunol* 211: 137–147
37 Tenen DG, Hromas R, Licht JD, Zhang D-E (1997) Transcription factors, normal myeloid development, and leukemia. *Blood* 90: 489–519
38 Pongubala JM, Nagulapalli S, Klemsz MJ, McKercher SR, Maki RA, Atchison ML (1992) PU-1 recruits a second nuclear factor to a site important for immunoglobulin κ 3′ enhancer activity. *Mol Cell Biol* 12: 368–378
39 Pongubala JM, Van-Beveren C, Nagulapalli S, Klemsz MJ, McKercher SR, Maki RA, Atchison ML (1993) Effect of PU-1 phosphorylation on interaction with NF-EM5 and transcriptional activation. *Science* 259: 1622–1625

40 Eisenbeis CF, Singh H, Storb U (1995) Pip, a novel IRF family member, is a lymphoid-specific, PU-1-dependent transcriptional activator. *Genes Dev* 9: 1377–1387
41 Hagemeier C, Bannister AJ, Cook A, Kouzarides T, Corden J, Wasylyk B, Buchwalder A, Sassone-Corsi P, Kedinger C, Chambon P (1993) The activation domain of transcription factor PU-1 binds the retinoblastoma (RB) protein and the transcription factor TFIID *in vitro*: RB shows sequence similarity to TFIID and TFIIB. *Proc Natl Acad Sci USA* 90: 1580–1584
42 Weintraub SJ, Chow KN, Luo RX, Zhang SH, He S, Dean DC (1995) Mechanism of active transcriptional repression by the retinoblastoma protein. *Nature* 375: 812–815
43 Ford AM, Bennett CA, Healy LE, Towatari M, Greaves MF, Enver T (1996) Regulation of the myeloperoxidase enhancer binding proteins Pu1, C-EBP α, *β*- and δ during granulocyte-lineage specification. *Proc Natl Acad Sci USA* 93: 10838– 10843
44 Wang CY, Petryniak B, Thompson CB, Kaelin WG, Leiden JM (1993) Regulation of the Ets-related transcription factor Elf-1 by binding to the retinoblastoma protein. *Science* 260: 1330–1335
45 Chen PL, Scully P, Shew JY, Wang JY, Lee WH (1989) Phosphorylation of the retinoblastoma gene product is modulated during the cell cycle and cellular differentiation. *Cell* 58: 1193–1198
46 Furukawa Y, DeCaprio JA, Freedman A, Kanakura Y, Nakamura M, Ernst TJ, Livingston DM, Griffin JD (1990) Expression and state of phosphorylation of the retinoblastoma susceptibility gene product in cycling and noncycling human hematopoiety cells. *Proc Natl Acad Sci USA* 87: 2770–2774
47 Scott EW, Simon MC, Anastasi J, Singh H (1994) Requirement of transcription factor PU-1 in the development of multiple hematopoietic lineages. *Science* 265: 1573–1577
48 McKercher SR, Torbett Be, Anderson KL, Henkel GW, Vestal DJ, Baribault H, Klemsz M, Feeney AJ, Wu GE, Paige CJ, Maki RA (1996) Targeted disruption of the PU-1 gene results in multiple hematopoietic abnormalities. *EMBO J* 15: 5647–5658
49 Landschulz WH, Johnson PF, McKnight SL (1988) The leucine zipper: a hypothetical structure common to a new class of DNA binding proteins. *Science* 240: 1759–1764
50 Natsuka S, Akira S, Nishio Y, Hashimoto S, Sugita T, Isshiki H, Kishimoto T (1992) Macrophage differentiation-specific expression of NF-IL-6, a transcription factor for interleukin-6. *Blood* 79: 460–466
51 Chumakov AM, Grillier I, Chumakova E, Chih D, Slater J, Koeffler HP (1997) Cloning of the novel human myeloid-cell-specific C/EBP-epsilon transcription factor. *Mol Cell Biol* 17: 1375–1386
52 Antonson P, Stellan B, Yamanaka R, Xanthopoulos KG (1996) A novel human CCAAT/enhancer binding protein gene, C/EBPepsilon, is expressed in cells of lymphoid and myeloid lineages and is localized on chromosome 14q11.2 close to the T cell receptor α/δ locus. *Genomics* 35: 30–38
53 Scott LM, Civin CI, Rorth P, Friedman AD (1992) A novel temporal expression pattern of three C/EBP family members in differentiating myelomonocytic cells. *Blood* 80: 1725– 1735
54 Wang ND, Finegold MJ, Bradley A, Ou CN, Abdelsayed SV, Wilde MD, Taylor LR, Wilson DR, Darlington GJ (1995) Impaired energy homeostasis in C/EBP α knock-out mice. *Science* 269: 1108–1112
55 Floby P, Barlow C, Kyelfjord H, Ahrlund-Richter L, Xanthopoulos KG (1996) Increased hepatic cell proliferation and lung abnormalities in mice deficient in CCAAT/enhancer binding protein α. *J Biol Chem* 271: 24753–24760
56 Zhang D-E, Zhang P, Wang N-D, Hetherington CJ, Darlington GJ, Tenen DG (1997) Absence of granulocyte colony-stimulating factor signaling and neutrophil development in CCAAT enhancer binding protein *α*-deficient mice. *Proc Natl Acad Sci USA* 94: 569–574
57 Tanaka T, Akira S, Yoshida K, Umemoto M, Yoneda Y, Shirafuji N, Fujiwara H, Suematsu S, Yoshida N, Kishimoto T (1995) Targeted disruption of the NF-IL-6 gene discloses its essential role in bacteria killing and tumor cytotoxicity by macrophages. *Cell* 80: 353–361
58 Screpanti I, Romani L, Musiani P, Modesti A, Fattori E, Lazzaro D, Sellitto C, Scarpa S, Bellavia D, Lattanzio G (1995) Lymphoproliferative disorder and imbalanced T-helper response in C/EBP beta-deficient mice. *EMBP J* 14: 1932–1941
59 Luscher B, Eisenman RN (1990) New light on Myc and Myb. Part I. Myc. *Genes Dev* 4: 2025–2035

60 Luscher B, Eisenman RN (1990) New light on Myc and Myb. Part II. Myb. *Genes Dev* 4: 2235–2241
61 Sheiness D, Gardinier M (1984) Expression of a proto-oncogene (proto-myb) in hemopoietic tissues of mice. *Mol Cell Biol* 4: 1206–1212
62 Gewirtz AM, Calabretta B (1988) A c-myb antisense oligodeoxynucleotide inhibits normal human hematopoiesis *in vitro*. Science 242: 1303–1306
63 Hoffman-Liebermann B, Liebermann DA (1991) Suppressiion of c-myc and c-myb is tightly linked to terminal differentiation induced by IL-6 or LIF and not growth inhibition in myeloid leukemia cells. *Oncogene* 6: 903–909
64 Anfossi G, Gewirtz AM, Calabretta B (1989) An oligomer complementary to c-myb-encoded mRNA inhibits proliferation of human myeloid leukemia cell lines. *Proc Natl Acad Sci USA* 86: 3379–3383
65 Mucenski ML, McLain K, Kier AB, Swerdlow SH, Schreiner CM, Miller TA, Pietryga DW, Scott WJ Jr, Potter SS (1991) A functional c-myb gene is required for normal murine fetal hepatic hematopoiesis. *Cell* 65: 677–689
66 Bainton DF, Farquhar MG (1966) Origin of granules in polymorphonuclear leukocytes. Two types derived from opposite faces of the Golgi complex in developing granulocytes. *J Cell Biol* 28: 277–301
67 Bainton DF, Ullyot JL Farquhar MG (1971) The development of neutrophilic polymorphonuclear leukocytes in human bone marrow. *J Exp Med* 134: 907–934
68 Oren A, Taylor JM (1995) The subcellular localization of defensins and myeloperoxidase in human neutrophils: immunocytochemical evidence for azurophil granule heterogeneity. *J Lab Clin Med* 125: 340–347
69 Damiano VV, Kucich U, Murer E, Laudenslager N, Weinbaum G (1988) Ultrastructural quantitation of peroxidase- and elastase-containing granules in human neutrophils. *Am J Pathol* 131: 235–245
70 Egesten A, Breton-Gorius J, Guichard J, Gullberg U, Olsson I (1994) The heterogeneity of azurophil granules in neutrophil promyelocytes: immunogold localization of myeloperoxidase, cathepsin G, leastase, proteinase 3, and bactericidal/permeability increasing protein. *Blood* 83: 2985–2994
71 Borregaard N, Sehested M, Nielsen BS, Sengelov H, Kjeldsen L (1995) Biosynthesis of granule proteins in normal human bone marrow cells. Gelatinase is a marker of terminal neutrophil differentiation. *Blood* 85: 812–817
72 Borregard N, Cowland JB (1997) Granules of the human neutrophilic polymorphonuclear leukocyte. *Blood* 89: 3503–3521
73 Gullberg U, Andersson E, Garwicz D, Lindmark A, Olsson I (1997) Biosynthesis, processing and sorting of neutrophil proteins: insight into neutrophil granule development. *Eur J Haematol* 58: 137–153
74 le Cabec V, Calafat J, Borregaard N (1997) Sorting of the specific granule protein, NGAL, during granulocytic maturation of HL-60 cells. *Blood* 89: 2113–2121
75 Sigurdsson F, Khanna-Gupta A, Lawson N, Berliner N (1997) Control of late neutrophil-specific gene expression: insights into regulation of myeloid differentiation. *Semin Hematol* 34: 303–310
76 Zimmer M, Medcalf RL, Fink TM, Mattmann C, Lichter P, Jenne DE (1992) Three human elastase-like genes coordinately expressed in the myelomonocyte lineage are organized as a single genetic locus on 19pter. *Proc Natl Acad Sci USA* 89: 8215–8219
77 Takahashi H, Nukiwa T, Yoshimura K, Quick CD, States DJ, Holmes MD, Whang-Peng J, Knutsen T, Crystal RG (1988) Structure of the human neutrophil elastase gene. *J Biol Chem* 263: 14739–14747
78 Fouret P, du-Bois RM, Bernaudin JF, Takahashi H, Ferrans VJ, Crystal RG (1989) Expression of the neutrophil elastase gene during human bone marrow cell differentiation. *J Exp Med* 169: 833–845
79 Hanson RD, Hohn PA, Popescu NC, Ley TJ (1990) A cluster of hematopoietic serine protease genes is found on the same chromosomal band as the human α/δ-cell receptor locus. *Proc Natl Acad Sci USA* 87: 960–963
80 Sturrock AB, Franklin KF, Rao G, Marshall BC, Rebentisch MB, Lemons RS, Hoidal JR (1992) Structure, chromosomal assignment, and expression of the gene for proteinase-3. The Wegener's granulomatosis autoantigen. *J Biol Chem* 267: 21193–21199

81 Friedman AD, Krieder BL, Venturelli D, Rovera G (1991) Transcriptional regulation of two myeloid-specific genes, myeloperoxidase and lactoferrin, during differentiation of the murine cell line 32D C13. *Blood* 78: 2426–2432
82 Suzow J, Friedman AD (1993) The murine myeloperoxidase promoter contains several functional elements, one of which binds a cell type-restricted transcription factor, myeloid nuclear factor 1 (MyNF1). *Mol Cell Biol* 13: 2141–2151
83 Khanna-Gupta A, Zibello T, Kolla S, Neufeld EJ, Berliner N (1995) CCAAT displacement protein (CDP/cut) recognizes a slilencer element within the lactoferrin gene promoter. *Blood* 90: 2784–2795
84 Salvesen G, Enghild JJ (1990) An unusual specificity in the activation of neutrophil serine proteinase zymogens. *Biochemistry* 29: 5304–5308
85 McGuire MJ, Lipsky PE, Thiele DL (1992) Purification and characterization of dipeptidyl peptidase I from human spleen. *Arch Biochem Biophys* 295: 2180–288
86 McGuire MJ, Lipsky PE, Thiele DL (1993) Generation of active myeloid and lymphoid granule serine proteases requires processing by the granule thiol protease dipeptidyl peptidase I. *J Biol Chem* 268: 2458–2467
87 Rao NV, Rao GV, Hoidal JR (1997) Human Dipeptidyl-peptidase I: gene characterization, localization, and expression. *J Biol Chem* 272: 10260–10265

Molecular Biology of the Lung
Vol. 1: Emphysema and Infection
ed. by R. A. Stockley

CHAPTER 7
Control of Connective Tissue Genes

Joel Rosenbloom

Department of Anatomy and Histology, School of Dental Medicine, University of Pennsylvania, Philadelphia, PA, USA

1. Introduction

The connective tissues of the lung consist of fibrous components such as the collagens, elastin, and nonfibrous components including proteoglycans, laminin, tenascin, and other proteins. The major goal of this chapter is to describe the ways in which the expression of these components is controlled, and the relationship of these control mechanisms to normal development and pathologic processes. This is a large area with an extensive literature and, because of space limitations, coverage cannot be comprehensive. Emphasis is, therefore, placed on consideration of type I collagen, elastin, and fibronectin as examples that illustrate general principles of regulation of gene expression. Expression of the macromolecular constituents of the extracellular matrix is tightly regulated both spatially and temporally. Although post-transcriptional mechanisms play an important role in some instances, the major focus of this chapter is on transcriptional control which is the most frequent way by which this regulation is achieved.

2. General Considerations of Transcription

All protein-encoding genes are transcribed by RNA polymerase II (Pol II), and these genes usually contain common core-promoter elements that are recognized by general transcription initiation factors, as well as gene-specific DNA elements, which are recognized by specific regulatory factors that modulate the function of the general initiation factors. Core-promoter elements are defined as those minimal DNA elements that are necessary and sufficient for accurate transcription initiation in reconstituted cell-free systems [1]. The most common of these elements are the TATA box (consensus TATAa/tAa/t and located at about position –30 relative to the transcription start site) and a pyrimidine-rich initiator (Inr, consensus YYANt/aYY)). Basal transcription is mediated through the assembly of an initiation complex containing Pol II and several general transcription factors which collectively interact with these *cis* elements. Currently, six general initiation factors, TATA-binding protein (TBP), TFIIA, TFIIB, TFIIE, TFIIF, and TFIIH, have been characterized and cloned [1, 2]. These factors probably assemble into a promoter initiation complex (PIC) in an ordered step-wise fashion. This process begins with the recognition and binding of TBP to the TATA box (Figure 1). TFIIB then interacts directly with TBP and with DNA sequences up- and down-stream of the TATA box. TFIIB plays an essential role in transcription start site selection [3]. TFIIA can enter the forming PIC at any time after TBP is bound and, although TFIIA is not essential for *in vitro* basal transcription, it probably has an important *in vivo* role in stabilization of weak TBP/TATA interactions. A Pol II/TFIIF preformed complex is then recruited. TFIIF has the critical function of targeting Pol II to legitimate initiator complexes and suppressing non-specific DNA binding [3, 4]. TFIIE then interacts directly with Pol II and possibly with TFIIF and TBP. A portion of TFIIE is localized near the start of transcription and it is essential for the recuitment of the last component, TFIIH [4]. TFIIH manifests helicase activity and the final result of PIC formation is the loosening of the DNA duplex and initiation of transcription [5, 6].

Although the basal elements are similar in almost all promoters and organisms, the regulatory elements through which specific gene expression is achieved are highly variable. These elements may be located near or at a great distance up-stream or down-stream of the core elements, and they interact with a wide variety of DNA-binding regulatory proteins. These proteins are the final common pathway whereby regulatory signals are transduced into effects on transcription. These transcription factors may enhance (activate) or inhibit (repress) transcription by targeted interactions with the general initiation factors. *In vivo*, TBP is not found as a free protein but bound to a number of TBP-associated factors (TAFs) to form a large complex designated TFIID. TFIID is the foremost target of the activators/repressors which act by modulating the binding of TFIID to DNA, with

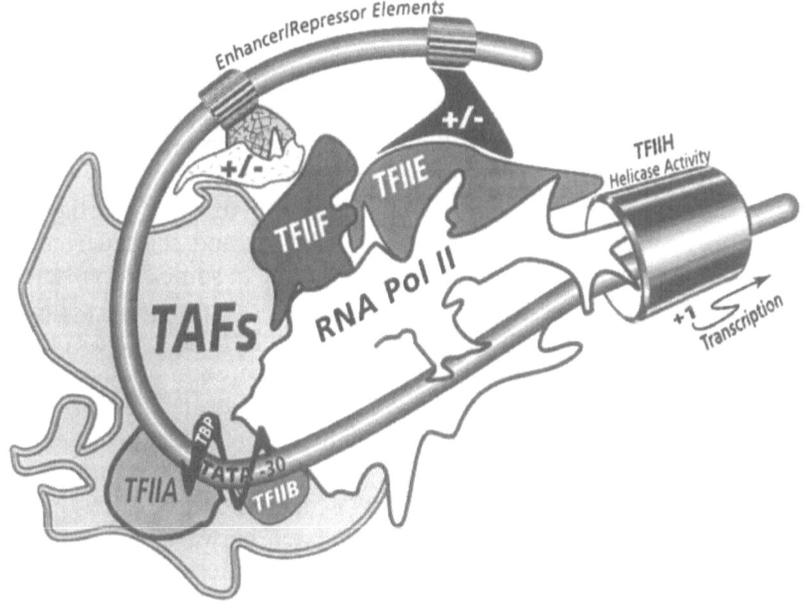

Figure 1. Diagrammatic model of preinitiation complex: This is a schematic illustration of the preinitiation complex composed of the general initiation factor and Pol II interacting with co-factors (TAFs and others) and activators/repressors. Note that such interactions may involve intermediary adaptor molecules interposed between the activator/repressor and TAFs or general factors.

subsequent alteration in the recruitment of other general factors and transcription rate [7, 8]. The interaction of these activators can involve either TBP or the TAFs that make up the TFIID complex [2, 9]. In this type of interaction, the TAFs can be regarded as co-activators and in some instances additional co-factors may be required as intermediaries between the activators and the target general factors, as illustrated in Figure 1 [10].

3. Regulation of Collagen Gene Expression

There are now at least 19 different types of collagen, the polypeptide chains of which are encoded by more than 30 genes [11], although only a limited number of these are quantitatively important in the lung. Within the parenchymal extracellular matrix, the most abundant is type I, with smaller amounts of types III, V, and VI being present. Type II is found within the supporting cartilage of the airways, whereas type IV forms a large portion of the basement membrane separating the epithelia from the underlying, mesenchymally derived tissue. As a result of its predominant role and because it was the first collagen to be cloned, the most information is available on the regulation of type I collagen expression.

3.1. Regulation of Type I Collagen Gene Promoters

Regulation of type I collagen expression must of necessity be complex because of the requirement for tight control during development and the widespread tissue distribution of the protein. Furthermore, expression of the $\alpha1$(I) and $\alpha2$(I) genes is modulated by a variety of cytokines, hormones, and pharmacological agents, and expression of type I collagen is disturbed in disorders such as pulmonary fibrosis and scleroderma. Although post-transcriptional mechanisms play a role in some circumstances, transcription is the major level at which regulation is usually achieved. Important *cis*-acting elements on either side of the transcription start site have been identified. A relatively short sequence between –220 and +116 of the $\alpha1$(I) promoter has been shown to exhibit strong transcriptional activity, whereas addition of more up-stream sequences tends to decrease activity [12]. Besides the general TATA box element, this short promoter fragment contains four *cis*-acting elements which bind three different transcription factors (Figure 2). The element located between –96 and –100 contains a CCAAT sequence which binds a multimeric activator called CBF. CBF is widely expressed and differs from other CCAAT-binding proteins such as CTF/NF1 and C/EB [13, 14]. To achieve specific expression of the $\alpha1$(I) gene, CBF must interact with other transcription factors. On either side of the CCAAT motif there are GC-rich 12-base-pair (bp) elements which bind a factor homologous to Sp1 [15]. Mutation of these sites abolishes Sp1 binding, resulting in a large increase in promoter activity, which suggests that these elements in some circumstances may act as an inhibitor of transcription [12]. Up-stream of CCAAT, there are G-rich elements which bind a member of a large family of transcription factors

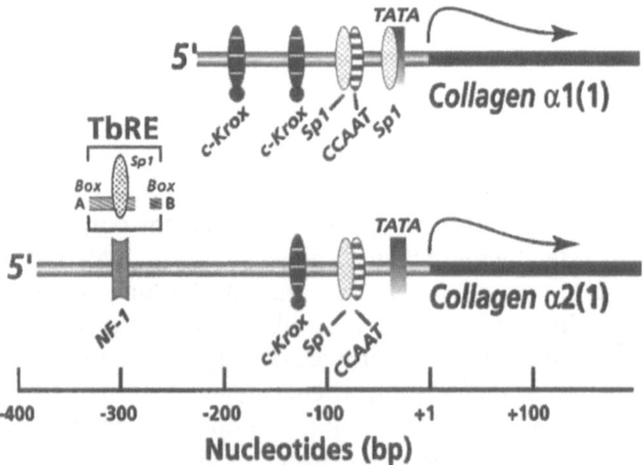

Figure 2. Diagram of the type I α chain promoters in which *cis* elements are identified. Both promoters contain contain TATA and CCAAT boxes. TbRE, TGF-β response element.

called Krox; these possess a zinc finger and are related to the *Drosophila* transcription factor, Krüppel [16]. This new factor has been called c-Krox and has been shown to increase transcription for the α1(I) promoter in co-transfection of fibroblasts [17]. Significantly, c-Krox is most abundant in skin, but appears to be absent in other collagen-producing tissues such as bone. This suggests that c-Krox may play a specific critical role in regulating type I collagen expression in the skin, in normal as well as in pathological situations. Its role in the lung, if any, remains to be determined.

Other segments of the type I collagen genes undoubtedly participate in regulation of expression in particular situations. Several *cis*-acting elements have been identified in the mouse α2(I) promoter. One, located at –250, acts as an activator of transcription as does a second located at –300 which binds nuclear factor 1 (NF1) [18]. A third element, located at –400, binds a factor that has not yet been characterized. In addition, results from several laboratories have indicated that both enhancer and silencer elements may be present within the first intron of the α1(I) gene [19, 20]. The most dramatic evidence for tissue-specific regulation came about when a transgenic strain of mice (Mov13), containing an inserted Moloney murine leukemia virus (M-MuLV) in the first intron of the collagen α1 gene, was found to have the α1 gene completely shut off in fibroblasts and other mesenchymal tissue [21]. Changes in chromatin conformation and methylation of proximal promoter sequences accompanied and perhaps caused the transcriptional block [22]. These findings support a regulatory role for the first intron. Surprisingly, odontoblasts and osteoblasts in the Mov13 strain continued to express α1 mRNA normally [23]. These data strongly suggest that odontoblasts and osteoblasts utilize *cis*-acting elements which are far up-stream from the proximal promoter. An element that apparently specifically regulates type I expression in osteoblasts has been identified in the α1(I) promoter between –1.7 kilobases and –2.3 kb [24].

3.2. Modulation of Expression by Hormones, Growth Factors, and Cytokines

Excessive collagen accumulation is the cardinal hallmark of all fibrotic diseases, including those affecting the lung [25]. The fibrotic pathophysiologic process is undoubtedly mediated by several cytokines which modulate the expression of a variety of matrix genes. However, transforming growth factor β (TGF-β) is preeminent among these cytokines because of its central and critical role in up-regulating expression of collagen and inhibitors of metalloproteinases (TIMPs) while down-regulating the expression of metalloproteinases themselves. In spite of numerous studies, the molecular mechanisms whereby TGF-β exerts its effects are only now becoming better understood. Based on transient transfection experiments of the mouse α2(I) promoter constructs, it was originally postulated that TGF-β acted through an NF1 site [26]. However, in these studies no difference in binding activity was observed between nuclear extracts prepared from control and TGF-β-treated cells, leaving unresolved the means by which the stimulation was achieved. More recent detailed studies of the human α2(I) promoter have clarified the mechanism [27]. Functional assays identified a 131-bp sequence (designated TGF-β response elements or TbRE, see Figure 2) containing two segments designated Box A and Box B which were absolutely required for the TGF-β response. The 3′ portion of Box A was shown to contain a Sp1 binding site, but the *trans*-acting factor binding to Box B has yet to be identified.

Interestingly, the same TbRE region appears to mediate the inhibitory effects of tumor necrosis factor α (TNF-α) [28]. Nuclear proteins prepared from cells treated with TNF-α bind to the TbRE more strongly than those from untreated cells. In addition, TNF-α increases binding of a second protein complex that recognizes a negatively *cis*-acting element located in the 5′ portion of Box A. However, the effects of TNF-α are complex and perhaps dependent upon the cell type, culture conditions, and state of differentiation. Many studies using fibroblasts [29, 30] or bone culture [31] have reported inhibition, whereas several others have found stimulation [32, 33]. In mouse silicosis and bleomycin models of pulmonary fibrosis, lung TNF-α mRNA levels (probably derived from macrophages) were found to be markedly elevated in association with increased collagen compared with controls [34, 35]. This elevation in collagen content was almost completely prevented by anti-TNF-α antibody administration. In addition, bleomycin caused a significantly smaller fibrotic reaction in lungs of mice deficient in TNF-α [36]. Although indirect and circumstantial, these studies argue strongly for a causal link between elevated TNF-α and collagen expression in an *in vivo* situation.

Interleukins IL-1α and IL-1β have been reported to increase collagen protein and mRNA levels in cultured skin and lung fibroblasts [32, 33, 37] as well as chondrocytes [38]. However, IL-1 induces the production of prostaglandin E_2 (PGE_2) which complicates the interpretation of the results because PGE_2 can itself modulate collagen expression [39]. Other studies have indicated that IL-1α can reduce collagen transcription [40], possibly acting through protein kinase C modulation of activator protein 1 (AP-1) activity [41].

Interferon-γ down-regulates type I collagen expression in all systems in which it has been tested, probably through a post-transcriptional mechanism involving mRNA destabilization because transcription appears to be unaffected [42]. In *in vivo* wound healing and fibrosis models, INF-γ inhibited the deposition of collagen [43, 44]. Although this could be an indirect effect by decreasing the inflammatory response and down-regulating other cytokines such as TGF-β [45], it does suggest that IFN-γ can inhibit fibrosis *in vivo*.

Glucocorticoids inhibit type I collagen production in cultured fibroblasts [46, 47], osteoblasts [48], and hepatocytes [49]. In some reports, type I transcription in the fibroblast cultures was unaffected and the inhibition appeared to be achieved by mRNA destabilization [46, 47], although in other cases transcriptional inhibition was observed [49, 50]. These diverse results suggest that, although glucocorticoids uniformly decrease collagen expression, the mechanism may vary depending upon the cell type and conditions.

4. Regulation of Elastin Gene Expression

4.1. Sequence and Functional Analysis of the Elastin Promoter

Unlike the collagens, the elastin promoter does not contain a canonical TATA sequence and it is likely that the CAAT sequence (located at −57 to −60 relative to the ATG translation start codon) is not functional (Figure 3). The proximal promoter region is also G+C-rich (66%) with a high frequency of CpG dinucleotides [51, 52]. These features have been previously associated with promoters of so-called "housekeeping genes", but more tissue-specific genes are being found to have them as well, so that the distinction between these classes is now breaking down [53]. As with many genes, the elastin promoter contains a remarkable constellation of potential binding sites for transcription regulatory factors indicative of complex regulation. These binding sites include multiple SP1- and AP-2-binding sites, glucocorticoid responsive elements (GREs), and tetradecanoyl phorbol acetate (TPA) and cyclic AMP (CRE) responsive elements. The ab-

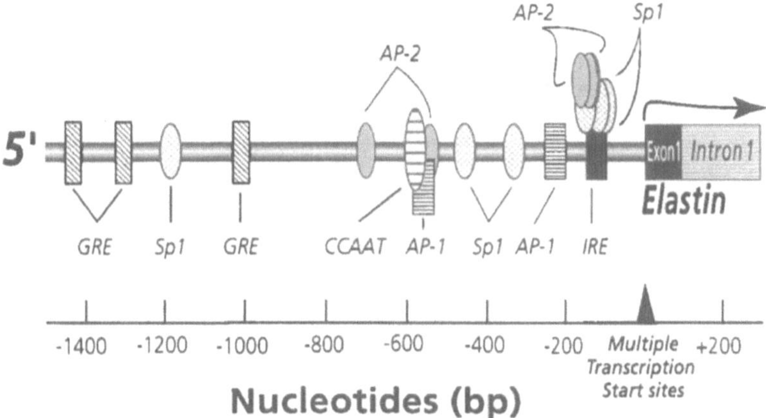

Figure 3. Diagram of the elastin promoter in which *cis* elements are identified. The promoter does not contain a TATA box and multiple transcription start sites have been identified. As a result of its distance from the start of transcription, it is unlikely that the indicated CCAAT box at −600 is functional. GRE, glucoocrticoid response element; IRE, insulin-like growth factor I response element.

sence of a TATA box in the putative promoter region suggested that there may be multiple sites of transcription initiation and S1 protection and primer extension analyses have shown this to be so [52]. It remains to be determined whether the multiple initiation has any physiologic significance, and whether there is any relationship between the position of transcript initiation and the pattern of alternative splicing.

Transient transfection analyses using promoter/reporter gene constructs have demonstrated the presence of multiple positive and negative regulatory elements within 5.2 kbp of the elastin promoter, and indicated that the core promoter necessary for basal expression is contained within the region –128 to –1 [54]. The positive regulatory and core-promoter activities may be explained, at least in part, by the presence of multiple SP1- and AP-2-binding sites within these regions, which may act as general enhancer elements, and DNAse footprinting experiments have indicated that SP1 and AP-2 sites interact with their respecitve *trans* factors. This notion is supported by the observation that deletion of the segment –134 to –87 containing three putative SP1-binding sites reduced the activity to 10–20% of the reference –475 to –1 construct. Significantly, when tissues of transgenic mice utilizing 5.2 kbp of the human elastin promoter were analyzed, there was reasonable correspondence between expression of the endogenous gene and the transgene within the tissues [55]. Nevertheless, because of some inconsistencies between expression of transfected or transgenes and the endogenous gene, these collective observations suggest that all elements for tissue- and development-specific expression of the elastin gene may not reside within the 5.2-kb promoter region tested. It has been observed in a number of genes, including three collagen genes, that the first intron contains segments that act as enhancer or silencer elements of promoter activity. Comparison of the intron sequences of the bovine, rat, and human elastin genes revealed regions of strong homology only in the first intron, suggesting that these regions may contain regulatory elements.

4.2. Modulation of Expression by Hormones, Growth Factors, and Cytokines

The elastin promoter contains three putative GREs which may be functionally active because glucocorticids were shown to increase elastin expression in the developing chick aorta, fetal rat lung, and cultured fetal bovine nuchal ligament fibroblasts [56–58]. Transient transfection of cell cultures of fetal bovine pulmonary smooth muscle with an elastin promoter/reporter construct containing these putative GREs resulted in a greater than three-fold increase in reported activity in response to dexamethasone treatment [57]. In agreement with these studies, transgenic mice possessing a –5200 to +2 elastin promoter/CAT reporter transgene exhibit significantly greater levels of CAT activity in lung tissue in response to the intraperitoneal injection of dexamethasone [59]. However, it is clear that glucocorticoid effects on elastin production are context dependent and the hormone can either up- or down-regulate elastin production, depending on the developmental stage and tissue. For example, glucocorticoids have been reported to down-regulate elastin synthesis in normal cultured human fibroblasts but not in those from keloids [60]. Direct proof that any of these effects are regulated at the transcriptional level is still lacking and Yee et al. [61] have presented evidence that glucocorticoids may act through modulation of production of TGF-β_3 in cultured fetal rat lung fibroblasts.

Insulin-like growth factor-I (IGF-I) has been shown significantly to enhance elastin gene expression in rat neonatal aortic smooth muscle cells both *in vitro* and *in vivo* [62]. Transient transfection experiments with elastin promoter constructs demonstrated that the IGF-I was acting at the transcriptional level [63]. Gel shift and DNA footprinting analyses suggested that IGF-I acts by releasing a transcriptional repressor, possibly Sp3, which binds to an element located between −137 and −123; this has homology to a retinoblastoma control element [64]. In contrast, recombinant TNF-α markedly suppressed elastin mRNA levels in cultured human skin fibroblasts and rat aortic smooth muscle cells, and also suppressed the expression of elastin promoter constructs in transiently transfected cells, again indicating regulation at the transcriptional level [65]. Detailed analyses of the mechanisms involved strongly suggested that the down-regulatory effect of TNF-α was mediated through jun/fos binding to an AP-1 site located at −223 to −229 in the elstin promoter. Basic fibroblast growth factor has also been shown to reduce elastin mRNA and protein levels significantly and the effect appears to be achieved at the transcriptional level [66]. Conflicting evidence has been presented on the effects of IL-1β. One group reported that the cytokine inhibited elastin synthesis and decreased elastin mRNA steady-state levels in cultures of a particular subtype of neonatal rat lung fibroblasts [67], whereas another group reported that the cytokine increased elastin gene expression in cultured human skin fibroblasts, apparently at the transcriptional level [68].

4.2.1. Post-transcriptional regulation: Currently, there is no evidence for translational control of elastin mRNA, but there is strong evidence for both up- and down-regulation of tropoelastin expression through alteration of elastin mRNA stability by several modulators. Elastin production, as determined by enzyme-linked immunosorbent assay (ELISA), was increased approximately threefold when porcine smooth muscle cells were incubated with TGF-β_1 [69]. Although the human promoter may respond to TGF-β [70], its major effect is to increase elastin production by message stabilization [71, 72]. Treatment of cultured human fetal lung fibroblasts with TGF-β produced a more than tenfold increase in steady-state elastin mRNA levels with no alteration in transcription, but with increased message stability

[72]. A phosphatidylcholine-specific phospholipase C and protein kinase C were involved in mediating the elastin message stabilization. When cultures of elastogenic fetal bovine chondrocytes were exposed to 0.1 µmol/l TPA, tropoelastin mRNA levels decreased more than tenfold and this was paralleled by a decline in the production of tropoelastin [73]. As determined by nuclear runoff assay and transient transfection with a human gene promoter-CAT construct, tropoelastin transcription was unaffected by exposure to TPA. The half-life of tropoelastin mRNA in conrol cells was estimated to be about 20 h, but exposure to TPA reduced the half-life to 2.2 h. Similarly, 0.1 µmol/l 1,25-dihydroxyvitamin D_3, a rather high non-physiologic dose, produced a marked decrease in steady-state and functional levels of tropoelastin mRNA, but transcription was not affected [74]. Collectively, these data indicate that tropoelastin expression can be controlled by post-transcriptional mechanisms.

5. Regulation of Fibronectin Gene Expression

Fibronectin is one of the most widely distributed and best characterized extracellular matrix molecules acting as a substrate for cell migration and adhesion through cell surface integrin receptors [75, 76]. Fibronectin and its receptors are involved in a wide variety of important biologic processes, including branching morphogenesis in the lung, response to injury and wound healing, and many fibroproliferative lesions resulting in profound alterations in lung structure and function. Expression of fibronectin is modulated by a variety of cytokines, growth factors, and hormones, which may themselves by involved in development and response to injury.

5.1. Promoter Structure and Function

The human, rat, and mouse genes have been cloned and the promoters shown to have segments of great homology to one another [77–79]. A TATA box is located at approximately position –25 and a CCAAT box at –150. The proximal promoter region is GC rich and contains several SP1 boxes at –102 and –45 and two AP-2 sites at –120 and –67 (Figure 4). Cyclic AMP-responsive elements are located at –170, –260, and –415. The –170 site may be important in maintaining basal transcription and has been shown to be responsible for the strong induction of fibronectin gene transcription by serum [80, 81]. It also appears that the site located at –170 is of higher affinity and appears to interact with the CCAAT box. Nuclear protein extracts from liver strongly protect the –150 CCAAT box when the –170 CRE is also occupied [82]. Disruption of binding to the –170 CRE results in deprotection of the CCAAT box, but not *vice versa*. This inter-

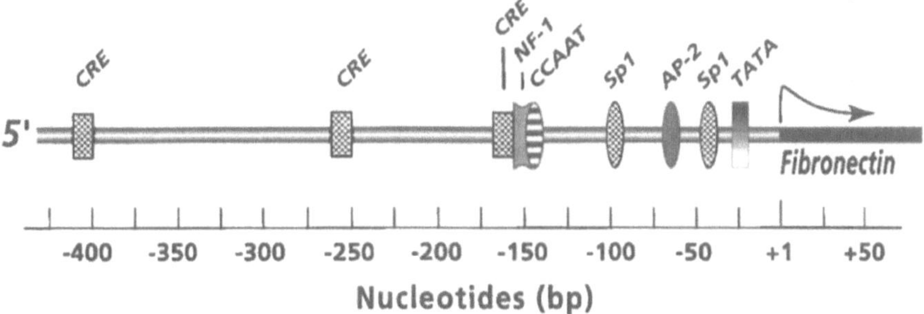

Figure 4. Diagram of the fibronectin promoter in which *cis* elements are identified. The promoter contains canonical TATA and CCAAT boxes. Interaction between the CRE at −170 and the CCAAT box may be an important feature of transcriptional regulation (see text).

action appears to be functionally important, because alteration of the spacing between the CCAAT and CRE also disrupted the cooperative binding and decreased the transcriptional efficiency of the promoter. The *trans*-acting factors involved in these interaction have yet to be characterized.

5.2. Modulation of Expression by Hormones, Growth Factors, and Cytokines

TGF-β stimulates transcription of the fibronectin gene, which is possible through an NF1 site located near the CCAAT element [83]. However, further work is necessary to substantiate this possibility and to define precisely the *trans*-acting factors and mechanisms involved. Fibronectin transcription is also enhanced by agents that raise cAMP levels and this effect appears to be mediated by one or more of the three CREs. Although each of these has been shown to confer cAMP responsiveness on a heterologous thymidine kinase promoter and form multiple complexes with nuclear protein extracts, only the −170 element has been extensively studied [84]. Currently, more than 20 CRE-binding proteins have been described which can form heterodimers, thus dramatically increasing the potential complexity. Several of these proteins have been well characterized [85]. Nuclear proteins from a variety of tissues and cells form different complexes with the −170 CRE which may contribute to tissue-specific regulation of expression [82, 86].

Glucocorticoids increase the biosynthesis of fibronectin and mRNA levels, but transcription appears to be unaltered [83]. Fibronectin mRNA is stabilized through a mechanism requiring protein synthesis, indicating that induction of one or more proteins is required. The nature of these proteins and the site of presumptive interaction on fibronectin mRNA have not been determined.

6. Role of Matrix Proteins in Lung Development

The complex process of lung development involves epithelial/mesenchymal interactions, many cytokines and growth factors, and a variety of matrix molecules. The matrix may function through cellular adhesion or modulation of cell motility, proliferation and differentiation. Several matrix components have been implicated in morphogenic events. Laminins are cell-adhesion glycoproteins found in basement membranes [87] and they have been shown to have a critical role in lung-branching morphogenesis. The region of the laminin mediating this activity has been localized to the globular segments of the β and γ chains [88]. The tenascins comprise a family of large matrix molecules characterized by epidermal growth factor (EGF) repeats, fibronectin type III-like repeats and a carboxyl-terminal fibrinogen domain. Antibodies to tenascin C also blocked branching morphogenesis as did recombinantly produced segments of tenascin C which consist of fibronectin type III repeats; this suggests a functional role for the protein [89]. It is also likely that fibronectin itself is involved in branching, because it is found at high levels at branch points during the pseudoglandular stage, and fibronectin fragments known to diminish fibronectin matrix assembly greatly in fetal lung fibroblasts cultures also prevented normal branching, whereas other fragments did not [90].

6.1. Role of Elastin

Although most of the available information concerning elastin expression in the lung comes from studies on experimental animals, particularly the rat, it is likely that the pattern of expression is similar in all mammals, including humans, at comparable stages of morphologic development. Elastin is produced primarily in the late fetal and neonatal periods. Expression of elastin starts in the pseudoglandular stage, increases in the canalicular and saccular stages, and reaches a maximal level during alveolarization in the neonate. Normally, there is little expression in the adult. Immunohistochemical and *in situ* hybridization techniques have localized expression to particular sites during the different developmental periods. In the pseudoglandular stage, minimal expression is seen in the loose mesenchymal connective tissue and in the smooth muscle of the intralobar pulmonary arteries. In the canalicular stage, smooth muscle cells subjacent to the differentiting airway epithelium express tropoelastin mRNA and fine elastic fibres can be detected surrounding terminal bronchioles. This process is accentuated in the saccular stage when clusters of cells close to the differentiating epithelium of terminal airspaces produce tropoelastin, resulting in a complex of well-developed elastic fibers which surround the terminal airspaces, particularly at branching sites. Subsequently, expression is highest in the forming alveolar walls, particularly at the tips of newly forming septa. At this stage, substantial elastic fibers are also found in the bronchioles and lamina of elastic arteries.

The localization of a condensed elastic matrix at the apex of forming alveolar septa suggested that this matrix might have a critical role in alveolar morphogenesis, as opposed to a purely structural one [91–93]. Recent studies in which the platelet-derived growth factor A chain (PDGF-A) has been knocked out have substantiated this idea [94]. Postnatally surviving PDGF-A-deficient mice developed emphysema secondary to failure of alveolar septation. The data suggested that PDGF-A synthesized by the alveolar epithelium is essential for the functional differentiation of PDGF receptor-α-positive alveolar myofibroblasts, which are responsible for the synthesis of the associated elastic fiber matrix. Thus, the deposition of elastic fibers in the prealveolar saccule wall may well be a critical morphogenic event.

The potential morphogenic role of elastin may be critical in developing strategies to treat complex destructive diseases affecting the lung. Masaro and Masaro [95] recently reported that treatmet with all-*trans*-retinoic acid reversed the destructive effects of pancreatic elastase administration in a rat emphysema model. It had previously been shown that retinoic acid could increase elastin production in neonatal rat lung fibroblast cultures [96].

7. Conclusions and Perspectives

Definition of the factors controlling the expression of genes that encode the extracellular matrix proteins is fundamental to understanding the role of these proteins in lung development and disease processes. Although the general features of the regulatory elements of the promoters of several of these genes have been reasonably well delineated, in most instances our understanding of many aspects of control is at a relatively primitive level. Considerably more studies are required to define the interactions of *trans*-acting factors and their cognate *cis*-acting-elements. It is very likely that, in many instances, more than one element is utilized to achieve a given effect (for example, see the modulation of transcription of the collagen α2(I) promoter by TGF-β). In *in vivo* situations, it is to be expected that multiple factors (cytokines, hormones, cell/matrix interactions) act in combination to achieve temporal and tissue-specific regulation of transcription of individual genes. Definition of such complex interactions is extremely challenging, but necessary, if we are to understand lung development and pathologic processes in molecular terms. An example of the potential practical usefulness of such knowledge is the effects of retinoids in treatment of emphysema.

Although transcriptional regulation has been stressed in this chapter, it is likely that other levels of control of gene expression (mRNA stability, alternative splicing) will assume greater importance as our understanding deepens.

Acknowledgements

The author would like to thank Dr William Abrams for the artwork in the figures and critical reading of the manuscript. Work from the author's laboratory was supported by National Institutes of Health Research Grants AR41474 and HL56401.

References

1 Roeder RG (1996) The role of general initiation factors in transcription by RNA polymerase II. *Trends Biochem Sci* 21: 327–335
2 Burley SK, Roeder RG (1996) Biochemistry and structural biology of transcription factor IID (TFIID). *Annu Rev Biochem* 65: 769–799
3 Zawel L, Reinberg D (1995) Common themes in assembly and function of eukaryotic transcription complexes. *Annu Rev Biochem* 64: 533–561
4 Leuther KK, Bushnell DA, Kornberg RD (1996) Two-dimensional crystallography of TGIIB- and IIE-RNA polymerase II complexes: implications for start site selection and initiation complex formation. *Cell* 85: 773–779
5 Conaway RC, Conaway JW (1993) General initiation factors for RNA polymerase II. *Annu Rev Biochem* 62: 161–190
6 Svejstrup JQ, Vichi P, Egly J-M (1996) The multiple roles of transcription/repair factor TFIIH. *Trends Biochem Sci* 21: 346–350
7 Workman JL, Abmayr SM, Cromish WA, Roeder RG (1988) Transcriptional regulation by the immediate early protein of pseudorabies virus during *in vitro* nucleosome assembly. *Cell* 55: 211–219
8 Horikoshi M (1988) Transcription factor ATF interacts with the TATA factor to facilitate establishment of a preinitiation complex. *Cell* 54: 1033–1042
9 Verrijzer CP, Tjian R (1996) TAFs mediate transcriptional activation and promoter selectivity. *Trends Biochem Sci* 21: 338–342
10 Kaiser K, Meisternst M (1996) The human general co-factors. *Trends Biochem Sci* 21: 342–345
11 Prockop DJ, Kivirikko KI (1995) Collagens: molecular biology, diseases, and potentials for therapy. *Annu Rev Biochem* 64: 403–434
12 Karsenty G, de Crombrugghe B (1990) Two different negative and one positive regulatory factors interact with a short promoter segment of the alpha 1(I) collagen gene. *J Biol Chem* 263: 9934–9942
13 Maity SN, Vuorio T, de Crombrugghe B (1990) The B subunit of a rat heteromeric CCAAT-binding transcription factor shows a striking sequence identity with the yeast Hap2 transcription factor. *Proc Natl Acad Sci USA* 87: 5378–5382
14 Maity SN, Golumbek PT, Karsenty G, de Crombrugghe B (1988) Selective activation of transcription by a novel CCAAT binding factor. *Science* 241: 582–585
15 Nehis M, Pippe R, Veloz L, Brenner DA (1991) Transcription factors nuclear factor I and Spl interact with the murine collagen alpha 1(I) promoter. *Mol Cell Biol* 11: 4065–4073
16 Knipple DC, Seifert E, Rosenberg UB, Preiss A, Jackle H (1986) Spatial and temporal patterns of Kruppel gene expression in early Drosophila embryos. *Nature* 317: 40–44
17 Galera P, Musso M, Ducy P, Karsenty G (1995) c-Krox, a transcriptional regulator of type I collagen gene expression, is preferentially expressed in skin. *Proc Natl Acad Sci USA* 9: 9372–9376
18 Karsenty G, Golumbek P, de Crombrugghe B (1988) Point mutations and small substitution mutations in three different upstream elements inhibit the activity of the mouse alpha 2(I) collagen promoter. *J Biol Chem* 263: 13909–13915

19 Rossouw CMS, Vergeer WP, duPlooy SS, Bernard MP, Ramirez F, de Wet W (1987) DNA sequences in the first intron of the human pro-α1(I) collagen gene enhance transcription. *J Biol Chem* 26: 15151–15157
20 Bornstein P, McKay J, Morishima JK, Devarayalu S, Galinas RE (1987) Regulatory elements in the first intron contribute to transcriptional control of the human α1(I) collagen gene. *Proc Natl Acad Sci USA* 84: 8869–8873
21 Hartung S, Jaenisch R, Breindl M (1986) Retrovirus insertion inactivates mouse α1(I) collagen gene by blocking initiation of transcription. *Nature* 320: 365–367
22 Jahner D, Jaenisch R (1985) Retrovirus-induced *de novo* methylation of flanking host sequences correlates with gene inactivity. *Nature* 315: 594–597
23 Kratochwil K, von der Mark K, Kollar EJ, Jaenisch R, Mooslehner K, Schwarz M, Haase K, Gmachl I, Harbers K (1989) Retrovirus-induced insertional mutation in Mov13 mice affects collagen I expression in a tissue-specific manner. *Cell* 57: 807–816
24 Pavlia D, Lichtler AC, Bedalar A, Kream BE, Harrison JR, Thomas HF, Gronowicz GA, Clark SH, Woody CO, Rowe DW (1992) Differential utilization of regulatory domains within the alpha 1(I) collagen promoter in osseous and fibroblastic cells. *J Cell Biol* 116: 227–236
25 Broekelmann TJ, Limper AH, Colby TV, McDonald JA (1991) Transforming growth factor beta 1 is present at sites of extracellular matrix gene expression in human pulmonary fibrosis. *Proc Natl Acad Sci USA* 88: 6642–6646
26 Rossi P, Karsenty G, Roberts AB, Roche NS, Sporn MB, de Crombrugghe B (1988) A nuclear factor 1 binding site mediates the transcriptional activation of a type I collagen promoter by transforming growth factor-beta. *Cell* 52: 405–414
27 Inagaki Y, Truter S, Ramirez F (1994) Transforming growth factor-β stimulates α2(I) collagen gene expression through a *cis*-acting element that contains an Sp1-binding site. *J Biol Chem* 269: 14828–14834
28 Inagaki Y, Truter S, Tanaka S, De Liberto M, Ramirez F (1995) Overlapping pathways mediate the opposing actions of tumor necrosis factor-α and transforming growth factor-β on α2(I) collagen gene transcription. *J Biol Chem* 270: 3353–3358
29 Mauviel A, Daireaux M, Redini F, Galera P, Loyau G, Pujol JP (1988) Tumor necrosis factor inhibits collagen and fibronectin synthesis in human dermal fibroblasts. *FEBS Lett* 236: 47–52
30 Solis-Herruzo JA, Brenner DA, Chojkier M (1988) Tumor necrosis factor alpha inhibits collagen gene transcription and collagen synthesis in cultured human fibroblasts. *J Biol Chem* 263: 5841–5845
31 Centrella M, McCarthy T, Canalis E (1988) Tumor necrosis factor-alpha inhibits collagen synthesis and alkaline phosphatase activity independently of its effect on deoxyribonucleic acid synthesis in osteoblast-enriched bone cell cultures. *Endocrinology* 123: 442–1448
32 Elias JA, Freundlich B, Adams S, Rosenbloom J (1990) Regulation of human lung fibroblast collagen production by recombinant interleukin-1, tumor necrosis factor, and interferon-gamma. *Ann NY Acad Sci* 580 : 233–244
33 Duncan MR, Berman B (1988) Differential regulation of collagen, glycosaminoglycan, fibronectin, and collagenase activity production in cultured human adult dermal fibroblasts by interleukin 1-alpha and beta and tumor necrosis factor-alpha and beta. *J Invest Dermatol* 92: 699–706
34 Piguet PF, Colart MA, Grau GE, Sappino AP, Vassalli P (1990) Requirement of tumour necrosis factor for development of silica-induced pulmonary fibrosis. *Nature* 344: 245–247
35 Piguet PF, Collart MA, Grau GE, Kapanci Y, Vassalli P (1989) Tumor necrosis factor/cachetin plays a key role in bleomycin-induced pneumopathy and fibrosis. *J Exp Med* 170: 655–663
36 Piguet PF, Kaufman S, Barazzone C, Muller M, Ryffel B, Eugster HP (1997) Resistance of TNF/LT-α double deficient mice to bleomycin-induced fibrosis. *Int J Exp Pathol* 78: 43–48
37 Postlethwaite AE, Raghow R, Stricklin GP, Poppleton H, Seyer JM, Kang AH (1988) Modulation of fibroblast functions by interleukin 1: increased steady-state accumulation of other functions but not chemotaxis by human recombinant interleukin 1 alpha and beta. *J Cell Biol* 106: 311–318
38 Goldring MB, Birkhead J, Sandell LJ, Kimura T, Krane SM (1988) Interleukin 1 suppresses expression of cartilage-specific types II and IX collagens and increases types I and III collagens in human chondrocytes. *J Clin Invest* 82: 2026–2037

39 Goldring MB, Krane SM (1987) Modulation by recombinant interleukin 1 of synthesis of types I and III collagens and associated procollagen mRNA levels in cultured human cells. *J Biol Chem* 262: 16724–16729
40 Harrison JR, Vargas SJ, Petersen DN, Lorenzo JA, Kream BE (1990) Interleukin-alpha and phorbol ester inhibit collagen synthesis in osteoblastic MC3T3-E1 cells by a transcriptional mechanism. *Mol Endocrinol* 4: 184–190
41 Muegge K, Williams TM, Kant J, Karin M, Chiu R, Schmidt A, Siebenlist U, Young HA, Durum SK (1989) Interleukin-1 co-stimulatory activity on the interleukin-2 promoter via AP-1. *Science* 246: 249–251
42 Czaja MJ, Winer FR, Eghbali M, Giambrone MA, Eghbali M, Zern MA (1987) Differential effect of γ-interferon on collagen and fibronectin expression. *J Biol Chem* 262: 13348–13351
43 Granstein RD, Deak MR, Jacques SL, Margolis RJ, Flotte TJ, Whitaker D, Long FH, Amento EP (1989) The systemic administration of gamma interferon inhibits collagen synthesis and acute inflammation in a murine skin wounding model. *J Invest Dermatol* 93: 18–27
44 Czaja MJ, Weiner FR, Takahashi S, Giambrone MA, van der Meide PH, Schellekens H, Bliempica L, Zern MA (1989) Gamma-interferon treatment inhibits collagen deposition in murine schistosomiasis. *Hepatology* 10: 795–800
45 Gurujeyalakshmi G, Giri SN (1995) Molecular mechanisms of antifibrotic effect of interferon gamma in bleomycin-mouse model of lung fibrosis: downregulation of TGF-β and procollagen I and III gene expression. *Exp Lung Res* 21: 791–808
46 Hamalainen L, Oikarinin J, Kivirikko KI (1985) Synthesis and degradation of type I procollagen mRNAs in cultured human skin fibroblasts and the effect of cortisol. *J Biol Chem* 260: 720–725
47 Raghow R, Gossag D, Kang AH (1986) Pretranslational regulation of type I collagen, fibronectin, and a 50-kilodalton noncollagenous extracellular protein by dexamethasone in rat fibroblasts. *J Biol Chem* 261: 4677–4684
48 Ng KW, Manji SS, Young MF, Findlay DM (1989) Opposing influences of glucoocorticoid and retinoic acid on transcriptional control in preosteoblasts. *Mol Endocrinol* 3: 2079–2085
49 Weiner FR, Czaja MF, Jefferson DM, Gliambrone MA, Tur-Kaspa R, Reid LM, Zern MA (1987) The effects of dexamethasone in *in vitro* collagen gene expression. *J Biol Chem* 262: 6955–6958
50 Cockayne D, Cutroneo KR (1989) Glucocorticoid coordinate regulation of type I procollagen gene expression and procollagen DNA-binding proteins in chick skin fibroblats. *Biochemistry* 27: 2736–2745
51 Yeh H, Anderson N, Ornstein-Goldstein N, Bashir MM, Rosenbloom JC, Abrams W, Indik Z, Yoon K, Parks W, Mecham R, Rosenbloom J (1989) Structure of the bovine elastin gene and S1 nuclease analysis of alternative splicing of elastin mRNA in the bovine nuchal ligament. *Biochemistry* 28: 2365–2370
52 Bashir MM, Indik Z, Yeh H, Ornstein-Goldstein N, Rosenbloom JC, Abrams W, Fazio M, Uitto J, Rosenbloom J (1989) Characterization of the complete human elastin gene. Delineation of unusual features in the 5′-flanking region. *J Biol Chem* 264: 8887–8891
53 Gardiner-Garden M, Frommer M (1987) CpG islands in vertebrate genomes. *J Mol Biol* 196: 261–282
54 Kahari V-M, Fazio MJ, Chen YQ, Bashir MM, Rosenbloom J, Uitto J (1990) Deletion analyses of 5′-flanking region of the human elastin gene: delineation of functional promoter and regulatory *cis*-elements. *J Biol Chem* 265: 9485–9490
55 Hsu-Wong S, Katchman SD, Ledo I, Wu M, Khillan J, Bashir MM, Rosenbloom J, Uitto J (1994) Tissue-specific and developmentally regulated expression of human elastin promoter activity in transgenic mice. *J Biol Chem* 269: 18072–18075
56 Eichner R, Rosenbloom J (1979) Collagen and elastin synthesis in the developing chick aorta. *Arch Biochem Biophys* 198: 414–423
57 Pierce RA, Mariencheck WI, Sandefur S, Crouch EC, Parks WC (1995) Glucocorticoids upregulate tropoelastin expression during late stages of fetal lung development. *Am J Physiol* 268: L491–L500
58 Mecham RP, Morris SL, Levy BD, Wrenn DS (1984) Glucocorticoids stimulate elastin production in differentiated bovine ligament fibroblasts but do not induce elastin synthesis in undifferentiated cells. *J Biol Chem* 259: 12414–12420

59 Ledo I, Wu M, Katchman S, Brown D, Dennedy S, Hsu-Wong S, Uitto J (1994) Glucocorticosteroids upregulate human elastin gene promoter activity in transgenic mice. *J Invest Dermatol* 103: 632–636
60 Russell SB, Trupin JS, Kennedy RZ, Russell JR, Davidson JM (1995) Glucocorticoid regulation of elastin synthesis in human fibroblasts: down-regulation in fibroblasts from normal dermis but not from keloids. *J Invest Dermatol* 104: 241–245
61 Yee W, Wang J, Liu J, Tseu I, Kuliszewski M, Post M (1996) Glucocorticoid-induced tropoelastin expression is mediated via transforming growth factor-β3. *Am J Physiol* 14: L992–L1001
62 Rich CB, Ewton DZ, Martin BM, Florini JR, Bashir M, Rosenbloom J, Foster JA (1992) IGF-1 regulation of elastogenesis: comparison of aortic and lung cells. *Am J Phys* 7: L276–L282
63 Wolfe BL, Rich CB, Goud HD, Terpstra AJ, Bashir M, Rosenbloom J, Sonenshein GE, Foster JA (1993) Insulin-like growth factor-I regulates transcription of the elastin gene. *J Biol Chem* 268: 12418–12426
64 Conn KJ, Rich CB, Jensen DE, Fontanilla MR, Bashir MM, Rosenbloom J, Foster JA (1996) Insulin-like growth factor-I regulates transcription of the elastin gene through a putative retinoblastoma control element. *J Biol Chem* 271: 28853–28860
65 Kahari V-M, Chen YQ, Bashir M, Rosenbloom J, Uitto J (1992) Tumor necrosis factor-α down-regulates human elastin gene expression. *J Biol Chem* 267: 26134–26141
66 Brettell LM, McGowan SE (1994) Basic fibroblast growth factor decreases elastin production by neonatal rat lung fibroblasts. *Am J Respir Cell Mol Biol* 10: 306–315
67 Berk JL, Franzblau C, Goldstein RH (1991) Recombinant interleukin-1β inhibits elastin formation by a neonatal rat lung fibroblast subtype. *J Biol Chem* 266: 3192–3197
68 Mauviel A, Chen YQ, Kahari V-M, Ledo I, Wu M, Rudnicka L, Uitto J (1993) Human recombinant interleukin-1β up-regulates elastin gene expression in dermal fibroblasts. *J Biol Chem* 268: 6520–6523
69 Liu J, Davidson JM (1989) The elastogenic effect of recombinant transforming growth factor-β on porcine aortic smooth muscle cells. *Biochem Biophys Res Commun* 154: 895–899
70 Marigo V, Volpin D, Vitale G, Bressan GM (1994) Identification of a TGF-beta responsive element in the human elastin promoter. *Biochem Biochys Res Commun* 199: 1049–1056
71 Kahari V-M, Olsen DR, Rhudy RW, Carrillo P, Chen YQ, Uitto J (1992) Transforming growth factor-β upregulates elastin gene expression in human skin fibroblasts. *Lab Invest* 66: 580–588
72 Kucich U, Rosenbloom JC, Abrams WR, Bashir MM, Rosenbloom J (1997) Stabilization of elastin mRNA by TGF-β: initial characterization of signaling pathway. *Am J Respir Cell Mol Biol* 17: 10–16
73 Parks WC, Kolodziej ME, Pierce RA (1992) Phorbol ester-mediated downregulation of tropoelastin expression is controlled by a posttranscriptional mechanism. *Biochemistry* 31: 6639–6645
74 Pierce RA, Kolodziej ME, Parks WC (1992) 1,23-Dihydroxyvitamin D_3 represses tropoelastin expression by a posttranscriptional mechanism. *J Biol Chem* 267: 11593–11599
75 Schwarzbauer J (1990) The fibronectin gene. In: LJ Sandell, CD Boyd (eds): *Extracellular matrix genes*. Academic Press, London, 195–220
76 Kornblihtt AR, Pesce CG, Alonso CR, Cramer P, Srebrow A, Werbajh S, Muro AF (1996) The fibronectin gene as a model for splicing and transcription studies. *FASEB J* 10: 248–257
77 Dean D, Bowlus C, Bourgeois S (1987) Cloning and analysis of the promoter region of the human fibronectin gene. *Proc Natl Acad Sci USA* 84: 1876–1880
78 Patel RS, Odermatt E, Schwarzbauer JE, Hines RO (1986) Organization of the rat fibronectin gene provides evidence for "exon shuffling" during evolution. *EMBO J* 6: 2565–2572
79 Polly P, Nicholson RC (1993) Sequence of the mouse fibronectin-encoding gene promoter region. *Gene* 137: 353–354
80 Miao S, Suri PK, Shu-Ling L, Abraham A, Cook N, Milos P, Zern MA (1993) Role of the cyclic AMP response element in rat fibronectin gene expression. *Hepatology* 17: 882–890
81 Dean DC, McQuillan JJ, Weintraub S (1990) Serum stimulation of fibronectin gene expression appears to result from rapid serum-induced binding of nuclear proteins to a cAMP response element. *J Biol Chem* 265: 3522–3527

82 Muro A, Bernath V, Kornblihtt A (1992) Interaction of the –170 cyclic AMP response element with the adjacent CCAAT box in the human fibronectin gene promoter. *J Biol Chem* 267: 12767–12774
83 Dean DC, Newby RF, Bourgeois (1988) Regulation of fibronectin biosynthesis by dexamethasone, transforming growth factor-β and cAMP in human cell lines. *J Cell Biol* 106: 2159–2170
84 Bowlus C, Dean DC (1991) Characterization of three different cAMP regulatory elements in the 5′ flanking region of the human fibronectin gene. *J Biol Chem* 266: 1122–1127
85 Ginty DD, Bonni A, Greenberg ME (1994) Nerve growth factor activates a Ras-dependent protein kinase that stimulates c-fos transcription via phosphorylation of CREB. *Cell* 77: 713–725
86 Dean DC, Blakely MS, Newby RF, Ghazal P, Henninghauser L, Bourgeois S (1989) Forskolin inducibility and tissue-specific expression of the fibronectin promoter. *Mol Cell Biol* 9: 1498–1506
87 Burgeson RE, Chiquet M, Deutzmann R (1994) A new nomenclature for the laminins. *Matrix Biol Chem* 263: 16536–16544
88 Schuger L, Skubitz APN, O'Shea KS, Chang JF, Varani J (1991) Identification of laminin domains involved in epithelial branching morphogenesis: effects of anti-laminin are differentially synthesized in mouse eggs and early embryos. *Dev Biol* 146: 531–541
89 Young SL, Chang L-Y, Erickson HP (1994) Tenascin-C in rat lung; distribution, ontogen and role in branching morphogenesis. *Dev Biol* 161: 615–625
90 Roman J, Crouch EC, McDonald JA (1991) Reagents that inhibit fibronectin matrix assembly of cultured cells also inhibit lung branching morphogenesis *in vitro*: implications for lung development, injury, and repair. *Chest* 99: 20S
91 Emery JL (1970) The postnatal development of the human lung and its implication for lung pathology. *Respiration* 27: 41–50
92 Burri PH, Weibel ER (1977) Ultrastructure and morphometry of the developing lung. In: WA Hodson (ed): *Development of the lung*, Part 1: *Structural development*, Marcel Dekker, New York, 215–268
93 Noguchi A, Reddy R, Kursar JD, Parks WC, Mecham RP (1989) Smooth muscle isoactin and elastin in fetal bovine lung. *Exp Lung Res* 4: 537–552
94 Bostrom H, Willetts K, Pekny M, Leveen P, Lindahl P, Hedstrand H, Pekna M, Hellstrom M, Gebre-Medhin S, Schalling M, Nilsson M, Kurland S, Törnell J, Hrath JK, Betsholtz C (1996) PDGF-A signaling is a critical event in lung alveolar myofibroblast development and alveogenesis. *Cell* 85: 863–873
95 Massaro GD, Massaro D (1997) Retinoic acid treatment abrogates elastase-induced pulmonary emphysema in rats. *Nature Med* 3: 675–677
96 Liu R, Harvey C, McGowan SE (1993) Retinoic acid increases elastin in neonatal rat lung fibroblast cultures. *Am J Physiol* 265: L430–L437

Infection

Molecular Biology of the Lung
Vol. 1: Emphysema and Infection
ed. by R. A. Stockley

CHAPTER 8
Genetic Models of Bacterial Lung Infection

Timothy J. Mitchell

Division of Infection and Immunity, Joseph Black Building, University of Glasgow, Glasgow, UK

1. Introduction

The lung is a point of intimate contact of the host with its environment and as such is a key point of interaction between animals and microbes. A range of host defence mechanisms exists to protect the lung from infection. These defence mechanisms include physical defences such as the filtration of air and the mucociliary escalator as well as the innate immune mechanisms such as the alveolar macrophage. The activity of these cells is augmented by the presence of various opsonins within the lung, including complement components and immunoglobulins. The inflammatory response and specific immune response in the lung are controlled by a range of cytokines and other immune mediators. To cause disease an invading pathogen must be able to subvert these normal defences.

Respiratory pathogens produce a range of virulence factors that interact with the immune system. To understand how pathogens and their products interact with the immune system in the lung it is useful to have mutants of both bacteria (as discussed in Chapter 9) and host. The use of genetic models to evaluate the contribution of host factors involved in protection can involve either the use of naturally occuring mutations (in either humans or animals) or the construction of mutations in animal systems via the use of transgenic technology.

Naturally occurring mutations are obviously of use in defining the role played by the immune response in humans. The role of the complement pathway and the importance of immunoglobulin in the protection against specific pathogens can be inferred from studies in deficient patients. The role of specific components of receptors can be studied in detail by use of appropriate manipulations of the genetic systems of animals for subsequent use in animal models. As the pathogenesis of respiratory infection in humans and animals depends on the interaction between the immune system and virulence factors of the pathogen, use can be made of mutants to probe these interactions. There is now a wide range of transgenic animals available for investigation of the pathogenesis of infection. However, there has been surprisingly little use of these animals in the study of pulmonary infection.

2. The Immune Response in the Lung

The immune response in the lung can be divided into innate immune defences, which clear microbes and prevent infection, and adaptive immunity which involves the production of specific antibody and cell-mediated responses to infection with the pathogen (Figure 1). The lung contains several protein components that are involved in defence including surfactants and proteinase inhibitors. One of the main mechanisms of innate immunity is the alternative complement pathway. This pathway can be considered as the first line of defence against many extracellular microbes [1]. Bronchoalveolar lavage fluid contains all the components of the alternative pathway [2, 3]. The classic complement pathway may also be activated by micro-organisms binding to antibody or other opsonins. Activation of the complement pathway leads to opsonization of pathogens and also to the generation of anaphylatoxins which have a range of biological activities including chemotaxis and vasodilatation. The exact role of antibody in protection of the lung from infection is less clear. The major antibody species in the lung is the immunoglobulin IgA, but the role played by this antibody in protection still remains to be defined. Activation of complement also leads to the generation of the membrane attack complex which is capable of destroying Gram-negative bacteria. During an immune response in the lung, cytokine production and the generation of chemotaxins result in the recruitment of cells to the site of infection via interaction with various cell adhesion molecules.

Once at the site of infection, cells interact with the opsonized particle via specific receptors and engulf and kill the invading microbe. Antigens asso-

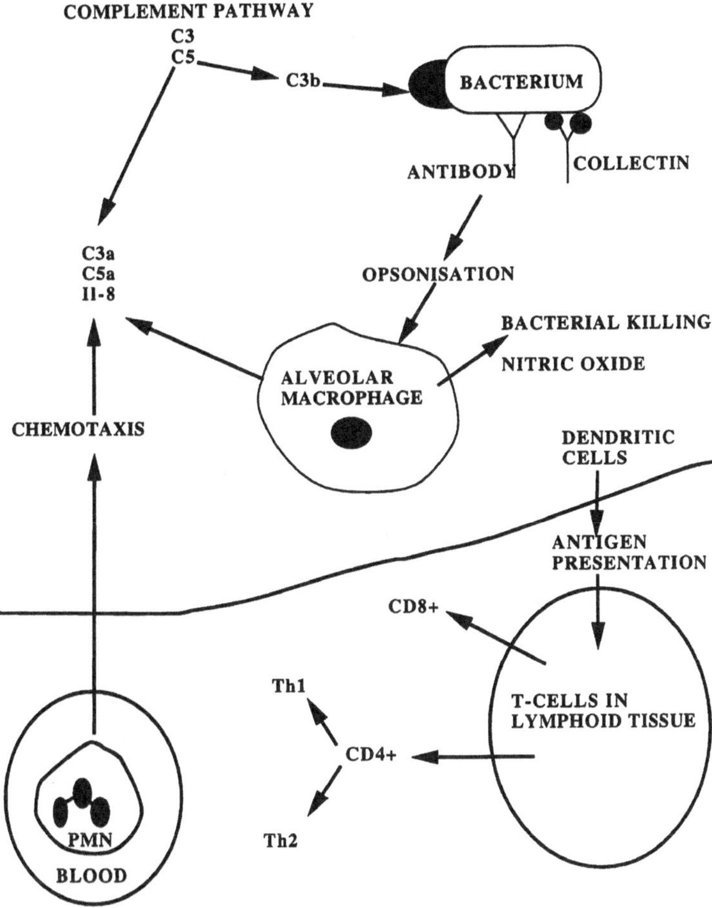

Figure 1. An outline of the immune response in lung. Bacteria entering the lung can be opsonized by complement components, collectins or antibody. The primary cell involved in immunity in the lung is the macrophage. Alveolar macrophages take up and kill bacteria. They also produce a range of cytokines which can be chemotactic (IL-8) or activate other cells (interferon-γ). Chemotaxic factors such as IL-8 and complement components result in the recruitment of polymorphonuclear cells (PMNS) from the bloodstream. Antigen draining from the lungs is presented to T cells which are either CD4 or CD8. CD4 cells will be activated by antigen presented in the context of MHC class II while CD8 cells are activated via the MHC class I pathway. CD4 cells can be further divided into Th1 and Th2 types. The Th1/Th2 profile will be determined by the cytokine milieu at the time of T cell activation.

ciated with pathogens in the lung are presented to T cells in associated lymphoid tissue by dendritic or other antigen-presenting cells. This leads to the production of adaptive immunity with the generation of antibody and specific cell-mediated immunity. Defects in all these processes are known and their study allows us to define their importance in the protection of the lung from infection. There are various transgenic models of infection, although these have not been widely used in the study of lung infections.

I use selected examples to define what systems are available for the study of each stage of the host-pathogen interaction in the lung.

3. Naturally Occurring Immune Deficiencies

3.1. The Complement Pathway

Many complement deficiencies exist in both humans and animal models of infection. There are genetic deficiencies in all components of the classic and alternative pathways except for factor B of the alternative pathway.

3.1.1. The role of complement C3: The most crucial component of the complement pathway is C3, and deficiency renders both classic and alternative pathways inactive. The role of C3 can be investigated in a variety of systems which include analysis in inherited complement deficiency, complement depletion models such as animals treated with cobra venom factor or transgenic knock-out mice.

Complement component C3 is important in protection from encapsulated bacteria such as *Streptococcus pneumoniae* (the pneumococcus). Animals depleted of C3 by treatment with cobra venom factor (CvF) show decreased ability to phagocytose encapsulated as opposed to non-encapsulated pneumococci. Using formalized pneumococci sensitized with rabbit anti-capsular antibody, it was shown that C1, C4, C2 and C3 are needed for optimal phagocytosis. There is complete abolition of phagocytosis in human serum depleted of C3. If guinea-pigs are depleted of C3 with CvF, clearance of pneumococci after intravenous injection is significantly delayed and the organisms replicate to the point of sustained bacteraemia leading to death. Depletion of C4 in these animals has no effect.

Studies performed using CvF-treated animals have shown that complement is one of the major factors contributing to the early clearance of pneumococci from the lungs [1, 4, 5]. After intratracheal challenge of depleted animals with pneumococci the clearance of organisms is reduced but not abolished. Mechanisms of clearance that do not involve complement, such as antibody-mediated clearance or surface phagocytosis, may be responsible for this effect [6]. After the initial stages of clearance, C3-depleted animals develop a more extensive pneumonia, more viable bacteria per lung and higher incidence and level of bacteraemia [5, 7, 8].

C3 deficiency is a rare condition in humans and can occur by a variety of mechanisms (Table 1). Inherited C3 deficiency can result from decreased mRNA levels of the C3 gene in some cases caused by abberant splicing of the RNA, decreased secretion of C3 or production of altered C3 [9]. There can be homozygous inheritance of a null gene on chromosome 19 which leads to decreased synthesis from the liver and levels of C3 ar 0.1% of control levels. This deficiency does not seem to affect extrahepatic

Table 1. Complement deficiencies of humans

Component	Defective function	Infectious disease
C1q, C1r, C1s	Activation of classic pathway	Susceptible to pyogenic infections
C4	Activation of classic pathway	Susceptible to pyogenic infections
C2	Activation of classic pathway	Susceptible to pyogenic infections
C3	Activation of classic and alternative pathways Defective opsonization and phagocytosis	Frequent and fatal pyogenic infections
Factor D	Activation of alternative pathway	Susceptible to pyogenic infections
Factor P	Activation of alternative pathway	Frequent pyogenic infection
C5, C6, C7, C8, C9	Membrane attack complex	Enhanced susceptibility to neisseria infection

synthesis of C3, so synthesis of complement components in the lung would not be affected. There can also be a genetic deficiency of regulatory factor I, which leads to continual activation of the alternative complement pathway and immediate degradation of C3 and factor B. Levels of C3 in these patients are 5% of normal and factor B is undetectable [10]. These patients suffer from recurrent pneumococcal and meningococcal infection. Aquired C3 deficiency has been implicated in increased susceptibility to infection in patients with alcoholic cirrhosis [11]. In this study there was a clear correlation between decreased levels of C3 and infection and the majority were pneumonia, caused in the main by *S. pneumoniae.*

There is a rarity of animal models for C3 deficiency, although C3-deficient guinea-pigs have been described. In these animals, the nucleotide sequence of the cDNA is normal, levels of C3 mRNA are normal, both pro-C3 and C3 proteins are secreted but the C3 lacks the reactive thiol-ester bond [12]. It has been suggested that there may be a deficiency in a specific enzyme required for the formation of the C3 thiol ester. However, whatever the cause, these animals are functionally deficient in C3.

A colony of beagles completely deficient in C3 has also been described [13, 14]. DNA sequence analysis of the C3 gene from the deficient animals showed that there is frameshift mutation which leads to a premature stop codon [15]. This mutation results in decreased levels of normal sized mRNA. The animals have an increased susceptibility to infection, including pneumonia.

3.1.2. The role of C5: Mice with a genetic deficiency of C5 are unable to clear *S. pneumoniae* from the lungs [16]. The role of C5 appears to be related to its role in generating chemotactic activity and a local inflammatory reaction. The bronchoalveolar lavage fluid of C5-deficient mice fails to generate as much chemotactic activity as that from C5-sufficient mice. Moreover, the number of polymorphonuclear leukocytes in the alveoli of C5-deficient mice is less than in C5-sufficient mice. However, this is in contrast to mice that have a defined deletion of the C5a receptor [17], and an increased recruitment of neutrophils after challenge with *Pseudomonas aeruginosa*.

3.1.3. Complement receptors: Complement receptor 3 (CR3) plays an important role in immune defence. The importance of CR3 in host defence against infection has been demonstrated by descriptions of patients with deficiencies in this receptor. Children with CR3 deficiency develop severe periodontitis, persistent leukocytosis, and fatal bacterial infections with organisms such as *Escherichia coli*, *P. aeruginosa* and *Salmonella* spp. [18 – 21]. The nature of the infections seen suggests that CR3 may play less of a role in primary defence against respiratory pathogens common in patients deficient in C3 (e.g. the pneumococcus).

3.2. Immunoglobulin

Studies of deficient patients suggest that immunoglobulin plays a critical role in protecting the mucosal surface from bacterial infection. Patients with panhypogammaglobulinaemia suffer from recurrent infections of the respiratory tract. Specific the immunoglobulins deficiencies in IgG2 and IgG4 [22] and IgG2 or IgG3 with IgA deficiency [23] also predispose to recurrent respiratory tract infections. The contribution of the different immunoglobulins to protection from infection may differ according to the site of the respiratory tract. For example, although IgA predominates in the upper respiratory tract [24], the major immunoglobulin in the lower respiratory tract is IgG [25]. Immunization can enhance antibacterial defences in the lower respiratory tract in animal models of bacterial infection. Immunization enhances the clearance of *P. aeruginosa*, *Proteus mirabelis* and *Haemophilus influenzae* from the lung [26–30], which correlated with the appearance of specific antibodies in the bronchoalveolar lavage [26–30]. Antibody derived from the serum contributes to the protection because it has been shown that bacterial proliferation in the lung can be prevented by passive systemic administration of IgG [30]. The permeability of the alveolar capillary barrier is known to change during bacterial infection and this may allow leakage of serum proteins into the air spaces. However, the local production of IgG also increases in the presence of bacterial colonization [31] and this may also play a role.

Immunoglobulin A is the major immunoglobulin found in the lung [24] and IgA deficiency is the most common primary immune deficiency [32]. IgA is present on the mucosa as secretory IgA, which is a dimer bound to secretory component. It has been suggested that secretory IgA binds to bacteria to inhibit their motility, or adherence to the mucosa. The fact that mucosal IgA is dimeric makes its role is host defence more difficult to understand. The lack of a free Fc domain precludes interaction with Fc receptors on phagocytic cells and may even serve to interfere with opsonization by other antibody classes. The role of IgA in protection of the lung remains an open question. Levels of IgA certainly increase after mucosal stimulation with antigen [32a] and the fact that mucosal pathogens produce proteases specific for human IgA [32b] also suggests that this immunoglobulin has a role to play. Immunoglobulin-deficient mice [33] may allow further investigation into the role of IgA in pulmonary infection.

4. Transgenic Mice in the Study of Lung Infection

The construction of transgenic mice allows defined mutations to be introduced into the genome to investigate the role of a particular gene product. Since the first generation of transgenic mice in 1980 [34], there has been a explosion in the use of these approaches in biomedical research. However, despite the impact of transgenic technology in many areas of biomedical research, its application to the study of the pathogenesis of lung infection still remains in its infancy. Transgenic mice can be produced by several different methods and there are several excellent reviews on the technical details [35–37]. Many lines of transgenic mice have been generated and their application of transgenic models for the study of lung biology and disease has been reviewed [38]. Some of the knock-out mice used in the study of lung infection are summarized in Table 2.

Table 2. Transgenic animal models used in the study of lung infection

Gene	Respiratory pathogen	Effect	References
SP-A	Group B streptococci	Exacerbation	[50]
Complement C3	Group B streptococci (systemic challenge)	Exacerbation	[51]
Complement C5a receptor	*Pseudomonas aeruginosa*	Exacerbation	[17]
IL-4	*C. trachomatis*	None	[52]
IFN-γ	*C. trachomatis*	Increased resistance	[52]
	M. tuberculosis	Exacerbation	[66]
	S. pneumoniae	Exacerbation	[64]
IgM	*M. tuberculosis*	Exacerbation	[63]
Perforin	*M. tuberculosis*	No effect	[59]
MHC class I	*M. tuberculosis*	Exacerbation	[58]
	C. trachomatis	No effect	[52]
MHC class II	*M. tuberculosis*	Exacerbation	[57]
	C. trachomatis	Exacerbation	[52]

4.1. Collectins

Collectins are a subgroup of the mammalian C-type lectin family and include surfactant proteins SP-A and SP-D and the serum proteins mannose-binding protein (MBP) and conglutinin. These lectins are structurally similar to the first component of the complement pathway (C1q) and are thought to play a role in host defence as part of the innate immunity [39–42]. Children deficient in MBP are susceptible to recurrent infection [43] and SP-A levels are reduced in patients with bacterial pneumonia [44] and children with respiratory failure [45]. SP-A gene transcription may also be reduced by tumour necrosis factor α (TNF-α) during the inflammatory process [46], which may predispose individuals to pneumonia and sepsis.

SP-A is produced by alveolar type II cells and Clara cells in the lung. The lectin binds to macrophages through specific cell receptors [47] and this enhances the binding of serum-opsonized *S. aureus* and non-serum-opsonized *S. aureus* and *E. coli* to alveolar macrophages [48, 49]. The binding of Sp-A to the carbohydrates present on *S. pneumoniae* and *S. aureus* is mediated through the lectin domain present in the C-terminal part of the molecule [41].

There is compelling evidence that SP-A binds to respiratory pathogens *in vitro* but its role *in vivo* is less clear. To assess the role of SP-A *in vivo*, SP-A knock-out mice have been generated [50]. When these animals were challenged by intratracheal instillation in group B streptococci, pulmonary infiltration was more severe and was associated with increased numbers of bacteria in the lung. The numbers of macrophages were similar in knock-out and control animals but the numbers of bacteria associated with macrophages was were decreased. Systemic dissemination of bacteria was greater in the knock-out mice compared with the controls.

4.2. The Complement System

4.2.1. C3 and C4: The first published studies of the construction of transgenic mice deficient in C3 or C4 involved the examination of the role of these components in innate and aquired immunity to group B streptococcal (GBS) infection [51]. This study used a systemic model of infection and showed that the alternative pathway is sufficient to mediate effective opsonophagocytosis and protective immunity to GBS in the presence of specific antibody. The increased susceptibility to infection of non-immune animals deficient in either C3 or C4 suggested that the classic pathway plays an essential role in host defence against GBS infection in the absence of specific immunity. The role of C3 and C4 in protection against pulmonary infection has not yet been investigated in these animals.

4.2.2 C5a receptor: The C5 molecule and its degradation products are important chemotaxins in the lung during inflammatory responses to

S. aureus, *S. pneumoniae*, *H. influenzae* and *P. aeruginosa*. The degradation product C5a has an important role in the inflammatory process as a vasodilator and a chemotaxin. The importance of the C5a chemoattractant receptor in mucosal defence has been demonstrated by Hopken et al. [17]. The murine C5a receptor (C5aR) gene was deleted by homologous recombination and when C5aR-deficient mice were challenged with *P. aeruginosa* the majority succumbed to the infection whereas none of the control animals died. The effect was dependent on challenge with viable bacteria because C5aR-deficient mice survived challenge with formalin- or heat-killed bacteria. Analysis of bacerial counts in the lungs of animals showed that the C5a receptor is essential for the clearance of bacteria from the lung. When the inflammatory response was examined it was clear that the number of neutrophils in the lungs of C5aR-deficient mice was higher. This is contrary to what would be expected if the function of C5a as a chemoattractant was critical and suggests that the recruitment of neutrophils is not dependent on C5a. It was also shown that there was increased vascular leak in the C5aR-deficient mice. Therefore, despite the large neutrophil influx and increased permeability of the alveolar capillary barrier, C5aR-deficient mice are unable to clear *P. aeruginosa* and there is progression to pulmonary injury and death.

C5aR-deficient mice were also susceptible to infection with other Gram-positive bacteria such as *Streptococcus* and *Staphylococcus* spp. after clearance of a sublethal infection with *P. aeruginosa.*

It is interesting to note from this study that, when mice were challenged with *P. aeruginosa* via the intraperitoneal route, both wild-type and C5aR-deficient mice cleared the infection within 24 h. Thus, the C5a receptor appears to be critical at the mucosal surface of the lung but not in the peritoneum.

4.3. Immunoglobulin

Transgenic mice with a mutation that deletes B cells have been constructed by targeted disruption of the membrane exon of the immunoglobulin μ chain [33]. These mice have not been used extensively to investigate the role of immunoglobulin in protection from lung infection. Studies using these mice have shown that immunoglobulins, including IgA, are not an absolute requirement for successful host defence in a model of pneumonitis caused by secondary infection with *Chlamydia trachomatis* [52].

4.4. T Cells

T cells are the central mediators of inflammation and recognize antigen through the T cell receptor (TCR). The TCR is a heterodimer composed of either an α and β chain or a γ and δ chain. Most (90%) T cells in humans and mouse are of the $\alpha\beta$ type. Transgenic mice lacking chains have been constructed so that mice are available which lack either $\alpha\beta$ T cells or $\gamma\delta$ T cells [53, 54]. Transgenic mice lacking CD4$^+$ T cell function (major histocompatability complex (MHC) class II function) [55] and CD8$^+$ T cell function (MHC class I function) have been generated [56]. To recognize a variety of antigens, a broad repertoire of TCR is required. The generation of this repertoire involves gene rearrangements via the recombinase-activating genes *RAG-1* and *RAG-2*. Deletions in *RAG-1* or *RAG-2* result in total loss of T and B cells [53, 54]. The mice can be used to define the roles played by different T cell subsets in the pathogenesis of infection. In the context of respiratory infection, these mice have been used mainly in the study of tuberculosis (see below).

4.5. Cytokines

Communication between cells of the immune system is mediated largely by cytokines. The nature of an immune response (humoral or cellular) is determined by the cytokine profile; $\alpha\beta$ T cells are divided into CD4 and CD8 phenotypes and CD4 T cells can be further divided into Th1 and Th2 (T-helper) types. Th1 cells promote cellular immunity and the production of interferon-γ (IFN-γ) and interleukin 2 (IL-2) while Th2 cells produce cytokines that promote humoral immunity, such as IL-4. The macrophage product IL-12 and the T cell products IFN-γ and IL-2 promote Th1 activities whereas the macrophage products IL-1 and IL-10 and the T cell product IL-4 promote Th2 activity. The use of cytokine or cytokine receptor knock-out mice allows this balance to be shifted in the Th1 or Th2 direction. However, although a range of cytokine- and cytokine receptor-deficient mice is now available, they have so far only been used in limited studies of pulmonary infection (see Table 2). Perhaps the most use of these mice has been made in the study of infection with *Mycobacterium tuberculosis*.

5. Specific Examples of Genetic Models Used to Study Lung Infection

5.1. Mycobacterium tuberculosis

The use of genetic models has greatly facilitated the study of pathogenesis of infection with *M. tuberculosis*. Studies with MHC class I- and class II-deficient mutants have been used to define the role of MHC restriction in infection with *M. tuberculosis*. Both MHC deficiencies dramatically impair immunity to *M. tuberculosis* infection [57, 58]. Interestingly, granulomas in MHC class I-deficient mice become necrotic and resemble the lesions from patients who have active tuberculosis (TB) [58]. The fact that MHC class I is essential for resistance to *M. tuberculosis* indicates an involvement of CD8+ cells. It is intruiging that mice with a disrupted perforin gene (perforin is involved in cytoxicity by CD8 cells) do not show any change in resistance to *M. tuberculosis*, suggesting that either perforin does not contribute to immunity to TB or that there is another pathway that can compensate for the lack of perforin [59]. During the course of TB, before the development of a specific T cell response, IFN-γ is produced (probably by natural killer (NK) cells or a subset of $\gamma\delta$ T cells). Production of IFN-γ by NK cells is promoted by IL-12 which is produced by infected macrophages [60]. IFN-γ and TNF-α stimulate the secretion of IL-12 by infected macrophages, thus creating a positive feedback loop for macrophage activation [61].

Administration of IL-12 to mice with TB prolonged survival of the animals, whereas the protective effect of IL-12 was not seen in transgenic mice defective for the production of IFN-γ [62]. Thus, the use of transgenic mice in the study of TB has shown that both CD4 and CD8 T cells are required for immunity and that immunity is not dependent on the production of perforin by CD8+ T cells. Protective immunity is provided by IL-12 and this is dependent on the ability to produce IFN-γ. It has also been suggested that B cells and/or antibody may play a role in immunity to *M. tuberculosis* because trangenic mice deficient for B cells and antibody production (μ chain knockouts) are significantly more susceptible to the development of disease [63]. It may be, therefore, that antibodies and B cells play a crucial role in antigen presentation in TB.

5.2. Streptococcus pneumoniae

Although INF-γ is critical to host defence against many intracellular bacteria (as for *M. tuberculosis* described above) it is now clear that it also regulates inflammatory responses to extracellular bacteria. IFN-γ plays an important role in the protection of mice from the extracellular pathogen *S. pneumoniae* [64]. INF-γ levels in the lung do not rise in response to pneumococcal infection and infection of IFN knock-out mice results in greater levels of bacteraemia. It may be that IFN-γ is having its effect in the serum rather than in the lung. It would be informative to evaluate bacterial growth in the lung and antibacterial activity of alveolar macrophages against *S. pneumoniae* in these animal models.

5.3. Chlamydia trachomatis

Genetic models have been used to probe the basis for humoral and cellular immunity in secondary infection caused by *C. trachomatis*. Mice deficient in CD4 T cells, CD8 T cells, B cells, IFN-γ or IL-4 have been used to define the nature of the immune response [52]. Resistance to infection with

C. trachomatis is heavily dependent on CD4 T cells and B cells are not essential for the development of immunity, indicating that antibody and antigen presentation by B cells is irrelevant in infection of the lung with this pathogen. It is possible that B-cell-deficient mice compensate for their deficiency by an increase in cell-mediated immune reponses (IFN-γ and TNF-α) as has been described in other models for B-cell-deficiency [65]. IL-4 appears to have no role in the development of protective immunity to *C. trachomatis*, suggesting that immunity is mediated by Th1-based mechanisms. Interestingly, however, mice deficient in IFN-γ are more resistant to infection with *C. trachomatis*, showing that IFN-γ is not an absolute requirement for resistance and implying the presence of a very effective compensatory system for overcoming the lack of IFN-γ.

6. Conclusion

There is now a range of genetic tools available for the investigation of infection in the lung. A wide range of genetically deficient animals exist including complement, antibody, a whole range of cytokines and cytokine receptors, T cells ($CD4^+$ and $CD8^+$), T cell receptors, surfactant proteins and other components of the immune system. The availability of these models, in conjunction with the availability of bacterial pathogen genome sequences that facilitate the construction of bacterial mutants, will allow study of the interaction of the host with pathogen during pulmonary infection. The study of respiratory infections using these approaches, however, still in its infancy.

References

1 Gross GN, Rehm SR, Pierce AK (1978) The effect of complement depletion on lung clearance of bacteria. *J Clin Invest* 21: 373–378
2 Robertson J, Cladwell JR, Castle JR, Waldman RH (1976) Evidence for the presence of components of the alternative (properdin) pathway of complement activation in respiratory secretions. *J Immunol* 117: 900–903
3 Coonrod JD, Yoneda K (1981) Complement and opsonins in alveolar secretions and serum of rats with pneumonia due to *Streptococcus pneumoniae*. *Rev Infect Dis* 3: 310–322
4 Heidbrink PJ, Toews GB, Gross GN, Pierce AK (1982) Mechanisms of complement mediated clearance of baccteria from the murine lung. *Am Rev Respir Dis* 125: 517–520
5 Coonrod JD, Yoneda K (1982) Comparative role of complement in pneumococcal and Staphylococcal pneumonia. *Infect Immun* 37: 1270–1277
6 Wood WB Jr (1951) Studies on the cellular immunology of acute bacterial infections. *Harvey Lect* 47: 72–98
7 Bakker-Woudenberg IAJM, deJong-Hoenderop JYT, Michel MF (1979) Efficacy of antimicrobial therapy in rat pneumonia: effects of impaired phagocytosis. *Infect Immun* 25: 366–375
8 Guckian JC, Christiansen GD, Fine DP (1980) The role of opsonins in recovery from experimental pneumococcal pneumonia. *J Infect Dis* 142: 175–190
9 Botto M, Fong KY, So AE, Rudge A, Walport MJ (1990) Molecular basis of hereditary C3 deficiency. *J Clin Invest* 86: 1158–1163

10 Alper CA, Abramson N, Johnson RB Jr, Jandel JH, Rosen FS (1970) Increased susceptibility to infection associated with abnormalities of complement-mediated functions and of the third component of complement (C3). *N Engl J Med* 282: 349–354
11 Homann C, Varming K, Hogasen K, Mollnes TE, Gradudal N, Thomsen AC, Garrod P (1997) Aquired C3 deficiency in patients with alcoholic cirrhosis predisposes to infection and increased mortality. *Gut* 40: 544–549
12 Auerbach HS, Burger R, Dodds A, Colten HR (1990) Molecular basis of complement C3 deficiency in guinea pigs. *J Clin Invest* 86: 96–106
13 Winkelstein JA, Cork LC, Griffin DE, Adams RJ, Price DL (1981) Genetically determined deficiency of the third component of complement in the dog. *Science* 212: 1169–1173
14 O'Neil KM, Ochs HD, Heller SR, Cork LC, Morris JM, Winkelstein JA (1988) Role of C3 in humoral immunity. *J Immunol* 140: 1939–1945
15 Ameratunga R, Winkelstein JA, Brody L, Binns M, Cork LC, Colombani P, Valle D (1998) Molecular analysis of the third component of canine complement (C3) and identification of the mutation responsible for hereditary canine C3 deficiency. *J Immunol* 160: 2824–2830
16 Toews GB, Vial WC (1984) The role of C5 in polymorphonuclear leukocyte recritment in response to *Streptococcus pneumoniae. Annu Rev Respir Dis* 129: 82–86
17 Hopken UE, Lu B, Gerard NP, Gerard C (1996) The C5a chemoattractant receptor mediates mucosal defence to infection. *Nature* 383: 86–89
18 Anderson DC, Schmalsteig FC, Kohl S, Arnaout MA, Hughes BJ, Towse MF, Bafoney GJ, Brinkley BR, Dickey WD, Abramson JS et al. (1984) Abnormalities of polymorphonuclear leukocyte function associated with a heritable deficiency of high molecular weight surface glycoprotein (gp138): common relationship to diminished cell adherence. *J Clin Invest* 74: 546–555
19 Arnaout MA, Pitt J, Cohen HJ, Melamed J, Rosen FS, Colten HR (1982) Deficiency in a granulocyte-membrane glycoprotein (gp150) in a boy with recurrent bacterial infections. *N Engl J Med* 305: 693–699
20 Bowen TJ, Ochs HD, Altman LC, Price HC, Van Epps DE, Brautigan DC, Rosin RE, Perkins WD, Babior BM, Klebanoff SJ et al. (1982) Severe recurrent bacterial infections associated with defective adherance and chemotaxis in two patients with neutrophils deficient in a cell-associated glycoprotein. *J Pediatr* 101: 932–940
21 Crowley CA, Curnutte JT, Rosin RE, Andre-Schwartz J, Gallin JI, Kiemphar M, Snyderman R, Southwick F, Stossel TP, Babior BM (1980) An inherited abnormality of neutrophil adhesion: its genetic transmission and its association with the missing protein. *N Engl J Med* 302: 1163–1168
22 Oxelius V-A (1974) Chronic infections in a family with hereditary deficiency of IgG2 and IgG4. *Clin Exp Immunol* 17: 19–24
23 Bjorkander J, Bake B, Oxelius V-A, Hanson LA (1985) Impaired lung function in patients with IgA deficiency and low levels of IgG2 or IgG3. *N Engl J Med* 313: 720–724
24 Morgan KL, Hussein AM, Newby TJ, Bourne FJ (1980) Quantification and origin of the immunoglobulins in procine respiratory tract secretions. *Immunology* 41: 729–736
25 Merrill WW, Naegel GP, Olchowski JJ, Reynolds HY (1985) Immunoglobulin subclass proteins in serum and lavage fluid of normal subjects: quantitation and comparison with immunoglobulin A and E. *Am Rev Respir Dis* 131: 584–587
26 Jakab GJ (1976) Factors influencing the immune enhancement of intrapulmonary bactericidal mechanisms. *Infect Immun* 14: 389–398
27 Dunn MM, Toews GB, Hart D, Pierce AK (1985) The effects of systemic immunization on pulmonary clearance of *Pseudomonas aeruginosa. Am Rev Respir Dis* 131: 426–431
28 Hansen EJ, Hart DA, McGehee JL (1988) Immune enhancement of pulmonary clearance of nontypable *Haemophilus influenzae. Infect Immun* 56: 182–190
29 Pennington JE, Hickey WF, Blackwood LL (1981) Active immunization with lipopolysaccharide Pseudomonas antigen for chronic Pseudomonas bronchopneumonia in guinea pigs. *J Clin Invest* 68: 1140–1148
30 Toews GB, Hart DA, Hansen EJ (1985) Effect of systemic immunisation on pulmonary clearance of *Haemophilus influenzae* type b. *Infect Immun* 48: 343–349
31 Hill SL, Mitchell JL, Burnett D, Stockley RA (1998) IgG subclasses in sputum from patients with bronchiectasis. *Thorax* 53: 463–468
32 Uderdown BJ, Schiff JM (1986) Immunoglobulin A: strategic defence at the mucosal surface: *Annu Rev Immunol* 4: 389–417

32a Orga PL, Karzou DT, Righthand F, MacGillivray M (1968) Immunoglobulin responses in serum and secretions after immunisation with live and inactivated polio vaccine and natural infection. *N Engl J Med* 279: 893–900

32b Plant AG (1983) The IgA proteases of pathogenic bacteria. *Ann Rev Microbiol* 37: 603–622

33 Kitamura D, Roes J, Kuhm R, Rajewsky K (1991) A B cell-deficient mouse by targeted disruption of the membrane exon of the immunoglobulin μ chain gene. *Nature* 350: 423–426

34 Gordon JW, Scangos GA, Plotkin DJ, Barbosa JA, Ruddle FH (1980) Genetic transformation of mouse embryos by microinjection of purified DNA. *Proc Natl Acad Sci USA* 77: 7380–7384

35 Hogan B, Constantini F, Lacy E (1986) *Manipulating the mouse embryo: A laboratory manual.* Cold Spring Harbor, New York

36 Field LJ (1993) Transgenic mice in cardiovascular research. *Annu Re Physiol* 55: 97–114

37 Gordon JW, Ruddle FH (1983) Gene transfer into mouse embryos: production of transgenic mice by pronuclear infection. *Methods Enzymol* 101: 411–433

38 Ho Y-S (1994) Transgenic models for the study of lung biology and disease. *Am J Physiol* 10: L319–L353

39 Friis-Christiansen P, Thiel S, Svehag S-E, Dessau R, Svendsen R, Andersen O, Lauren SB, Jensenius JC (1990) *In vivo* and *in vitro* antibacterial activity of conglutinin, a mammalian plant lectin. *Scand J Immunol* 31: 453–460

40 Ezekowitz RAB, Kuhlman M, Groopman JE, Byrn RA (1989) A human-serum mannose-binding protein inhibits *in vitro* infection by the human immunodeficiency virus. *J Exp Med* 169: 185–196

41 McNeeley TB, Coonrod JD (1993) Comparison of the opsonic activity of human surfactant protein A for *Staphylococcus aureus* and *Streptococcus pneumoniae* with rabbit and human macrophages. *J Infect Dis* 167: 91–97

42 Kuan SF, Rust K, Crouch E (1992) Interactions of surfactant protein D with bacterial lipopolysaccharide. *J Clin Invest* 90: 97–106

43 Super M, Thiel JS, Lu J, Levinsky RJ, Turner MW (1989) Association of low levels of mannan binding protein with a common defect of opsonisation. *Lancet ii*: 1236–1239

44 Baughman RP, Sternberg RI, Hull W, Buchsbaum JA, Whitsett J (1993) Decreased surfactant protein A in patients with bacterial pneumonia. *Am Rev Respir Dis* 147: 653 – 657

45 LeVine AM, Lotze A, Stanley S, Stroud C, O'Donnell R, Whitsett J, Pollack MM (1996) Surfactant content in children with inflammatory lung disease. *Crit Care Med* 24: 1062– 1067

46 Wispe JR, Clark JC, Warner BB, Fajardo D, Hull WE, Holtzman RB, Whitsett JA (1990) Tumor necrosis factor alpha inhibitx expression of pulmonary surfactant protein. *J Clin Invest* 86: 1954–1960

47 Pison U, Wright JR, Hawgood S (1992) Specific binding of surfactant protein apoprotein SP-A to rat alveolar macrophages. *Am J Physiol* 262: L412–L417

48 Manz-Keinke H, Plattner H, Schlepper-Schafer J (1992) Lung surfactant protein A (SP-A) enhances serum independent phagocytosis of bacteria by alveolar macrophages. *Eur J Cell Biol* 57: 95–100

49 Van Iwaarden F, Welmers B, Verhoef J, Haagsman HP, van Golde LMG (1990) Pulmonary surfactant protein A enhances the host defence mechanism of rat alveolar macrophages. *Am J Respir Cell Mol Biol* 2: 91–98

50 LeVine AM, Bruno MD, Huelsman KM, Ross GF, Whitsett JA, Korfhagen TR (1997) Surfactant protein A-deficient mice are susceptible to group B streptococcal infection. *J Immunol* 158: 4336–4340

51 Wessels MR, Butko P, Ma M, Warren HB, Lage AL, Carroll MC (1995) Studies of group B streptococcal infection in mice deficient in complement component C3 or C4 demonstrate an essential role for complement in both inate and aquired immunity. *Proc Natl Acad Sci USA* 92: 11490–11494

52 Williams DM, Grubbs BG, Pack E, Kelly K, Rank RG (1997) Humoral and cellular immunity in secondary infection due to murine *Chlamydia trachomatis. Infect Immun* 65: 2876–2882

53 Mombaerts P, Clarke AR, Hooper ML, Tonegawa S (1991) Creation of a large genomic deletion at the T cell antigen receptor beta-subunit locus in mouse embryonic stem-cells by gene targetting. *Proc Natl Acad Sci USA* 88: 3084–3087

54 Itohara S, Mombaerts P, Lafaille J, Iacomi J, Nelson J, Clarke AR, Hooper ML, Farr A, Tonegawa S (1993) T-cell receptor delta-gene mutant mice-independet generation of alpha-beta T-cells and programmed rearrangements of gamma-delta TCR genes. *Cell* 72: 337–348

55 Grusby MJ, Johnson RS, Papaioannou VE, Glimcher LH (1991) Depletion of CD4$^+$ T cells in major histocompatability complex II-deficient mice. *Science* 253: 1417–1420

56 Koller BH, Smithies O (1989) Inactivating the β_2-microglobulin locus in mouse embryonic stem cells by homologous recombination. *Proc Natl Acad Sci USA* 86: 8932–8935

57 Kaufmann SHE, Ladel CH (1994) Application of knock-out mice to the experimental analysis of infections with bacteria and protozoa. *Trends Microbiol* 2: 235–242

58 Flynn JL, Goldstein MM, Triebold KJ, Koller BBRB (1992) Major histocompatiability complex class-I restricted T cells are required for resistance to *Mycobacterium tuberculosis* infection. *Proc Natl Acad Sci USA* 89: 12013–12017

59 Laochumroomvorapong P, Wang J, Chau-Ching L, Ye W, Moreira AL, Elkon KB, Freedman VH, Kaplan G (1997) Perforin, a cytotoxic molecule which mediates cell necrosis, is not required for the control of early mycobacterial infection in mice. *Infect Immun* 65: 127–132

60 Flesch IE, Hess JH, Huang S, Aguet M, Rothe J, Bluethmann H, Kaufmann SHE (1995) Early interleukin 12 production by macrophages in response to mycobacterial infection depends on interferon γ and tumor necrosis factor α. *J Exp Med* 181: 1615–1621

61 Fulton SA, Johnson JM, Wolf SF, Sieburth DS, Bloom WH (1996) Interleukin-12 production by human monocytes infected with *Mycobacterium tuberculosis*: Role of phagocytosis. *Infect Immun* 64: 2523–2531

62 Cooper AM, Roberts AD, Rhoades ER, Callahan JE, Getzy DM, Orme IM (1995) The role of interleukin-12 in aquired immunity to *Mycobacterium tuberculosis* infection. *Immunology* 84: 423–432

63 Vordmeier HM, Kenkataprasad N, Harris DP, Ivanyi J (1996) Increase of tuberculous infection in the organs of B-cell-deficient mice. *Clin Exp Immunol* 106: 312–316

64 Rubins JB, Pomeroy C (1997) Role of gamma interferon in the pathogenesis of bacteremic pneumococcal pneumonia. *Infect Immun* 65: 2975–2977

65 Taylor-Robinson AW, Phillips RS (1996) Reconstitution of B-cell depleted mice with B-cells restores the Th2-type immune response during *Plasmodium chabaudi chaubdi* infection. *Infect Immun* 64: 366–370

66 Cooper AM, Dalton DK, Stewart TA, Griffin JP, Russell DG, Orme IM (1993) Disseminated tuberculosis in interferon-gamma gene-disrupted mice. *J Exp Med* 178: 2243–2247

Molecular Biology of the Lung
Vol. 1: Emphysema and Infection
ed. by R. A. Stockley

CHAPTER 9
Genetics of Bacteria: Role in Pathogenesis of Infection of the Respiratory Tract

Karin L. Klingman[1] and Timothy F. Murphy[2]

[1] *State University of New York at Buffalo, Erie County Medical Center, Buffalo, NY, USA*
[2] *State University of New York at Buffalo, Buffalo VANC, Buffalo, NY, USA*

1. Introduction

A strong relationship exists between specific bacterial species and the ability to cause infection of the lower respiratory tract in human hosts with particular underlying conditions. For example, *Pseudomonas aeruginosa* causes potentially devastating infections in people with cystic fibrosis. Chronic bronchitis is strongly associated with infections caused by *Haemophilus influenzae*, *Branhamella catarrhalis*, and *Streptococcus pneumoniae*. Pneumonia caused by *Staphylococcus aureus* is seen after influenza but is rarely seen in other clinical settings.

The striking relationships between specific bacterial respiratory pathogens and particular hosts indicates that a high degree of specificity exists in the interaction between the two. The application of powerful molecular techniques to studies of bacterial pathogenesis has led to the identification and initial characterization of some of the surface bacterial molecules which mediate various steps in the pathogenesis of infection and account for the specificity observed in the relationships between pathogen and host.

2. Nontypable *Haemophilus influenzae*

Nontypable *H. influenzae* colonizes the lower respiratory tract of adults with chronic obstructive pulmonary disease (COPD) and causes periodic episodes of lower respiratory tract infections in these patients [1]. The lower airways of healthy adults remain free of colonization with nontypable *H. influenzae*. Of interest, *H. influenzae* neither colonizes nor naturally causes infection in other mammalian species; therefore, *H. influenzae* is an exclusively human pathogen. These observations illustrate the high degree of the specificity of the interaction of nontypable *H. influenzae* with the human respiratory tract in patients with COPD.

Studies of the molecular mechanisms of pathogenesis of infection caused by nontypable *H. influenzae* and the human immune response to the bacterium have led to the identification of several classes of surface molecules, which account for the remarkable ability of nontypable *H. influenzae* to cause persistent colonization and intermittent infection of the lower respiratory tract of adults with COPD.

In this chapter, we use nontypable *H. influenzae* as a model human respiratory tract pathogen to discuss four concepts dealing with molecular mechanisms of bacterial pathogenesis:

1. Expression of redundant adhesin molecules with a variety of binding specificities conferring the ability to bind to host cells.
2. Features of a major outer membrane protein which accounts for the ability of the bacterium to persist in the respiratory tract, including a high degree of antigenic heterogeneity among strains, the presence of an immunodominant epitope, and the ability to undergo mutations under immune selective pressure.
3. Phase variation and sialylation of surface glycolipid molecules and the concept of molecular mimicry of host molecules.
4. The availability of the sequence of the genome of a strain of *H. influenzae* and the effect of this information on approaches to the study of molecular pathogenesis.

3. Expression of Multiple Adhesion Molecules

The paradigm of infection can be broadly thought to occur in three steps: attachment of the organism to the surface of the host, colonization, and invasion. A respiratory tract pathogen must be able to survive in the respiratory tract secretions, and then colonize by adhering to the surface of the epithelial cells and replicating there. The mechanisms of bacterial adherence to the respiratory epithelial cell have been elucidated only in the last 10 years.

Adherence of *H. influenzae* involves several different interactions with the host. *H. influenzae* expresses pili (also known as fimbriae), fibrils, and adhesin proteins which mediate adherence of the organism to the epithelial cell surface. The strain phenotype and function of these various components may be redundant or complementary, depending on the local environment in which the bacterium resides and the genetic capability of the organism.

The respiratory tract secretions function as a nonspecific host defence mechanism. The most abundant constituents of these secretions are the mucins, a class of high-molecular-weight glycoproteins. Mucins may serve to facilitate the removal of bacteria by binding bacteria and promoting removal by ciliary action. The production of mucins in guinea-pig tracheal explant models is stimulated by some strains of *H. influenzae* [2]. The interaction between mucins and *H. influenzae* are specific. Three outer membrane proteins (P2, P5, and a third, as yet unidentified, protein) bind mucins [3]. Sialic acid containing oligosaccharides of human mucins might also be the receptors for *H. influenzae* [3].

The bacterium-mucin interaction promotes adherence of *H. influenzae* to respiratory tract cells *in vitro* [4]. Bacterial cells of many species, including *H. influenzae*, express surface appendages called pili or fimbriae. Piliated strains of *H. influenzae* adhere better to mucins *in vitro*, than do non-piliated strains [5]. Piliated strains incubated with mucins showed increased binding to nasopharyngeal cells compared with piliated strains that were not pre-incubated with mucins [4]. Therefore, pili may facilitate the interaction of *H. influenzae* with mucin and subsequent epithelial binding.

Pili cause hemagglutination by specifically binding to the blood group antigen, AnWj [6]. Piliated strains of *H. influenzae* show differential adherence to cell lines, binding directly to a variety of respiratory cell lines *in vitro*, but not, for instance, to HeLa cells, which are not derived from the respiratory tract. These observations illustrate the specificity of adherence with host cells.

Phase variation occurs in the expression of pili on the bacterial surface. In natural infection, isolates of *H. influenzae* type b recovered from mucosal surfaces are usually piliated whereas isolates from systemic sites are generally not piliated [7]. The ability to turn off expression of pili is an adaptive mechanism because pili are advantageous for the bacterium when it is on the mucosa but are potentially detrimental in the bloodstream or cerebrospinal fluid.

The genetic basis of this phenotypic change has been elucidated recently. There are five genes, *hifA* to *E*, in the pilus gene cluster [8]: the gene *hifA* encodes the major structural protein, *hifB* a periplasmic chaperone, *hifC* an outer membrane usher and *hifD* and *hifE* encode minor protein subunits and participate in the biogenesis of pili. Although similar to pilus gene clusters found in other organisms, the *H. influenzae* gene cluster is unique in its regulation by multiple repetitive palindromic sequences. The promoter sites of *hifA* and *hifB* are overlapping and the two genes are divergently transcribed. In the overlapping promoter regions there are repeating TA units. Variation in the number of repeating units alters the spacing between the promoter regions. If there are 10 or 11 TA units, both promoters function properly and pili are formed. If the number of TA units is changed from 10 or 11, by slipped-strand mispairing, pili are not expressed [7, 9].

Strains of nontypable *H. influenzae* isolated from children with otitis media express a nonhemagglutinating surface appendage, which has been called fimbriae by Sirakova et al. [10]. This 36-kDa protein (fimbrin) shares homology with the OmpA family of proteins and is therefore distinct from pili or what is referred to as fimbriae by other authors. Disruption of fimbrin gene expression reduced adherence to human oropharyngeal cells, and reduced induction of otitis media in the chinchilla model. Passive and active immunization of chinchillas was protective in the animals challenged with the homologous strain [10].

Nonpiliated and pilin-deficient mutant strains are still capable of attachment to human epithelial cells in tissue culture. Using electron microscopy, St Geme and Cutter [11] described short, thin structures on the surface of *H. influenzae* type b. These structures, named fibrils, are distinct from pili and are composed of an approximately 240-kDa protein, which is the *hsf* gene product. The *hsf* gene is found in all type b strains and a quarter of nontypable strains of *H. influenzae*. Low-level homology exists with other bacterial adhesins, although there is a highly conserved N-terminal domain of 24 amino acids shared among some of these adhesins. Fibrils may be important for adherence in the lower respiratory tract or the middle ear [12, 13].

Several outer membrane proteins function as adhesins without forming surface appendage structures. Barenkamp and Bodor [14] described two high-molecular-weight outer membrane proteins, HMW1 and –2, with molecular masses of 125 and 120 kDa, respectively. The sequences of HMW1 and -2 are about 80% identical to one another and share sequence homology with the filamentous hemagglutinin (FHA) of *Bordetella pertussis* [15]. These proteins are involved in the binding of *H. influenzae* to the surface of epithelial cells and macrophages, similar to FHA-mediated macrophage interactions with *B. pertussis*. Unlike FHA, HMW-dependent binding to the macrophage is not mediated by the CR3 receptor [16]. Immunoelectron microscopy of *H. influenzae* reveals that these two proteins tend to aggregate or cap and these caps are released into the medium as disk-like aggregates, similar to FHA. The human oropharyngeal cell membrane has a desmosome-like structure associated with a bacterial protein cap in tissue culture [17]. FHA is involved in the entry of *B. pertussis* into eukaryotic cells. Nontypable *H. influenzae* enter human epithelial cells [18, 19]. Bakaletz and Barenkamp [17] infer, given the similarities between the HMW proteins of *H. influenzae* and the FHA of *B. pertussis*, that eukaryotic cell entry of *H. influenzae* may be mediated by these proteins. Viable intracellular *H. influenzae* is present in adenoidal tissue from children with chronic otitis media or adenoidal hypertrophy [20]. These observations indicate that epithelial cell invasion occurs *in vivo*. Bacteria residing intracellularly are protected from the host immune response. This may explain the extended periods of nasopharyngeal colonization seen in adults with chronic bronchitis or otitis-prone children.

Table 1. Adhesins of *Haemophilus influenzae*

Adhesin	Gene	Structural characteristics	References
Pili	*hifA-E*	Hair-like appendages Hemagglutination	[7–9, 54, 55]
Haemophilus surface fibrils	*hsf*	Surface fibrils by electron microscopy 240-kDa protein	[11–13]
Fimbrin (outer membrane protein P5)	*omp P5*	36-kDa OMPA-like protein surface structure	[10]
HMW1, HMW2	*hmw1*, *hmw2*	125 and 120-kDa outer membrane proteins. Adherence to epithelial cells and macrophages	[16, 17, 56, 57]
Hia (*H. influenzae* adhesin)	*hia*	114-kDa outer membrane protein Allele of *hsf*	[21]
Hap (Haemophilus adherence and penetration)	*hap*	160-kDa outer membrane protein Homology with IgA protease	[22]

HMW1 and HMW2 are present in 70–75% of strains of nontypable *H. influenzae*. Most strains that lack these proteins express another protein adhesin called Hia (*H. influenzae* adhesin) [21]. The *hia* gene encodes a 114-kDa protein which binds avidly to Chang conjunctival cells. The *hia* gene may be an allele of the *hsf* gene described above [12].

Another gene, which encodes a 160-kDa nonpilus adhesin called Hap (*haemophilus* adhesion and penetration), was described by St Geme et al. [22]. Hap is involved in bacterial adherence and internalization. The sequence shows homology with the immunoglobulin A (IgA) protease of *Neisseria gonorrhoeae* but the *hap* gene is distinct from the IgA protease gene of *H. influenzae*. Although the role of Hap on the cell surface is not yet clear, a protease that is present on the bacterial cell surface or secreted may alter the eukaryotic cell surface to promote bacterial cell entry [22].

The adherence of *H. influenzae* to the respiratory tract epithelial cell is a complex interaction which utilizes multiple adhesin molecules and appendages (summarized in Table 1). The precise function of and interaction among these various factors remain an intense area of research. Lessons learned from *H. influenzae* will be applicable to other pathogens, just as motifs from *B. pertussis*, *Escherichia coli*, and other pathogens have been found repeated in *H. influenzae*.

4. Mechanisms of Antigen Variation of Surface Protein Antigens

Nontypable *H. influenzae* expresses six to eight major proteins in its outer membrane. Studies in the 1980s demonstrated that a high degree of variability in the molecular weights of these outer membrane proteins existed among strains of nontypable *H. influenzae* [23, 24]. Outer membrane protein P2, which comprises about half the protein content of the outer membrane, showed a particularly high degree of size variability among strains [24]. P2 is the major porin protein of *H. influenzae*, allowing small hydrophilic molecules to pass through the outer membrane [25]. Analysis of the sequence of the gene that encodes P2 revealed that portions of the protein which are buried within the outer membrane are relatively conserved among strains, but several of the eight loops that are exposed on the bacterial surface show a high degree of sequence variability among strains [26–28]. As antibodies to P2 elicit strain-specific protection [29–31], these observations suggested that antigenic heterogeneity of the major surface protein plays a role in the ability of nontypable *H. influenzae* to cause recurrent respiratory tract infections in humans.

Analysis of outer membrane protein patterns from strains of nontypable *H. influenzae* recovered prospectively from patients with COPD reveals a high degree of turnover of strains in some patients and persistent infection by the same strain in other patients [32]. Among the strains that show persistence in the respiratory tract, variants which have changes in the molecular weight of P2 but identical DNA fingerprints are observed [29, 32]. To determine the mechanism of this antigenic drift, Duim et al. [33] studied the sequences of the genes encoding the P2 of these variants. The antigenic drift resulted from single base changes in the P2 gene, all generating amino acid changes in surface-exposed loops of the P2 protein [33]. Similar single base changes were observed in the P2 gene from variants selected in subcutaneous cages implanted in rabbits and from a variant that survived antibody-mediated killing *in vitro* [33–35]. All of the point mutations in the P2 gene were non-synonymous because they resulted in amino acid changes. As all of the substitutions resulted in amino acid changes, these mutations produced a selective advantage for the bacterium. These observations strongly suggested that the accumulation of point mutations under immune-selective pressure resulted in antigenic drift of surface-exposed regions of a major outer membrane protein. This mechanism of evading an immune response by the host could allow persistent *H. influenzae* infection.

Outer membrane protein P2 is strongly immunogenic in experimental animals and humans [29, 36–38]. Analysis of monoclonal antibodies to P2, which were generated by immunizing mice with whole bacterial cells, revealed that most antibodies were directed toward a single surface-exposed loop on the P2 protein [39, 40]. All of these antibodies were highly specific for the immunizing strain. This observation suggested that nontypable *H. influenzae* expresses an immunodominant, strain-specific epitope on the bacterial surface. To test the hypothesis that the expression of such epitopes on the bacterial surface induces a strain-specific immune response, mice and rabbits were challenged with whole cells of a strain of nontypable *H. influenzae* [37]. Analysis of the antibody response with immunoblot, bactericidal, and immunoprecipitation assays revealed a prominent antibody response almost exclusively to a single surface-exposed loop of the P2 molecule [37]. These observations, along with those involving non-synonymous point mutations in the P2 gene described above [33], support the notion that the surface-exposed loops of the P2 protein are under intense immune-selective pressure. The expression of strain-specific, immunodominant epitopes represents a mechanism by which the bacterium induces antibodies that will protect against recurrent infection by the homologous strain but will not protect against infection by heterologous strains. Point mutations in the P2 gene which correspond to the immunodominant loops provide a mechanism for the bacterium to evade the host immune response and persist in the respiratory tract.

Recent studies of an Aboriginal community in the Northern Territory of Australia reveal a second mechanism by which nontypable *H. influenzae* alters its P2 molecule to evade host defenses. Rural Aboriginal children are heavily colonized by nontypable *H. influenzae* in the nasopharynx at an early age [41]. Ribotyping of prospectively recovered isolates has revealed that the children are colonized by multiple strains of *H. influenzae* simultaneously, and that strains are acquired and cleared frequently resulting in a high rate of turnover [42]. By determining the sequences of P2 genes from selected strains, Smith-Vaughn et al. [43] demonstrated the presence of identical P2 genes in strains with different genetic backgrounds. In view of the wide diversity of P2 gene sequences, the authors concluded that horizontal transfer of the P2 gene occurred among strains. The presence in the human respiratory tract of simultaneous, multiple strains of a bacterium that is competent for DNA uptake provides a powerful mechanism for the bacterium to alter expression of surface molecules. This phenomenon is likely to occur in other settings in which multiple strains of nontypable *H. influenzae* colonize the respiratory tract such as cystic fibrosis [44] and chronic bronchitis (our unpublished observations).

In summary, antigenic heterogeneity of P2 among strains, expression of immunodominant epitopes, point mutations in the P2 gene, and horizontal transfer of the P2 gene among strains are adaptive molecular traits which allow the bacterium to evade the host immune response and persist in the human respiratory tract.

5. Phase Variation and Sialylation of Surface Glycolipid Molecules

Endotoxin, or lipopolysaccharide (LPS), is the major glycolipid in the outer membrane of Gram-negative bacteria and is essential to the integrity and functioning of the bacterial cell wall. Non-enteric Gram-negative mucosal pathogens, including *H. influenzae*, express an endotoxin molecule which lacks the long, repeating polysaccharide side chains that are typical of lipopolysaccharide of enteric Gram-negative bacteria as *E. coli* and *Salmonella* spp. Therefore, the endotoxin of *H. influenzae* is more accurately called lipooligosaccharide (LOS).

LOS is involved at several stages in the pathogenesis of infection, including colonization of the respiratory tract and cytotoxic injury to target tissues. The importance of LOS in pathogenesis has generated considerable interest in studies of the biosynthesis and structure of the molecule. Such studies are complicated because it is necessary to study tertiary products of genes which are turned on and off at high frequencies. Nevertheless, considerable amounts of new information have been learned about LOS biosynthesis and structure in the past decade.

LOS is composed of a membrane-anchoring lipid A portion which is responsible for its endotoxic-like properties, including mitogenicity, pyrogenicity, platelet aggregation, cytokine activation, and adjuvant activity. Lipid A is linked by a single 2-keto-3-deoxyoctulosonic acid (KDO) molecule to a heterogeneous oligosaccharide made up of glucose, galactose and heptose. Marked intrastrain and interstrain variation in the size of LOS is observed in sodium dodecylsulfate polyacrylamide gel electrophoresis (SDS-PAGE). This variation is a result of differences in the quantity and assembly of the neutral sugars, particularly galactose [45].

Surface determinants, which are essential for the organism at one stage of colonization or infection, may be unnecessary or even detrimental at a later stage of infection. Bacteria have evolved adaptive mechanisms for phenotypic variation of surface molecules, including LOS [46].

The LOS of *H. influenzae* shows considerable structural heterogeneity both between strains and within a clonal population derived from a single strain. This heterogeneity occurs as a result of several mechanisms. LOS is the end-product of a complex biosynthetic process and some variation occurs as a result of factors that influence interaction of enzymes, regulatory proteins, and substrates [46]. Such factors may determine the number of phosphate substitutions, anomeric linkages, saccharide branching chains, and other structural modifications, so that LOS is expressed as a family of molecules on the bacterial surface. A variety of environmental factors influence LOS structure as well, including: exposure to serum; exposure to mixtures of glucose, lactate, urea, and bicarbonate *in vitro*; alteration of growth rate; and cystine limitation.

Another mechanism by which *H. influenzae* alters its LOS is phase variation, which is the ability to regulate the expression of molecules by turning on and off the expression of selected genes. The LOS of *H. influenzae* demonstrates phase variation which occurs through a mechanism known as slipped strand mispairing [47]. The *lic* locus, which is responsible for synthesis of oligosaccharide structures, contains open reading frames which are preceded by multiple tandem repeats of the tetramer 5′-CAAT-3′. Alterations in the number of repeats through the nonrecombinational mechanism of slipped strand mispairing shift upstream initiation codons into or out of frame, creating a translational switch that results in phase variation [47]. Multiple oligosaccharide structures undergo phase variation in a complex pattern. Some genes vary independently and some vary in a coordinate fashion with other genes. As a result, the bacterium has the ability to display a varied array of LOS structures on its surface. This ability enables *H. influenzae* to adapt to its environment in the various stages of colonization and infection.

The LOS of many strains of *H. influenzae* contains a terminal digalactoside, Gal-α-(1–4)-β-Gal, which is also present in human glycosphingolipids in the urinary tract, intestinal epithelium, and erythrocytes [48]. The mimicry of host tissue may be an adaptive mechanism which promotes bacterial survival in the respiratory tract of the host.

The LOS components which resemble moieties in human tissue can be altered by the addition of sialic acid both *in vitro* and *in vivo* [48]. Indeed, many strains of *H. influenzae* contain sialylated LOS [49]. The oligosaccharide portion of sialylated LOS may also resemble sialylated oligosaccharides present in human glycosphingolipids. Sialylated LOS may play a variety of potential roles in the pathogenesis of colonization and infection by *H. influenzae* [48]. These include: the anti-recognition of bacterial surface antigens by the host; the down-regulation of opsonophagocytosis by bacteria because bacteria with sialylated LOS are more resistant to phagocytosis; the decreased adherence of bacteria to host cells or to other bacteria; the intracellular survival of bacteria; and the alteration of bacterial or host cell signaling pathways.

In summary, *H. influenzae* has an enormous capacity to alter the expression of its LOS by a variety of mechanisms. The mechanisms that have evolved illustrate some of the adaptive potential of surface bacterial determinants and their role in colonization and infection of the human respiratory tract.

6. The Genome of *Haemophilus Influenzae* and the Birth of Genomics

In 1995, the DNA sequence of the entire genome of *H. influenzae*, strain Rd, was published in *Science* [50] and placed into computerized databases. The 1.83 megabase-pair (Mbp) DNA sequence is accessible to any person with access to the Internet or to the printed version in the journal. This accomplishment launched, in earnest, a new form of scientific inquiry called genomics. Genomics is the study of the DNA sequence of an organism. Before genomics, science could determine the function of a protein by studying its structure or devising experiments to determine its function. By the 1980s, genomics in the form of computer-assisted analysis of DNA sequence databases began. DNA sequences of individual genes could be compared with sequences of other genes in a database. This DNA sequence analysis helped to reveal a structure or function based on homology with other sequences in the database, but revealed less about mechanisms of control of gene expression or relationships of genes upstream or downstream from the gene being studied. Now, scientists can look at the entire

DNA sequence of organisms and infer homology with known genes, look for genes that appear to be linked together in a biosynthetic pathway, and devise experiments to show if the function or structure of the unknown genes is similar to that of known genes.

A genomics-based approach relies on the observation that functional and structural motifs recur in biological processes [51]. For example, the DNA sequence of an active site of an enzyme in a bacterium may be conserved across species or even kingdoms of living things. Pattern analysis of sequences can be used to analyze physiologic processes of the organism by determining which enzyme pathways are present or absent in the genome. For instance, *H. influenzae*, strain Rd, is missing three of the enzymes needed to complete the tricarboxylic acid cycle. This surprising information could be used to determine the substrates that the bacterium needs to survive within the human host environment. Furthermore, based on the assumption that an important function requires more space in the genome, one can infer the relative importance of particular capabilities of the organism by identifying the amount of genome devoted to a specific function [51]. Use of the complete genome sequence of *H. influenzae* allowed Hood et al. [52] to identify and clone 25 genes involved in LOS biosynthesis.

One can analyze codon usage of the genome to learn about genomic structure and function. Repeating patterns or variations in codon usage can be identified and studied. For example, phase variation of LOS of *H. influenzae* is mediated by slipped strand mispairing of multiple tandem repeats of CAAT tetramers and phase variation of pili is related to repeats of TA. As phase variation is a mechanism of regulation of virulence factors, searching the genome for such motifs may identify virulence factors [53]. This approach was used by Hood et al. [53] who analyzed the *H. influenzae* genome for tandem repeats of the tetranucleotides CAAT or GACA. Twelve loci with multiple tetranucleotide repeats were identified, six of which were not previously known to be virulence genes. One of these genes, designated the *lgtC* homolog, was investigated. In *Neisseria meningitidis, lgtC* is a glycosyltransferase involved in LOS biosynthesis. Its function was investigated in *H. influenzae* by transposon mutagenesis; the mutant strain had an altered LOS molecule and was less virulent in an infant rat model. This observation illustrates the power of genomics. By applying recognized virulence motif-tandem repeats, to an organism with a known DNA sequence, hitherto unrecognized genes were found and a function was identified.

Analysis of codon usage can also be used to determine whether portions of the genome have been acquired from other organisms. Bacterial virulence factors are known to be grouped in the genome in areas called pathogenicity islands. These islands may display codon usage which is different from the rest of the genome. This difference implies that these islands may have been acquired from other organisms. Genes encoding virulence factors which move among bacterial species may result in entirely new disease manifestations. By evaluating a genome for distinct areas of different codon usage, putative pathogenicity islands can be identified and studied [51].

Genomics saves time, provides clues to gene function, and can lead to the discovery of new virulence genes, but it cannot ultimately substitute for studies of cellular protein function and interaction with the host. Sequence homology implies but does not confirm that the genes are functional homologs. The biological function may be entirely different from that of the genetic homolog. For example, enzymatic binding sites may have different substrates, even though the DNA sequences may be similar, and the opposite may also occur. Similar motifs or strategies in pathogenesis may be found in different organisms, but the proteins involved in these similar strategies share little to no DNA homology [51].

The use of genomics has just begun. One promise of genomics in the study of bacterial pathogenesis lies in the ability to identify new genes that encode virulence factors which are expressed exclusively during human infection and not during *in vitro* growth. Newer techniques of probing gene expression in the host or other environmental milieus of the pathogen life cycle can then be applied. The impact of environmental factors on gene expression of a bacterial pathogen and survival strategies of the pathogen in different environments will lead to a better understanding of pathogenesis of infections. Besides leading to better treatments and vaccines, this information will lead to understanding of the impact of environmental changes (perhaps caused by human intervention) which may create the opportunities for new infectious diseases to emerge [51].

References

1 Murphy TF, Sethi S (1992) Bacterial infection in chronic obstructive pulmonary disease. *Am Rev Respir Dis* 146: 1067–1083

2 Adler KB, Hendley DD, Davis GS (1986) Bacteria associated with obstructive pulmonary disease elaborate extracellular products that stimulate mucin secretion by explants of guinea pig airways. *Am J Pathol* 125: 501–514

3 Reddy MS, Murphy TF, Faden HS, Bernstein JM (1997) Middle ear mucin glycoprotein: purification and interaction with nontypable *Haemophilus influenzae* and *Moraxella catarrhalis. Otolaryngol Head Neck Surg* 116: 175–189

4 Davies J, Carlstedt I, Nilsson A-K, Hakansson A, Sabharwal H, van Alphen L, van Ham M, Svanborg C (1995) Binding of *Haemophilus influenzae* to purified mucins from the human respiratory tract. *Infect Immun* 63: 2485–2492

5 Barsum W, Wilson R, Read RC, Rutman A, Todd HC, Houdret N, Roussel P, Cole PJ (1995) Interaction of fimbriated and nonfimbriated strains of unencapsulated *Haemophilus influenzae* with human respiratory tract mucus *in vitro. Eur Respir J* 8: 709–714

6 van Alphen L, van Ham SM (1994) Adherence and invasion of *Haemophilus influenzae. Rev Med Microbiol* 5: 245–255

7 van Ham SM, van Alphen L, Mooi FR, van Putten JPM (1993) Phase variation of *H. influenzae* fimbriae: Transcriptional control of two divergent genes through a variable combined promoter region. *Cell* 73: 1187–1196

8 van Ham SM, van Alphen L, Mooi FR, van Putten JPM (1994) The fimbrial gene cluster of *Haemophilus influenzae* type b. *Mol Microbiol* 13(4): 673–684
9 Gilsdorf JR, McCrea KW, Marrs CF (1997) Role of pili in *Haemophilus influenzae* adherence and colonization. *Infect Immun* 65: 2997–3002
10 Sirakova T, Kolattukudy PE, Murwin D, Billy J, Leake E, Lim D, DeMaria T, Bakaletz L (1994) Role of fimbriae expressed by nontypeable *Haemophilus influenzae* in pathogenesis of and protection against otitis media and relatedness of the fimbrin subunit to outer membrane protein A. *Infect Immun* 62: 2002–2020
11 St Geme III JW, Cutter D (1995) Evidence that surface fibrils expressed by *Haemophilus influenzae* type b promote attachment to human epithelial cells. *Mol Microbiol* 15: 77–85
12 St Geme III JW, Cutter D, Barenkamp SJ (1996) Characterization of the genetic locus encoding *Haemophilus influenzae* type b surface fibrils. *J Bacteriol* 178: 6281–6287
13 St Geme III JW, Cutter D (1996) Influence of pili, fibrils, and capsule on *in vitro* adherence by *Haemophilus influenzae* type b. *Mol Microbiol* 21: 21–31
14 Barenkamp SJ, Bodor FF (1990) Development of serum bactericidal activity following nontypable *Haemophilus influenzae* acute otitis media. *Pediatr Infect Dis J* 9: 333–339
15 Barenkamp SJ, Leininger E (1992) Cloning, expression, and DNA sequence analysis of the genes encoding nontypable *Haemophilus influenzae* high-molecular-weight surface-exposed proteins related to filamentous hemagglutinin of *Bordetella pertussis. Infect Immun* 60: 1302–1313
16 Noel GJ, Barenkamp SJ, St Geme III JW, Haining WN, Mosser DM (1994) High-molecular-weight surface-exposed proteins of *Haemophilus influenzae* mediate binding to macrophages. *J Infect Dis* 169: 425–429
17 Bakaletz LO, Barenkamp SJ (1994) Localization of high-molecular-weight adhesion proteins of nontypable *Haemophilus influenzae* by immunoelectron microscopy. *Infect Immun* 62: 4460–4468
18 St Geme III JW, Falkow S (1991) Loss of capsule expression by *Haemophilus influenzae* type b results in enhanced adherence to and invasion of human cells. *Infect Immun* 59: 1325–1333
19 St Geme III JW, Falkow S (1990) *Haemophilus influenzae* adheres to and enters cultured human epithelial cells. *Infect Immun* 58: 4036–4044
20 Forsgren J, Samuelson A, Borrelli S, Christensson B, Jonasson J, Lindberg AA (1996) Persistence of nontypable *Haemophilus influenzae* in adenoid macrophages: a putative colonization mechanism. *Acta Oto-Laryngol* 116(5): 766–773
21 Barenkamp SJ, St Geme III JW (1996) Identification of a second family of high-molecular-weight adhesion proteins expressed by non-typable *Haemophilus influenzae. Mol Microbiol* 19(6): 1215–1223
22 St Geme III JW, de la Morena ML, Falkow S (1994) A *Haemophilus influenzae* IgA protease-like protein promotes intimate interaction with human epithelial cells. *Mol Microbiol* 14: 217–233
23 Barenkamp SJ, Munson RS Jr, Granoff DM (1982) Outer membrane protein and biotype analysis of pathogenic nontypable *Haemophilus influenzae. Infect Immun* 36: 535–540
24 Murphy TF, Dudas KC, Mylotte JM, Apicella MA (1983) A subtyping system for nontypable *Haemophilus influenzae* based on outer-membrane proteins. *J Infect Dis* 147: 838–846
25 Vachon V, Kristjanson DN, Coulton JW (1988) Outer membrane porin protein of *Haemophilus influenzae* type b pore size and subunit structure. *Can J Microbiol* 34: 134–140
26 Sikkema DJ, Murphy TF (1992) Molecular analysis of the P2 porin protein of nontypable *Haemophilus influenzae. Infect Immun* 60: 5204–5211
27 Duim B, Dankert J, Jansen HM, van Alphen L (1993) Genetic analysis of the diversity in outer membrane protein P2 of non-encapsulated *Haemophilus influenzae. Microb Pathog* 14: 451–462
28 Bell J, Grass S, Jeanteur D, Munson RS Jr (1994) Diversity of the P2 protein among nontypable *Haemophilus influenzae* isolates. *Infect Immun* 62: 2639–2643
29 Groeneveld K, van Alphen L, Voorter C, Eijk PP, Jansen HM, Zanen HC (1989) Antigenic drift of *Haemophilus influenzae* in patients with chronic obstructive pulmonary disease. *Infect Immun* 57: 3038–3044
30 Karasic RB, Trumpp CE, Gnehm H, Rice PA, Pelton SI (1985) Modification of otitis media in chinchillas rechallenged with nontypable *Haemophilus influenzae* and serological response to outer membrane antigens. *J Infect Dis* 151: 273–279

31 Troelstra A, Vogel L, van Alphen L, Eijk P, Jansen H, Dankert J (1994) Opsonic antibodies to outer membrane protein P2 of nonencapsulated *Haemophilus influenzae* are strain specific. *Infect Immun* 62: 779–784
32 Groeneveld K, van Alphen L, Eijk PP, Jansen HM, Zanen HC (1988) Changes in outer membrane proteins of nontypable *Haemophilus influenzae* in patients with chronic obstructive pulmonary disease. *J Infect Dis* 158: 360–365
33 Duim B, van Alphen L, Eijk P, Jansen HM, Dankert J (1994) Antigenic drift of non-encapsulated *Haemophilus influenzae* major outer membrane protein P2 in patients with chronic bronchitis is caused by point mutations. *Mol Microbiol* 11: 1181–1189
34 Vogel L, Duim B, Geluk F, Eijk P, Jansen H, Dankert J, van Alphen L (1996) Immune selection for antigenic drift of major outer membrane protein P2 of *Haemophilus influenzae* during persistence in subcutaneous tissue cages in rabbits. *Infect Immun* 64: 980–986
35 Duim B, Vogel L, Puijk W, Jansen HM, Meloen RH, Dankert J, van Alphen L (1996) Fine mapping of outer membrane protein P2 antigenic sites which vary during persistent infection by *Haemophilus influenzae. Infect Immun* 64: 4673–4679
36 Murphy TF, Bartos LC (1988) Human bactericidal antibody response to outer membrane protein P2 of nontypable *Haemophilus influenzae. Infect Immun* 56: 2673–2679
37 Yi K, Murphy TF (1997) Importance of an immunodominant surface-exposed loop on outer membrane protein P2 of nontypable *Haemophilus influenzae. Infect Immun* 65: 150–155
38 Srikumar R, Chin AC, Vachon V, Richardson CD, Ratcliffe MJH, Saarinen L, Kayhty H, Makela PH, Coulton JW (1992) Monoclonal antibodies specific to porin of *Haemophilus influenzae* type b: localization of their cognate epitopes and tests of their biological activities. *Mol Microbiol* 6(5): 665–676
39 Haase EM, Campagnari AA, Sarwar J, Shero M, Wirth M, Cumming CU, Murphy TF (1991) Strain-specific and immunodominant surface epitopes of the P2 porin protein of nontypable *Haemophilus influenzae. Infect Immun* 59: 1278–1284
40 Haase EM, Yi K, Morse GD, Murphy TF (1994) Mapping of bactericidal epitopes on the P2 porin protein of nontypable *Haemophilus influenzae. Infect Immun* 62: 3712–3722
41 Leach AJ, Boswell JB, Asche V, Nienhuys TG, Mathews JD (1994) Bacterial colonization of the nasopharynx predicts very early onset and persistence of otitis media in Australian Aboriginal infants. *Pediatr Infect Dis J* 13: 983–989
42 Smith-Vaughan HC, Leach AJ, Shelby-James TM, Kemp K, Kemp DJ, Mathews JD (1996) Carriage of multiple ribotypes of non-encapsulated *Haemophilus influenzae* in Aboriginal infants with otitis media. *Epidemiol Infect* 116: 177–183
43 Smith-Vaughan HC, Sriprakash KS, Mathews JD, Kemp DJ (1997) Nonencapsulated *Haemophilus influenzae* in aboriginal infants with otitis media: prolonged carriage of P2 porin variants and evidence for horizontal P2 gene transfer. *Infect Immun* 65: 1468–1474
44 Moller LVM, Regelink AG, Grasselier H, Dankert-Roelse JE, Dankert J, van Alphen L (1995) Multiple *Haemophilus influenzae* strains and strain variants coexist in the respiratory tract of patients with cystic fibrosis. *J Infect Dis* 172: 1388–1392
45 Weiser JN (1992) The oligosaccharide of *Haemophilus influenzae. Microb Pathog* 13: 335–342
46 Roche RJ, Moxon ER (1995) Phenotypic variation of carbohydrate surface antigens and the pathogenesis of *Haemophilus influenzae* infections. *Trends Microbiol* 3: 304–309
47 High NJ, Jennings MP, Moxon ER (1996) Tandem repeats of the tetramer 5′-CAAT-3′ present in *lic2A* are required for phase variation but not lipopolysaccharide biosynthesis in *Haemophilus influenzae. Mol Microbiol* 20: 165–174
48 Mandrell RE, Apicella MA (1993) Lipo-oligosaccharides (LOS) of mucosal pathogens: molecular mimicry and host-modification of LOS. *Immunobiology* 187: 382–402
49 Mandrell RE, McLaughlin R, Abu Kwaik Y, Lesse A, Yamasaki R, Gibson B, Spinola SM, Apicella MA (1992) Lipooligosaccharides (LOS) of some *Haemophilus* species mimic human glycosphingolipids, and some LOS are sialylated. *Infect Immun* 60: 1322–1328
50 Fleischmann RD, Adams MD, White O, Clayton RA, Kirkness EF, Kerlavage AR, Bult CJ, Tomb J-F, Dougherty BA, Merrick JM et al. (1995) Whole-genome random sequencing and assembly of *Haemophilus influenzae* Rd. *Science* 269: 496–512
51 Strauss EJ, Falkow S (1997) Microbial pathogenesis: genomics and beyond. *Science* 276: 707–712

52 Hood DW, Deadman ME, Allen T, Masoud H, Martin A, Brisson JR, Fleischmann R, Venter JC, Richards JC, Moxon ER (1996) Use of the complete genome sequence information of *Haemophilus influenzae* strain Rd to investigate lipopolysaccharide biosynthesis. *Mol Microbiol* 22(5): 951–965
53 Hood DW, Deadman ME, Jennings MP, Bisercic M, Fleischmann RD, Venter C, Moxon ER (1996) DNA repeats identify novel virulence genes in *Haemophilus influenzae*. *Proc Natl Acad Sci USA* 93: 11121–11125
54 McCrea KW, Watson WJ, Gilsdorf JR, Marrs CF (1994) Identification of *hifD* and *hifE* in the pilus gene cluster of *Haemophilus influenzae* type b strain Eagan. *Infect Immun* 62: 4922–4928
55 Gilsdorf JR, Marrs CF, McCrea KW, Forney LJ (1990) Cloning, expression, and sequence analysis of the *Haemophilus influenzae* type b strain M43p$^+$ pilin gene. *Infect Immun* 58: 1065–1072
56 St Geme III JW, Falkow S, Barenkamp SJ (1993) High-molecular-weight proteins of nontypable *Haemophilus influenzae* mediate attachment to human epithelial cells. *Proc Natl Acad Sci USA* 90: 2875–2879
57 Barenkamp SJ, St Geme III JW (1994) Genes encoding high-molecular-weight adhesion proteins of nontypable *Haemophilus influenzae* are part of gene clusters. *Infect Immun* 62: 3320–3328

Molecular Biology of the Lung
Vol. 1: Emphysema and Infection
ed. by R. A. Stockley

CHAPTER 10
Polymerase Chain Reaction in the Diagnosis of Respiratory Tract Infections

Neil W. Schluger

Division of Pulmonary, Allergy, and Critical Case Medicine
College of Physicians and Surgeons, Columbia University, New York, NY, USA

1. Introduction

For many years, the cornerstone of the diagnostic armamentarium for respiratory infections has been culture, whether for bacteria, mycobacteria, fungi, or viruses. Relatively more recently, adjunctive tests, such as antibody-based detection of microbial antigens in sptum, bronchoalveolar lavage fluid, and other biological specimens, have also been applied [1]. The limitations of these techniques for sensitive and specific diagnosis of upper and lower respiratory tract infections are well known. For example, many series have demonstrated that, despite extensive laboratory investigation, only about 50% of cases of community-acquired pneumonia can be ascribed to a specific pathogen [2, 3]. For this reason, the evolution of the polymerase chain reaction (PCR) as a potential diagnostic tool in clinical medicine has been followed with great interest by those in pulmonary medicine [4]. Potentially, PCR offers unmatched diagnostic sensitivity and specificity: this technique can create millions of identical copies of unique DNA sequences from a single template (a single bacteria or virus, for example) in only a few hours.

The need for improved diagnostic techniques in pulmonary infectious disease is clear. The range of pathogens now commonly encountered in clinical practice is wider than ever before, for a variety of reasons. The increasing numbers of immunocompromised patients (whether as a direct result of an illness such as AIDS or as a complication of treatment for another condition, such as immune suppression used to treat organ transplantation or collagen vascular disease) has greatly expanded the range of microorganisms that are commonly associated with respiratory illness. In addition, frequent travel and migration of populations bring previously less commonly encountered illnesses to a variety of settings. Many of these respiratory infections (*Pneumocystis carinii* pneumonia and tuberculosis, to name just two) can cause significant morbidity and mortality, and require specific therapy, making prompt and accurate diagnosis important in clinical practice.

A strong argument can be made that specific diagnosis even of common bacterial pneumonias is urgently needed. Although some have urged a reduced emphasis on making precise etiologic diagnosis in community-acquired pneumonia, favoring instead the use of relatively broad-spectrum empiric antibiotic therapy chosen after considering clinical and demographic features of a given patient, this strategy probably reflects the limitations of currently available diagnostic techniques rather than a true ideal of medical practice [5, 6]. In fact, the routine administration of broad-spectrum antibiotics is largely responsible for the emergence of drug-resistant pathogens such as penicillin-resistant *Streptococcus pneumoniae* [7]. Accurate and rapid bacterial diagnosis could allow narrowly tailored therapy which might slow the appearance of antibiotic resistance among common microorganisms.

In addition to identifying specific causes of respiratory infection, there are instances in which an ideal diagnostic tool is needed to determine whether in fact any pulmonary infection is present at all. The patient receiving mechanical ventilation in the intensive care unit, who has fever and infiltrates on a chest radiograph, may or may not have pneumonia, but currently available techniques are poor at determining this [8]. As a result, broad-spectrum antibiotics are often administered, perhaps without efficacy but, again, undoubtedly contributing to the problem of drug resistance in virulent pathogens such as Gram-negative bacilli.

As the foregoing discussion suggests, rapid and accurate diagnosis of pulmonary infectious diseases is not an end in and of itself. It must be demonstrated that improvements in diagnosis lead to improved patient outcomes, either directly by decreasing morbidity and mortality, or more indirectly perhaps, by retarding the development of drug-resistant microorganisms. It is against these measures that PCR diagnosis of respiratory infections will be judged in this chapter.

2. The Polymerase Chain Reaction

This chapter is not intended to be a detailed review of PCR technology, but a general overview of the principles of the technique and important considerations concerning sample preparation and selection of DNA templates is appropriate.

The PCR, as mentioned earlier, is a process by which literally millions of identical copies of specific nucleic acid sequences can be created through DNA amplification [9]. The steps involved in a typical PCR reaction are demonstrated in Figure 1. First, the sample that contains the DNA to be analyzed is heated so that double-stranded DNA denatures into single-stranded DNA. Then, short pieces of previously synthesized DNA (primers), which are complementary to the portion of DNA to be amplified and which have been previously added to a sample containing the target DNA, bind to the target of interest in a process known as annealing. Using a specific thermostable DNA polymerase and free nucleotides, which are present in the reaction mixture, the primers are extended to form long complementary strands of DNA. In this manner, each PCR cycle doubles the number of preexisting DNA templates and the number of amplified copies grows exponentially, so that 30 cycles of PCR amplification results in 230 copies of the original region of interest. The amplified DNA is easily detected by agarose gel electrophoresis (or a variety of other methods), and the presence of the DNA target in the original sample is verified (Figure 2). The PCR products (amplicons) should be the same size as the target that was amplified; conformation of the result can also be obtained with restriction enzyme analysis or DNA sequencing, although this is usually only carried out when the reaction is initially standardized.

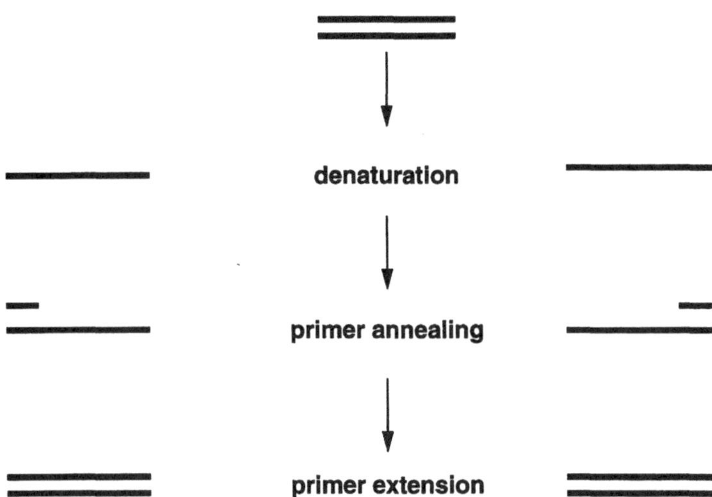

Figure 1. To amplify specific DNA sequences (templates) using the polymerase chain reaction, the template DNA is first denatured by heating, to a temperature between 92 and 95°C. Primers are annealed to the template at temperatures ranging from 45 to 60°C, and primer extension is carried out using a heat-stable DNA polymerase operating typically at a temperature of 72°C. Each step takes between 30 and 60 seconds. The steps together constitute a single cycle, and in a typical assay, 30–40 cycles are performed.

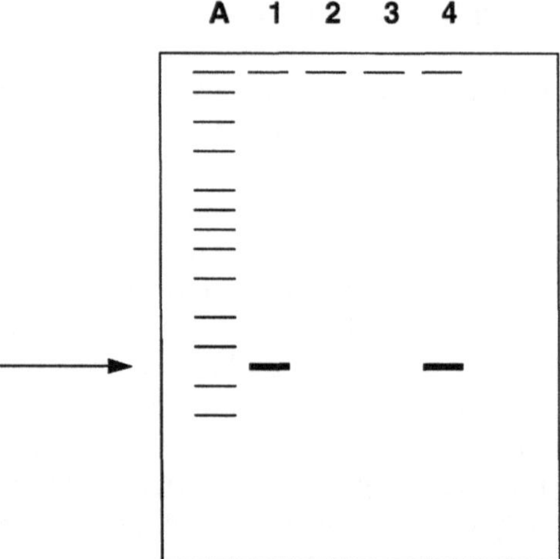

Figure 2. After the PCR reaction is performed, PCR products are typically detected with agarose gel electrophoresis. In this schematic example, lane A contains a DNA ladder to be used as a size marker. Lane 1 contains positive control template DNA which yields an amplicon of the desired size, as indicated by the arrow. Lanes 2–4 contain clinical samples: lane 4 shows a positive result, whereas lanes 2 and 3 are negative.

Although PCR is a technique of DNA amplification, it can also be used to assess the presence of RNA in a sample through a process known as reverse transcriptase PCR (RT-PCR). In this technique, RNA in a sample is first extracted and converted into cDNA using the enzyme reverse transcriptase. This cDNA is then used as the template for a PCR reaction which proceeds in the manner described above.

The ability of PCR to detect specific microorganisms depends on the ability to use primers which will bind DNA sequences that occur uniquely in particular organisms. For example, a DNA sequence known as IS6110 has been shown to occur in *Mycobacterium tuberculosis*, but not in any other mycobacteria or other class of microbe [10]. Thus, the sequence is a useful amplification target of a PCR reaction: if the IS6110 DNA sequence is present in a biological sample, *M. tuberculosis* must be present in that sample. It follows therefore that, before PCR reactions can be used in diagnosis, unique DNA sequences from a variety of pathogens must be identified. This has in fact been carried out for a large number of bacteria, viruses, parasites, and other microorganisms that cause respiratory tract illness [4]. The specificity of the reaction can also be affected by several of the reaction conditions, including the temperature at which the primers anneal to the template and the composition of the buffer solution in which the reaction takes place.

The sensitivity of the assay is exquisite in theory: under optimal conditions, a single copy of DNA can be identified and amplified to create more than 10 million identical copies which can easily be seen on gel electrophoresis. In actual practice, however, biological specimens such as sputum or blood often contain PCR inhibitors, so that the sensitivity of the assay is less than ideal. The amount of target DNA in the sample and the presence of inhibitors can also be affected by methods used to extract that DNA for use in PCR (for example, heating, freeze-thawing, organic extraction). Thus, in creating an optimal PCR assay many technical details need to be worked out before clinical utility can even be considered.

3. Use of PCR in Diagnosis of Respiratory Infections

The remainder of the chapter addresses the utility of PCR in diagnosis of specific pulmonary infectious diseases and highlights the caveats for using the test in routine clinical practice.

3.1. Tuberculosis

PCR technology has generated great interest as a potential advance in the diagnostic approach to tuberculosis. Despite the magnitude of the public health problem caused by tuberculosis (nearly 2 billion people infected world wide and 8–12 million new cases of active disease each year), methods of diagnosis have changed little (in a qualitative sense) since the tubercle bacillus was first identified by Robert Koch in 1882 [11]. In developed countries culture is routinely performed, and 85% of cases of pulmonary tuberculosis are eventually confirmed in this manner, with the remainder being clinically diagnosed after a response to therapy. Advances in culture techniques, particularly the introduction of broth-based culture, has had a significant impact on diagnosis, because a substantial number of cases of smear-positive tuberculosis can be confirmed with broth-based culture in 7–14 days. In poor countries, however, culture is not routinely performed, and cases are diagnosed based on a combination of symptoms, chest radiographs, and acid-fast smears. Thus, potential applications of PCR diagnosis in wealthy countries would primarily allow more rapid diagnosis, whereas, in poor countries, overall case detection rates and diagnostic accuracy might be expected to improve, assuming that the technology for PCR could be put in place and is affordable (two rather substantial assumptions).

As noted above, most early work in PCR diagnosis of tuberculosis was based on amplification of the DNA insertion sequence IS6110 [10]. This DNA sequence is common to be *M. tuberculosis* complex of organisms (*M. tuberculosis*, *M. bovis*, *M. africanum*, and *M. microti*), but is not found in any other species of mycobacteria, making it a useful amplification target for potential clinical use. More recently developed commercial PCR assays for diagnosis of tuberculosis amplify ribosomal RNA (rRNA) genes whose specificity is equal to that of IS6110. In theory, rRNA sequences are much more abundant in cells than single copy DNA sequences and are therefore attractive as DNA templates in PCR assays. However, the published literature indicates little difference in diagnostic performance of PCR for tuberculosis with these two amplification targets, and they will be discussed interchangeably.

A large number of studies have been published concerning the use of PCR assays for the detection of *M. tuberculosis* [12–17]. The vast majority of these studies have focused on the laboratory perspective rather than the clinical perspective, making the results somewhat difficult to translate into routine clinical use, and this has been a concern of expert panels assembled to evaluate the role of currently available DNA amplification tests in actual practice. In addition, published studies to date (as well as unpublished data presented to licensing agencies such as the US Food and Drug Administration) span a wide range of DNA amplification techniques. Remarkably, however, there has been fairly substantial agreement among several studies regarding the overall sensitivity and specificity of these assays, so that reference to the two commercially available assays, the GenProbe MTD and the Roche Amplicor, can stand as typical values [18]. Overall sensitivity with these two assays ranges from 77% to 80%, with specificity ranging from 98% to 99%. However, the performance characteristics of the tests differ in smear-positive and smear-negative tuberculosis. In smear-positive cases, sensitivity and specificity of the commercial PCR assays are in the 95–100% range, but in smear-negative tuberculosis, sensitivity of PCR is of the order of 48–53% (specificity remains in the 96–99% range). For these reasons, in the USA, these commercial assays are felt to be indicated only for rapid confirmation that a smear-positive sample is in fact *M. tuberculosis* and not an atypical mycobacterium. This may be a useful application, particularly in areas where isolation of *M. avium* complex organisms is common.

Put in other terms, PCR wil reliably and rapidly detect nearly all cases of smear-positive tuberculosis and about half of the smear-negative, culture-positive cases. Although there has been some disappointment that PCR does not detect all culture-positive tuberculosis, it should be kept in mind that the overal sensitivity of PCR for tuberculosis is considerably better than acid-fast bacillus (AFB) smear alone, which is currently the only other widely available, rapid, diagnostic test for tuberculosis. If PCR were to replace sputum smear examination completely for the diagnosis of active, previously untreated cases of tuberculosis, more patients would be accurately diagnosed in less time than with any other currently available test. However, several limitations prevent PCR from replacing AFB smears at this moment. These limitations include not only the cost of the assay but also the lack of data regarding the use of the assay to determine infectiousness of a given patient and response to therapy, two major uses of acid-fast smears. Several small studies indicate that PCR assays may remain positive long after smears and cultures have become negative, and these issues need to be evaluated prospectively in large clinical trials [19–21]. Finally, the optimal number of samples to be collected and assayed by PCR per patient remains to be determined [22].

Several small clinical studies have suggested that PCR can be used in novel ways to diagnose both pulmonary and extrapulmonary tuberculosis. Peripheral blood samples (often easier to obtain than sputum) from patients with pulmonary tuberculosis have been reported to contain *M. tuberculosis* DNA detectable by PCR, although the consistency of this finding is not clear, with studies reporting a sensitivity of between 35% and 89% using this approach [23–25]. Extrapulmonary cases of tuberculosis, often culture negative using current technology (especially cases of tuberculous meningitis), can certainly be diagnosed using PCR, although the exact overall sensitivity of DNA amplification in these settings requires further study [26]. Recently, Pfyffer and colleagues reported that, when applied to 322 non-respiratory specimens (including cerebrospinal fluid), a commercial PCR assay had a sensitivity and specificity of 93.1% and 97.7%, respectively [27]. It seems safe to say at this point in time that a positive PCR result on a non-respiratory specimen can reliably be taken as presumptive evidence of extrapulmonary tuberculosis.

3.2. Pneumocystis carinii *pneumonia*

In developed countries, *P. carinii* pneumonia (PCP) remains the most common opportunistic pulmonary infection in patients with the acquired immune deficiency syndrome (AIDS) [28]. In addition, widespread use of immunosuppressive therapy for organ transplantation and other disorders has made PCP a more common problem in a variety of clinical settings [29]. As a good deal of evidence suggests that early treatment is associated with significant benefit, in terms of reducing morbidity and mortality, prompt diagnosis is important [30].

Diagnosis of PCP in patients with AIDS is usually straighforward. Patients generally present with bilateral diffuse interstitial infiltrates, although a variety of radiographic manifestations, including cystic lesions, localized infiltrates, a miliary pattern, or pleural effusions, have been described [31]. Early on in the AIDS epidemic, PCP was frequently diagnosed with open lung biopsy, but bronchoalveolar lavage (BAL) with or without transbronchial biopsy quickly became the diagnostic procedure of choice, with a sensitivity of more than 95% [32]. More recently, staining of an induced sputum specimen (collected according to rigorous standards) with a variety of staging techniques or monoclonal antibodies has been able almost to match BAL for sensitivity [33]. It is in this setting that PCR assays for PCP have been developed. As bronchoscopy with BAL has an extremely high yield using conventional staining techniques, the greatest impact of PCR would be on sputum samples, either induced or expectorated, which can be collected with less cost and risk to the patient than lavage specimens.

A large number of PCR studies for diagnosis of PCP have been published, a small number of representative studies are discussed here. Skot et al. [34] found a sensitivity of 85% and a specificity of 100% for PCR in 117 HIV-positive patients (40 of whom were eventually diagnosed with PCP) undergoing BAL; in a second group of 33 patients, PCR performed as well on induced sputum samples as on BAL fluid. These results were not as good as those obtained with conventional staining. In a study that attempted to examine the utility of PCR on induced sputum samples, Chouaid and colleagues [35] studied 49 HIV-positive patients who had sputum induction which, if negative, was followed by BAL. In a blinded fashion, PCR was performed on all induced sputum samples. With standard staining, six induced sputum samples and seven BAL samples revealed PCP, so that sensitivity of standard staining on induced sputum samples was 46.5% (6 of 13). All 13 cases of PCP were detected using PCR in the induced sputum samples, for a sensitivity of 100%. It should be noted, however, that several other studies have demonstrated a higher yield of conventional staining on induced sputum than was reported by Chouaid et al., although their experience may actually be more representative of results in hospitals generally. In a smaller study involving a mix of induced and expectorated sputum, Eisen and colleagues [36] also found that PCR had a higher sensitivity than conventional staining. Cartwright and colleagues compared PCR with fluorescent antibody staining for *P. carinii* and found that DNA amplification was again the more sensitive technique [37].

PCR for *P. carinii* has also been applied to serum samples of patients with presumed pneumonia, and several groups have reported that respiratory illness can be accurately diagnosed in this matter, a finding that is also supported by animal models of this infection [38–40]. However, only relatively small studies have been published, and there is a lack of agreement regarding the optimal PCR amplification targets and techniques for detection of *P. carinii* in peripheral blood samples.

An interesting application of PCR in the study of *P. carinii* has been in the investigation of whether PCP results from direct transmission of the causative organism or by reactivation of long dormant pathogens that have colonized the host previously. Serological testing had suggested that most people are infected with *P. carinii* at a young age, but as the organism has been virtually impossible to grow reliably in culture, confirmation of the early colonization study has been lacking [41]. Peters and colleagues [42] performed PCR for *P. carinii* on lung tissues samples taken from autopsies of 15 non-immunosuppressed individuals, aged 15–70, and were unable to detect the presence of the pathogen in any specimen. More recently, Leigh and co-worker [43] studied 90 subjects in an effort to address this same issue. Induced sputum samples were obtained from 20 HIV-positive men with respiratory symptoms without PCP, 10 HIV-positive men with $CD4^+$ cell counts of less than $60/mm^3$ receiving PCP prophylaxis, 20 HIV-positive men with $CD4^+$ cell counts of less than $400/mm^3$ not receiving PCP prophylaxis, 20 HIV-positive men with $CD4^+$ cell counts of more than $400/mm^3$, 10 HIV-negative homosexuals, and 10 HIV-negative heterosexuals. No *P. carinii* could be detected using PCR in either of the two HIV-negative control groups. Colonization (without any signs of illness) was detected in 40% of those with a $CD4^+$ count of less than 60, 20% of those with a $CD4^+$ count of less than 400, and 10% of those with a $CD4^+$ count of over 400. The authors concluded that colonization with PCP is more common with increasing immunosuppression. It seems possible, however, that the failure to detect *P. carinii* in induced sputum samples from healthy controls may be still related to the level of detection of the assay as performed on respiratory samples, so that the hypothesis that colonization occurs in healthy persons cannot be discarded with complete confidence.

Overall, it has been demonstrated that PCR for detection of *P. carinii* in clinical samples, including induced sputum, is a sensitive and specific means of making the diagnosis of PCP. However, the exact role of this diagnostic approach has not been evaluated alongside current diagnostic and treatment algorithms, and no reliable estimate of the impact of this test on outcome can be made at present.

3.3. Community-Acquired Pneumonia

As stated above, recent trends in management of community-acquired pneumonia have led to a reduced emphasis on extensive diagnostic investigations. This has occurred because currently available diagnostic techniques are successful in identifying a specific etiology in only about 50% of cases, and the availability of relatively safe, broad-spectrum antibiotic therapy leads to a good outcome in most cases, even if an exact diagnosis is not made [44]. Thus, the true test of the value of PCR diagnostics for community-acquired pneumonia will be an improvement in outcome or a reduction in the development of drug-resistant bacteria. No studies addressing the efficacy of PCR for these two goals have been published, so the discussion below focuses only on the ability of PCR to make an accurate diagnosis.

3.3.1. Chlamydial respiratory infections: In recent years, pneumonia resulting from *Chlamydia pneumoniae* has been recognized with increasing frequency, and in some series this pathogen accounts for 10% of cases of community-acquired illness [45]. *C. pneumoniae* seems to occur more frequently in adults than in children. The clinical and radiographic presentations are non-specific, and diagnosis is made (though not reliably) with immunofluorescent serologic techniques. Culture is not widely available. Treatment is with tetracyclines, macrolides, or quinolones.

Several studies have demonstrated the feasibility of detection of *C. pneumoniae* in resporatory specimens obtained from both adults and children. In an early study from Japan, Ouchi and colleagues [46] compared PCR with the standard diagnostic technique (serum microimmunofluorescence) in 156 children between the ages of 2 months and 15 years admitted with lower respiratory tract symptoms. *C. pneumoniae* was detected in five children by microimmunofluorescence and in four of those five by PCR. Pruckl et al. [47] tested PCR performed on gargled water samples from 193 children with a variety of acute and chronic respiratory illnesses, and detected chlamydial organisms in three children, two of whom had chest radiographic changes consistent with pneumonia. These two studies do not allow firm conclusions about the use of PCR as an epidemiologic or diagnostic tool for *C. pneumoniae* in children.

Several larger studies have been carried out in adult populations. Thom et al. [48] studied 743 patients (mean age 40.5 years) with respiratory illness and found 21 with positive serology by immunofluorescence. PCR was positive in 15 of the 21, and in no additional patients. Dalhoff and Maass [49] prospectively studied 57 HIV-negative patients hospitalized with community-acquired pneumonia and performed extensive diagnostic evaluations for a variety of common pathogens on all of the subjects. This study also included 47 patients with HIV infection and 100 controls with non-infectious pulmonary illness. All patients underwent BAL to obtain samples for evaluation. *C. pneumoniae* was detected by PCR in 16% of HIV-negative patients, 13% of HIV-positive subjects, and in none of the controls (total of 15 cases). Only four cases were decteted by culture, and the authors concluded that PCR was superior to culture as a diagnostic aid.

Although the aforementioned studies do not establish a firm role for PCR in routine clinical diagnosis of *C. pneumoniae* respiratory infections, it seems that the test might be roughly as sensitive as microimmunofluorescence (MIF), the current standard. In addition, the criteria for making a diagnosis with MIF include collection of acute and convalescent serum (or a single IgM titer of 1:16 or greater, or an IgG of 1:512 or greater). PCR can make a diagnosis in one sitting and can thus potentially be a more rapid means of detection. Routine clinical use of PCR in this setting will, however, require more definitive clinical studies.

3.3.2. Pneumonia caused by Legionella *spp.*: *Legionella pneumophila* is said to cause no more than 1% of community-acquired pneumonia, although it is recognized as a somewhat more common cause of severe respiratory illness, accounting for as much as 10% of infections requiring hospitalization [50]. In several series, it is the second or third most common cause of pneumonia severe enough to warrant admission to the intensive care unit. Although originally described as a cause of pneumonia in outbreak settings, many sporadic cases of legionella infections have been described.

Several methods of diagnosing pneumonia caused by *L. pneumophila* are available. Direct fluorescent antibody staining of sputum is positive in about 50% of cases [51]. Indirect immunofluorescence to detect antibodies in serum has a greater sensitivity, but the collection of acute and convalescent titers makes this an impractical approach in the acute setting. Direct culture of the organism is possible using selective media. Culture should detect 80% of cases if enough specimens are collected and properly grown in the laboratory. The more recently developed urinary antigen detects *L. pneumophila* serogroup I only (which accounts for 80–90% of important *L. pneumophila* infections) with greater than 90% sensitivity and 99% specificity [52].

PCR assays for *L. pneumophila* have been developed and are commercially available, although extensive clinical investigation of the assays has not been done. Murdoch and colleagues used a PCR assay for a tRNA gene of *L. pneumophila* to detect the organism in stored serum and urine samples collected as part of a prospective investigation of the etiology of pneumonia [53]. The sensitivity of the legionella PCR was 64% (18 of 28 patients in whom a diagnosis of legionella infection was made by other methods), which improved to 73% if samples collected more than 4 days after the onset of symptoms were not tested. The specificity of PCR was 100%. In another study, Ramirez and co-workers [54] detected five of six cases of legionella infection by performing PCR on throat swabs of patients with pneumonia. Overall, data are insufficient to make recommendations for widespread introduction of legionella PCR into clinical practice. Specifically, a prospective comparison of PCR and urinary antigen detection should be done in patients with severe community-acquired pneumonia. PCR may have a role in infection control independent of diagnosis of pneumonia, because one study has demonstrated that the assay can be used to identify infected water supplies which may the source of outbreaks.

3.3.3. Mycoplasma pneumoniae *pneumonia*: Another of the so-called atypical pneumonias, mycoplasma pneumonia, is believed to be common, yet is fairly difficult to diagnosis routinely [55]. Culture is difficult and unreliable; the most widely used method of diagnosis is serologic testing. A fourfold increase in titers (using the complement fixation method) from acute to convalescent serum is believed to be diagnostic, although this is obviously a retrospcetive method of diagnosis. Other serologically based methods, including enzyme-linked immunosorbent assays (ELISA), have been developed as well.

Direct species-specific probes for rRNA of *Mycoplasma* spp. have been developed and have sensitivities reported to be in the 75–100% range [56]. More recently, true DNA amplification assays using PCR have also become available, although clinical experience has been variable. In a study of 155 patients with lower respiratory illness who underwent extensive diagnostic evaluations, PCR performed on a single throat swab specimen detected eight of nine cases of serologically proven myocoplasma pneumonia [54]. Using samples obtained by transthoracic needle aspiration (a technique not routinely performed in most hospitals), Falguera and colleagues [57] diagnosed mycoplasma pneumonia using PCR in eight patients; however, an additional 10 patients were PCR negative and were diagnosed on serologic grounds. No false-positive diagnoses were made using PCR, so that the sensitivity was only 45%, although the specificity was high. Blackmore and colleagues [58] studied 99 patients hospitalied for pneumonia and found that 24 adults and 25 children had *Mycoplasma pneumoniae* detected from throat swab specimens using PCR. Although the overall sensitivity and specificity of this study were 92% and 98%, respectively, acute and convalescent serum samples were not available for all patients, so that some cases were diagnosed only with a combination of a single serum titer and clinical criteria.

As *M. pneumoniae* pneumonia is usually a relatively benign illness easily treated with macrolide antibiotics that are commonly prescribed for pneumonia, routine PCR diagnostic testing does not seem warranted at present in view of the lack of standardized assays and the variability of results in reported studies.

3.3.4. Other bacterial pneumonias: Common pneumonia pathogens such as *S. pneumoniae* and *Haemophilus influenzae* are routinely covered by broad-spectrum antibiotics used to treat community-acquired pneumonia, so improvements in outcome that are associated with more rapid and sensitive PCR assays for these organisms might be difficult to demonstrate or even postulate. A limited experience with PCR has been published in these settings. Rudolph et al. [59] detected *S. pneumoniae* DNA in buffy coat samples of five of eight patients with known pneumococcal bacteremia, and detected no DNA in samples from 13 of 14 patients with pneumonia from other causes (sensitivity 63%, specificity 93%). Hassan-King and colleagues [60] from the Gambia screened blood cultures of 295 children with pneumonia using a multiplex technique (i.e. two different PCR reactions carried out simultaneously) for detection of *S. pneumoniae* and *H. influenzae* and found that PCRs compared favorably with blood culture results and were positive in four cases of *H. influenza* pneumonia with negative blood cultures. Using sputum samples, Gillespie and colleagues [61] detected *S. pneumonia* DNA in sputum from 13 and 14 patients with a heavy growth of pneumococci; a C-polysaccharide enzyme-linked immunosorbent assay (ELISA) was also positive in the same number of patients.

Other than demonstrating the technical feasibility of PCR for detecting common bacterial pneumonia pathogens, no clinical indications for routine use can be gleaned from the literature published to date.

3.4. Viral Pneumonias

Viral pneumonias occur in two settings: immunocompetent hosts who may become infected with respiratory syncytial virus (RSV), adenovirus, influenza virus, or, less commonly, measles or varicella virus; and immunocompromised hosts, who may develop disease as a result of cytomegalovirus (CMV) or other opportunists. Distinguishing viral pneumonias from other causes of infection or inflammation is usually made on clinical and radiographic grounds. Laboratory diagnosis of these infections has rested on a variety of tests, including direct and indirect fluorescent antibody staining, cultures, and ELISA [62]. In normal hosts, little specific therapy of great efficacy is available, although amantadine and ribavarin are occasionally used. For cytomegalovirus pneumonitis in patients with bone marrow transplantation, specific therapy has been shown to improve survival markedly, and timely and accurate diagnosis is of considerable importance [63].

3.4.1. Viral infections affecting normal hosts: PCR assays have been developed for detection of adenovirus, RSV, and influenza virus in a variety of clinical specimens, although most studies have focused on nasopharyngeal swab samples, because these are easy to obtain, particularly from children. Straightforward PCR technology has been used, although in the case of RNA viruses such as RSV, an RT-PCR method is needed. The published clinical experience with PCR in these settings has to date been fairly limited. Morris and colleagues [64] attempted rapid diagnosis of adenoviral upper respiratory infections in adults and found that the sensitivity of the PCR method was 76% compared with culture of a variety of adenoviral subtypes. Some subtypes were more readily detected than others in this study, implying that genetic variability among various subtypes was responsible for false-negative results. Throat swabs or nasopharyngeal aspirates were used as substrates in this study.

Studies of the utility of PCR for diagnosis of influenza and RSV infections, particularly in children, have shown somewhat better results. In several relatively small studies, PCR has been found to have sensitivity for diagnosis in the 95–100% range, compared with viral culture, which has been used as the gold standard in most trials. Two larger studies merit more detailed mention. Freymuth and co-workers [65] obtained nasal aspirates from 238 infants hospitalized with acute respiratory infections and compared PCR for RSV with viral isolation (culture) and immunofluorescence. PCR was found to have a sensitivity as high as 97.5% and a specificity of 63.9% compared with the other methods. The positive predictive value of the assay was only 57.8%, however. In a similar study of influenza diagnosis, Claas and colleagues evaluated 342 children in the Netherlands and found that PCR was at least as sensitive as culture for diagnosis, but could yield results in as little as 2 days, whereas culture combined with immunofluorescence took up to 14 days [66].

3.4.2. Viral infections affecting immunocompromised hosts: A substantial advance in the treatment and outcome of patients with CMV pneumonitis was made several years ago when investigators at Memorial-Sloan Kettering Cancer Center established criteria for diagnosis, which combined clinical and radiographic findings with results of monoclonal antibody staining of cells recovered by BAL [63]. With this approach, early diagnosis and treatment could be accomplished and mortality rates fell substantially. Since then, many efforts have been made to speed and refine diagnosis of CMV using PCR further. In an early study, Cathomas and colleagues from Memorial-Sloan Kettering extended their earlier work and compared PCR, viral culture, and immunostaining of BAL cells in bone marrow transplant recipients [67]. Seventy-five transplant recipients with clinical and radiographic evidence of pneumonitis were studied, and the results of the diagnostic assays were correlated with outcome. Ultimately, seven patients were determined to have true CMV pneumonitis and eight others were found to have CMV infection without disease. PCR detected all cases of infection and disease, but monoclonal antibody immunostaining of BAL cells was more specific for actual pneumonitis. The excellent sensitivity of PCR for detecting CMV in lavage fluid of patients with CMV pneumonitis has been confirmed by several subsequent studies, and it seems likely that this approach to diagnosis will become clinically important in the coming years. Detection of CMV by PCR of serum samples from at-risk patients has also been a promising approach, although the reported experience with this avenue of diagnosis has been limited [68–71].

4. Conclusion

The development of the PCR has generated great excitement as new possibilities for rapid, sensitive, and specific diagnosis of respiratory infection have become apparent. The first phase of development of diagnostic PCR assays has been concluded, and it has been demonstrated that such assays are technically feasible and can be used to detect microorganisms in a wide variety of biological specimens under ideal laboratory conditions. On the other hand, the second phase of development, namely the large-scale evaluation of PCR-based diagnostics for routine clinical use, is only just beginning. In addition, in areas where PCR assays seem to offer genuine clinical benefit, such as for improved diagnosis of tuberculosis, cost, and technology transfer to poor countries where the disease is common, remain significant issues. Nevertheless, it is likely that the next four years will see PCR assays move into more routine clinical use for a wide variety of respiratory pathogens.

References

1 Woodhead MA, Arrowsmith J, Chamberlain-Webber R, Wooding S, Williams I (1991) The value of routine microbial investigation in community acquired pneumonia. *Respir Med* 85: 313–317
2 Fang GD, Fine M, Orloff J, Arisumi D, Yu VL, Kapoor W, Grayston JT, Wang SP, Kohler R, Muder RR et al. (1990) New and emerging etiologies for community acquired pneumonia with implication for therapy: a prospective multicenter study of 359 cases. *Medicine* 69: 307–316
3 Garibaldi RA (1985) Epidemiology of community-acquired respiratory tract infections in adults: incidence, etiology, and impact. *Am J Med* 78: 32S–37S
4 Schluger NW, Rom WN (1995) The polymerase chain reaction in the diagnosis and evaluation of pulmonary infections. *Am J Respir Crit Care Med* 152: 11–15
5 Niederman MS, Bass JB, Campbell GD, Fein AM, Grossman RF, Mandell LA, Marrie TJ, Sarosi GA, Torres A, Yu V (1993) Guidelines for the initial management of adults with community-acquired pneumonia: diagnosis, assessment of severity, and initial antimicrobial therapy. *Am Rev Respir Dis* 148: 1418–1426
6 Bartlett JG, Mundy LM (1995) Community-acquired pneumonia. *N Engl J Med* 333: 1618–1624
7 Breiman RF, Butler JC, Tenover FC, Elliott JA, Facklam RR (1994) Emergence of drug-resistant pneumococcal infections in the United States. *JAMA* 271: 1831–1835
8 Marquette CH, Copin MC, Wallet F, Neviere R, Saulnier F, Mathieu D (1995) Diagnostic tests for pneumonia in ventilated patients: prospective evaluation of diagnostic accuracy using histology as a diagnostic gold standard. *Am J Respir Crit Care Med* 151: 1878–1888
9 Saiki RK, Gelfand DH, Stoffel S, Scharf SJ, Higuchi R, Horn GT, Mullis KB, Erlich HA (1988) Primer-directed enzymatic amplification of DNA with a thermostable DNA polymerase. *Science* 239: 487–491
10 Hermans PWM, Schuitema ARJ, Van Soolingen D, Verstynen CP, Bik EM, Kolk AH, van Embden (1990) Specific detection of *Mycobacterium tuberculosis* complex strains by polymerase chain reaction. *J Clin Microbiol* 28: 1204–1213
11 Schluger N, Rom WM (1994) Current approaches to the diagnosis of active pulmonary tuberculosis. *Am J Respir Crit Care Med* 149: 264–267
12 Eisenach KD, Sifford MD, Cave MD, Bates JH, Crawford JT (1991) Detection of *Mycobacterium tuberculosis* in sputum samples using a polymerase chain reaction. *Am Rev Respir Dis* 144: 1160–1163
13 Forbes BA, Hicks KES (1993) Direct detection of *Mycobacterium tuberculosis* in respiratory specimens in a clinical laboratory by polymerase chain reaction. *J Clin Microbiol* 31: 1688–1694
14 Clarridge JE, Shawar RM, Shinnick TM, Plikaytis BB (1993) Large-scale use of polymerase chain reaction for detection of *Mycobacterium tuberculosis* in a routine mycobacteriology laborators. *J Clin Microbiol* 31: 2049–2056
15 Pierre C, Olivier C, Lecossier D, Boussougant Y, Yeni P, Hance AJ (1993) Diagnosis of primary tuberculosis in children by amplification and detection of mycobacterial DNA. *Am Rev Respir Dis* 147: 420–424
16 Marshall BG, Shaw RJ (1996) New technology in the diagnosis of tuberculosis. *Br J Hosp Med* 55: 491–534
17 Dalovisio JR, Montenegro-James S, Kemmerly SA, Genre CF, Chambers R, Greer D, Pankey GA, Failla DM, Haydel KG, Hutchinson L et al. (1996) Comparison of the amplified *Mycobacterium tuberculosis* (MTB) direct test, Amplicor MTB PCR, and IS6110-PCR for detection of MTB in respiratory specimens. *Clin Infect Dis* 23: 1099–1106
18 Forbes BA (1997) Critical assessment of gene amplification approaches on the diagnosis of tuberculosis. *Immunol Invest* 26: 105–116
19 Schluger NW, Kinney D, Harkin TJ, Rom WN (1994) Clinical utility of the polymerase chain reaction in the diagnosis of infections due to *Mycobacterium tuberculosis*. *Chest* 105: 1116–1121
20 Yuen KY, Chan KS, Ho BSW, Dai LK, Chau PY, Ng MH (1993) Use of PCR in routine diagnosis of treated and untreated pulmonary tuberculosis. *J Clin Pathol* 46: 318–322

21 Yuen KY, Chan KS, Chan CM, Ho PL, Ng MH (1997) Monitoring the therapy of pulmonary tuberculosis by nested polymerase chain reaction assay. *J Infect* 32: 29 – 33
22 Catanzaro A, Davidson B, Fujiwara P, Goldberger M, Gordin F, Salfinger M, Schluger NW, Sierra M, Woods GL (1997) Proceedings of an American Thoracic Society Workshop, "Rapid Diagnostics Tests for Tuberculosis. What is the Appropriate Use?" *Am J Respir Crit Care Med* 155: 1804–1814
23 Condos R, McClune A, Rom WN, Schluger NW (1996) Identification of patiens with active pulmonary tuberculosis using a peripheral blood-based polymerase chain reaction assay. *Lancet* 347: 1082–1085
24 Rolfs A, Beige J, Finckh U, Kohler B, Schaberg T, Lokies J, Lode H (1995) Amplification of *Mycobacterium tuberculosis* from peripheral blood. *J Clin Microbiol* 33: 3312–3314
25 Folgueira L, Delgado R, Palenque E, Aguado JM, Noriega AR (1996) Rapid diagnosis of *Mycobacterium tuberculosis* bacteremia by PCR. *J Clin Microbiol* 34: 512–515
26 Kaltwasser G, Garcia S, Salinas AM, Montiel F (1993) Enzymatic DNA amplification (PCR) in the diagnosis of extrapulmonary *Mycobacterium tuberculosis* infection. *Mol Cell Probes* 7: 465–470
27 Pfyffer Ge, Kissling P, Jahn EM, Welscher HM, Salfinger M, Weber R (1996) Diagnostic performance of amplified *Mycobacterium tuberculosis* direct test with cerebrospinal fluid, other nonrespiratory, and respiratory specimens. *J Clin Microbiol* 34: 834–841
28 Rosen MJ (1996) Overview of pulmonary complications [of AIDS]. *Clin Chest Med* 17: 621–631
29 Sepkowitz KA, Brown AE, Armstrong D (1995) *Pneumocystis carinii* pneumonia without acquired immunodeficiency syndrome. More patients, same risk. *Arch Intern Med* 155: 1125–1128
30 Fernandez P, Torres A, Miro JM, Vieigas C, Mallolas J, Zamora L, Gatell JM, Valls ME, Riquelme R, Rodriguez-Roisin R (1995) Prognostic factors influencing the outcome in *Pneumocystis carinii* pneumonia in patients with AIDS. *Thorax* 50: 668–671
31 Safrin S (1993) Pneumocystis carinii pneumonia in patients with the acquired immunodeficiency syndrome. *Semin Respir Infect* 8: 96–103
32 Pisani RJ, Wright AJ (1992) Clinical utility of bronchoalveolar lavage in immunocompromised hosts. *Mayo Clinic Proc* 67: 221–227
33 Blumenfeld W, Kovacs JA (1988) Use of a monoclonal antibody to detect *Pneumocystis carinii* in induced sputum and bronchoalveolar lavage flud by immunoperoxidase staining. *Arch Pathol Laboratory Med* 112: 1233 – 1236
34 Skot J, Lerche AG, Kolmos HJ, Nielsen JO, Mathiesen LR, Lundgren JD (1995) *Pneumocystis carinii* in bronchoalveolar lavage and induced sputum: detection with a nested polymerase chain reaction. *Scand J Infect Dis* 27: 363–367
35 Chouaid C, Roux P, Lavard I, Poirot JL, Housset B (1995) Use of the polymerase chain reaction technique on induced-sputum samples for the diagnosis of *Pneumocystis carinii* pneumonia in HIV-infected patients. A clinical and cost-analysis study. *Am J Clin Pathol* 104: 72–75
36 Eisen D, Ross BC, Fairbairn J, Warren RJ, Baird RW, Dwyer B (1994) Comparison of *Pneumocystis carinii* detection by toluidine blue O staining, direct immunofluorescence and DNA amplification in sputum specimens from HIV positive patients. *Pathology* 26: 198–200
37 Cartwright CP, Nelson NA, Gill VJ (1994) Development and evaluation of a rapid and simple procedure for detection of *Pneumocystis carinii* by PCR. *J Clin Microbiol* 32: 1634–1638
38 Sepkowitz K, Schluger N, Godwin T, Cerami A, Bucala R (1993) DNA Amplification in experimental pneumocystosis: characterization of serum *P. carinii* DNA and potential *P. carinii* carrier states. *J Infect Dis* 168: 421–426
39 Schluger N, Godwin T, Sepkowitz K, Armstrong D, Rifkin M, Bernard E, Cerami A, Bucala R (1992) Application of the polymerase chain reaction to pneumocystosis and frequent detection of *Pneumocystis carinii* in serum of patients with Pneumocystis pneumonia. *J Exp Med* 176: 1327–1333
40 Miyawaki H, Fujita J, Hojo S, Harada M, Yamaji Y, Suguri S, Takahara J (1996) Detection of *Pneumocystis carinii* sequences in serum by polymerase chain reaction. *Respir Med* 90: 153–157

41 Masur H, Lane HC, Kovacs JA, Allegra CJ, Edman JC (1989) NIH conference. Pneumocystis pneumonia: from bench to clinic. *Ann Intern Med* 111: 813–826
42 Peters SE, Wakefield AE, Sinclair K, Millard PR, Hopkin JM (1992) A search for *Pneumocystis carinii* in post-mortem lungs by DNA amplification. *J Pathol* 166: 195–198
43 Leigh TR, Kangro HO, Gazzard BG, Jeffries DJ, Collins JV (1993) DNA amplification by the polymerase chain reaction to detect sub-clinical *Pneumocystis carinii* colonization in HIV-positive and HIV-negative male homosexuals with and without respiratory symptoms. *Respir Med* 87: 525–529
44 Fine MJ, Auble TE, Yealy DM, Hanusa BH, Weissfeld LA, Singer DE, Coley CM, Marrie TJ, Kapoor WN (1997) A prediction rule to identify low-risk patients with community-acquired pneumonia. *N Engl J Med* 336: 243–250
45 Grayston JT, Kuo CC, Wang S (1988) A new chlamydia psittaci strain TWAR, isolated in acute respiratory tract infections. *N Engl J Med* 315: 161–168
46 Ouchi K, Nakazawa T, Karita M, Kanehara Y (1994) Prevalence of *Chlamydia pneumoniae* in acute lower respiratory infection in the pediatric population in Japan. *Acta Paediatr Jap* 36: 256–260
47 Pruckl PM, Aspock C, Makristathis A, Rotter ML, Wank H, Willinger B, Hirschl AM (1995) Polymerase chain reaction for detection of *Chlamydia pneumoniae* in gargled-water specimens of children. *Eur J Clin Microbiol Infect Dis* 14: 141–144
48 Thom DH, Grayston JT, Campbell LA, Kuo CC, Diwan VK, Wang SP (1994) Respiratory infection with *Chlamydia pneumoniae* in middle-aged and older adult outpatients. *J Clin Microbiol Infect Dis* 13: 785–792
49 Dalhoff K, Maass M (1996) *Chlamydia pneumoniae* pneumonia in hospitalized patients. Clinical characteristics and diagnostic value of polymerase chain reaction detection in BAL. *Chest* 110: 351–356
50 Falco V, Fernandez de Sevilla T, Alegre J, Ferrer A, Vasquez J (1991) L. pneumophila-a cause of severe community acquired pneumonias. *Chest* 100: 1007–1011
51 Joly JR, Ramsay D (1985) Use of monoclonal antibodies in the diagnosis and epidemiologic studies of legionellosis. *Clin Lab Med* 5: 561–574
52 Kazandjian D, Chiew R, Gilbert GL (1997) Rapid diagnosis of *Legionella pneumophila* serogroup 1 infection with the Binax enzyme immunoassay urinary antigen test. *J Clin Microbiol* 35: 954–956
53 Murdoch DR, Walford EJ, Jennings LC, Light GJ, Schousboe MI, Chereshsky AY, Chambers ST, Town GI (1996) Use of the polymerase chain reaction to detect Legionella DNA in urine and serum samples from patients with pneumonia. *Clin Infect Dis* 23: 475–480
54 Ramirez JA, Ahkee S, Tolentino A, Miller RD, Summersgill JT (1996) Diagnosis of *Legionella pneumophila*, *Mycoplasma pneumoniae*, or *Chlamydia pneumoniae* lower respiratory infection using the polymerase chain reaction on a single throat swab specimen. *Diagn Microb Infect Dis* 24: 7–14
55 Luby JP (1991) Pneumonia caused by *Mycoplasma pneumoniae* infection. *Clin Chest Med* 12: 237–244
56 Dular R, Kajioka R, Kasatiya S (1988) Comparison of Gen-Probe commercial kit and culture technique for the diagnosis of *Mycoplasma pneumoniae* infection. *J Clin Microbiol* 26: 1068–1069
57 Falguera M, Nogues A, Ruiz-Gonzalez A, Garcia M, Puig T (1996) Detection of *Mycoplasma pneumoniae* by polymerase chain reaction in lung aspirates from patients with community-acquired pneumonia. *Chest* 110: 972–976
58 Blackmore TK, Reznikov M, Gordon DL (1995) Clinical utility of the polymerase chain reaction to diagnose *Mycoplasma pneumoniae* infection. *Pathology* 27: 177–181
59 Rudolph KM, Parkinson AJ, Black CM, Mayer LW (1993) Evaluation of polymerase chain reaction for diagnosis of pneumococcal pneumonia. *J Clin Microbiol* 31: 2661–2666
60 Hassan-King M, Baldeh I, Adegbola R, Omosigho C, Usen SO, Oparaugo A, Greenwood BM (1996) Detection of *Haemophilus influenzae* and *Streptococcus pneumoniae* DNA in blood culture by a single PCR assay. *J Clin Microbiol* 34: 2030–2032
61 Gillespie SH, Ullman C, Smith MD, Emery V (1994) Detection of *Streptococcus pneumoniae* in sputum samples by PCR. *J Clin Microbiol* 32: 1308–1311
62 Leland DS, Emanuel D (1995) Laboratory diagnosis of viral infections of the lung. *Semin Respir Infect* 10: 189–198

63 Emanuel D, Cunningham I, Jule-Elysee K, Brochstein JA, Kernan KA, Laver J, Stover D, White DA, Fells A, Polsky B et al. (1988) Cytomegalovirus pneumonia after bone marrow transplantation successfully treated with the combination of ganciclovir and high-dose intravenous immune globulin. *Ann Intern Med* 109: 777–782
64 Morris DJ, Cooper RJ, Barr T, Bailey AS (1996) Polymerase chain reaction for rapid diagnosis of respiratory adenovirus infection. *J Infect* 32: 113–117
65 Freymuth F, Eugene G, Vabret A, Petitjean J, Gennetay E, Brouard J, Duhamel JF, Guillois B (1995) Detection of respiratory syncytial virus by reverse transcription-PCR and hybridization with a DNA enzyme immunoassay. *J Clin Microbiol* 33: 3352–3355
66 Claas EC, van Milaan AJ, Sprenger MJ, Ruiten-Stuiver M, Arron GI, Rothbarth PH, Masurel N (1993) Prospective application of reverse transcriptase polymerase chain reaction for diagnosing influenza infections in respiratory samples from a children's hospital. *J Clin Microbiol* 31: 2218–2221
67 Cathomas G, Morris P, Pekle K, Cunningham I, Emanuel D (1993) Rapid diagnosis of cytomegalovirus pneumonia in marrow transplant recipients by bronchoalveolar lavage using the polymerase chain reaction, virus culture, and the direct immunostaining of alveolar cells. *Blood* 81: 1909–1913
68 Watanabe N, Takeda M, Ishigaki S, Tsuji N, Sakamaki S, Kato J, Kohda K, Mori Y, Niitsu Y (1995) CMV viraemia demonstrated in the serum of a patient with cytomegalovirus pneumonia. *Br J Haematol* 90: 457–458
69 Tokimatsu I, Tashiro T, Nasu M (1995) Early diagnosis and monitoring of human cytomegalovirus pneumonia in patients with adult T cell leukemia by DNA amplification in serum. *Chest* 107: 1024–1027
70 Flint A, Frank TS (1994) Cytomegalovirus detection in lung transplant biopsy samples by polymerase chain reaction. *J Heart Lung Transplant* 13: 38–42
71 Eriksson BM, Brytting M, Zweygberg-Wirgart B, Hillerdal G, Olding-Stenkvist E, Linde A (1993) Diagnosis of cytomegalovirus in bronchoalveolar lavage by polymerase chain reaction, in comparison with virus isolation and detection of viral antigen. *Scand J Infect Dis* 25: 421–427

Molecular Biology of the Lung
Vol. 1: Emphysema and Infection
ed. by R.A. Stockley

CHAPTER 11
Cystic Fibrosis

Uta Griesenbach[1], Duncan M. Geddes[2] and Eric W.F.W. Alton[1]

[1] *Imperial College School of Medicine at the National Heart & Lung Institute, London, UK*
[2] *Royal Brompton Hospital, London, UK*

1. Introduction

Cystic fibrosis (CF) is the most common lethal autosomal recessive single gene disorder in Caucasians, with an incidence of 1 in 1500 to 1 in 6500 in various populations [1]. The phenotype is complex with involvement of multiple organs. Chronic obstruction and infection of the respiratory tract, exocrine pancreatic insufficiency and elevated sweat electrolytes are typical features of the disease. The transport of sodium (Na^+) and chloride (Cl^-) ions, particularly the latter, is central to the basic defect in CF.

2. Clinical Manifestations

CF affects a number of epithelial-lined organs, the most important being the lungs, responsible for most of the morbidity in this disease, and eventually the usual cause of death from respiratory failure. Progressive mucus obstruction, infection and inflammation of the lower airways are the major pathological changes seen in the CF lung. Hypertrophy of submucosal glands and an increased number of goblet cells are mainly responsible for the increased mucus production.

The lungs of CF patients are often colonized with *Staphylococcus aureus* and *Haemophilus influenzae*, but most characteristically with *Pseudomonas aeruginosa* [2]. Bacterial colonization usually occurs in childhood and progresses to episodes of overt infection and subsequent lung damage. In addition to chronic infection, inflammation is a major contributing factor in the pathogenesis of the lung disease in CF. Unusually high numbers of neutrophils in the airways cause lung destruction and an increase in pro-inflammatory and a decrease in anti-inflammatory cytokines in the CF lung has been observed [3].

Exocrine pancreatic insufficiency occurs in the vast majority of CF patients [4]. Obstruction and dilation of ducts and acini by mucus leads to suboptimal secretion of pancreatic enzymes in about 85% of the patients [5]. Pancreatic enzyme supplementation is therefore necessary in most patients. Liver disease and gallbladder abnormalities are also frequently seen in CF patients but severity varies widely [6]. More than 95% of male CF patients are infertile because the vas deferens, tail and body of the epididymis and seminal vesicles are atrophic, fibrotic or completely absent [7]. Although a significant number of female CF patients are fertile (>15% [8], the overall reduced fertility appears to result from menstrual irregularities, as well as thick mucus plugs in the cervix preventing normal sperm migration [9].

In addition to the classic CF phenotype, several can be classified as atypical or mild cystic fibrosis. Infertile males, as a result of a congenital bilateral absence of the vas deferens (CBAVD), have a high incidence (80%) of mutations of CFTR, the gene product of cystic fibrosis. Specifically the mutation R117H is more frequent in CBAVD than in the general population [1]. Recently it has been reported that azoospermic males (those not having CBAVD) also have an increased frequency of CFTR mutations [10], and an increased incidence of CFTR mutations has also been found in patients with classic bronchiectasis [11].

3. Cystic Fibrosis Transmembrane Conductance regulator (CFTR): The Gene Product

The human CF gene was identified in 1989 through positional cloning approaches [12, 13]. It is located on chromosome 7q31.3 [14], spans 250 kilobase-pairs (kb) of genomic DNA and contains 27 exons [15]. The mRNA is 6.2 kb and encodes a polypeptide of 1480 amino acids with a molecular mass of about 170 kDa [12]. Alternative splicing of the mRNA has been noted in several tissues [16], but the physiological role of the alternatively spliced products, if any, is not known [17].

The gene product was named the cystic fibrosis transmembrane conductance regulator (CFTR). The amino acid sequence of CFTR suggests a tandem repeat structure with two identical halves, each consisting of six putative transmembrane α-helices and an intracellular nucleotide-binding domain. The two halves are linked through a highly charged intracellular R-domain which contains numerous potential phosphorylation sites (Figure 1) [12]. Numerous studies have indicated its role as a cAMP-regulated chloride channel (see below).

More than 600 mutations have been detected in the *CFTR* gene [18]. The major mutation, present in about 70% of CF chromosomes worldwide, is a deletion of phenylalanine at position 508 (ΔF508). The relative frequency of the other mutations varies among different populations, but most of them are very rare.

Several factors might account for the high incidence of CF in the caucasian population. Increased fertility [19] and increased resistance to tuberculosis [20] or cholera [21] of heterozygote carriers have been suggested. However, founder effects and inbreeding have been shown to account for the high incidence of CF in some populations [22].

CFTR mutations can be divied into five classes [23]. Class I mutations are nonsense, frameshift and splice mutations that lead to truncations or absence of CFTR protein synthesis. Class II mutations, including ΔF508, are mutations that interfere with correct post-translational processing. The

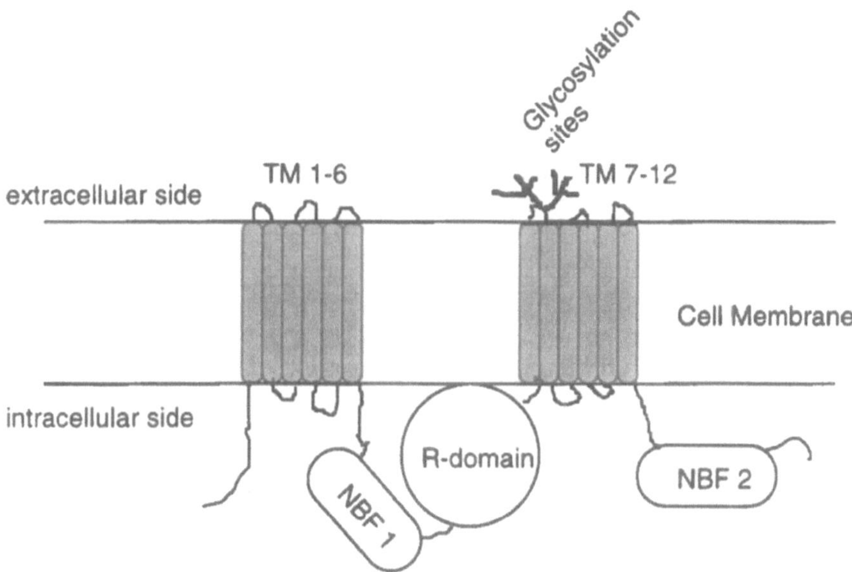

Figure 1. Topology of the CFTR protein. The *CFTR* gene encodes a protein of 1480 amino acids. The amino acid sequence suggests a tandem repeat structure with two identical halves, each consisting of six putative transmembrane α-helices (TM1–6 and TM7–12) and an intracellular nucleotide-binding domain (NBF1 and 2). Two consensus N-linked glycosylation sites are present between membrane spanning segments 7 and 8. The two halves of the protein are linked through a highly charged intracellular domain (R-domain). The R-domain contains multiple phosphorylation sites and is important for chloride channel regulation.

vast majority of mutant protein does not reach the apical membrane, although the protein itself is likely to retain normal function [24]. Class III mutations, such as G551D, give rise to Cl^- channels that show a reduced response to cAMP stimulation. Class IV mutations alter the ion selectivity or conductance of CFTR Cl^- channels and class V mutations interfere with correct transcription or translation, resulting in reduced levels of functional CFTR.

4. Chloride Channel and Other Functions of CFTR

The predicted structure of CFTR shows homology with a large superfamily of proteins known as ABC (ATP-binding cassette) transporters which function as ATP-requiring pumps, exporting macromolecules from the cell interior [25]. Well-characterized members of this family include the multidrug resistance (MDR) gene product P-glycoprotein [26] and the yeast α-mating factor STE6 [27]. Initially, several aspects of CFTR suggested that it would not itself be a Cl^- channel, including its lack of resemblance to any known channel, the homology with known transporters and the presence of ATP-binding sites generally not associated with, or required by, channels.

To study its function, CFTR was expressed in a variety of cells known not to produce this protein endogenously. These included mammalian (fibroblasts, HeLa, Chinese hamster ovary) as well as non-mammalian (oocytes of *Xenopus*, Cf9, vero) cells. These studies unanimously demonstrated that CFTR expression produces a Cl^- conductance which can be regulated through the cAMP-dependent protein kinase (PKA) pathway [28–33]. This strongly suggested that CFTR was actually a Cl^- channel, or the more remote possibility that, in the presence of CFTR, these cells expressed a Cl^- channel that had previously lain dormant. To distinguish these two possibilities, site-directed mutagenesis was used to mutate basic lysine to acidic amino acids at sites within the predicted membrane-spanning region of CFTR [34]. If CFTR is a Cl^- channel, these changes should alter its ability to conduct Cl^-. In particular the anion selectivity of the channel (relative permeability for example of Cl^- and I^-) depends on both the hydrated size of the ion and the electrostatic forces between the interior of the channel and the ion. These mutations reversed this permeability sequence from $Cl^- > I^-$ for unaltered CFTR, to $I^- > Cl^-$ for the mutated protein, clearly indicating that CFTR itself is a Cl^- channel. Confirmation of this was provided by the purification of the protein and its incorporation into lipid bilayers where it functions as a cAMP/PKA-regulated Cl^- channel [35].

The CFTR Cl^- channel is regulated through cycles of protein phosphorylation and dephosphorylation and of ATP hydrolysis [36]. In normal epithelial cells, hormonal stimulation of G protein-linked receptors leads to activation of CFTR Cl^- channels via phosphorylation by PKA [37]. Multiple consensus phosphorylation sites are located in the R-domain of the CFTR protein [12] and site-directed mutagenesis studies are under way to determine the importance of individual putative phosphorylation sites [38].

Apart from functioning as a Cl^- channel, CFTR has been implicated in the regulation of a number of other epithelial ion channels (Figure 2). Sodium absorption in CF tissues is two- to threefold higher than in normal controls [39] and can be corrected through transient expression of CFTR [40]. After cloning of the amiloride-sensitive epithelial Na^+ channel (ENaC) [41], co-transfection of CFTR and ENaC directly demonstrated the negative modulation of ENaC by CFTR [42]. CFTR decreases the open probability of ENaC, rather than altering the channel number [43].

The outward-rectifying Cl^- channel (ORCC) [44] in epithelial membranes is regulated through cAMP and ATP, as well as by CFTR, which decreases Cl^- transport by the ORCC [45]. Furthermore, Ca^{2+}-dependent Cl^- secretion appears to be up-regulated in certain cells in the absence of CFTR [46]. Finally, K^+ channels present on the basolateral surface of epithelial cells are probably also regulated by CFTR [47].

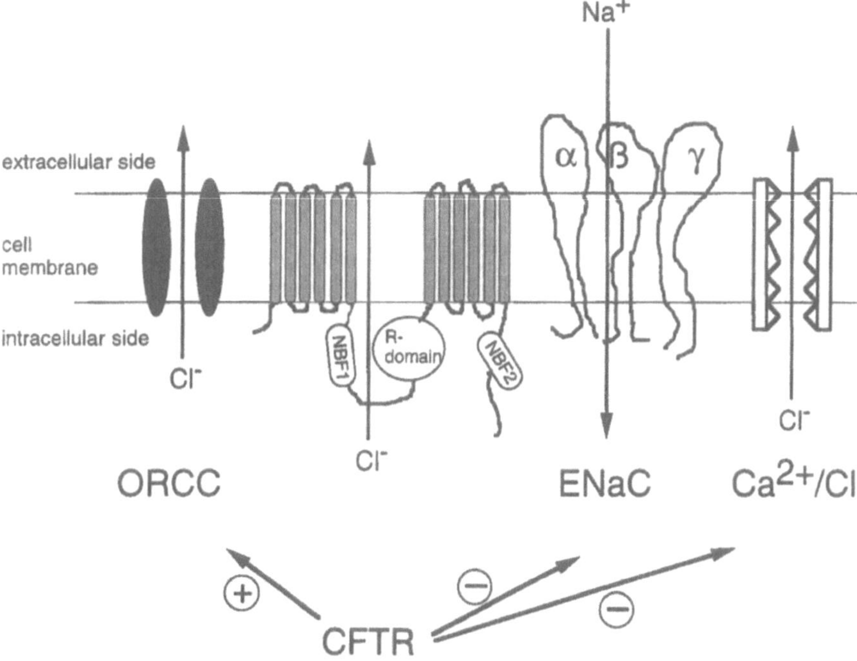

Figure 2. Regulatory function of CFTR. CFTR has been shown to regulate the activity of other ion channels in the apical membrane of epithelial cells. CFTR inhibits sodium transport through amiloride-sensitive Na^+ channels (ENaC) and chloride transport through calcium-dependent Cl^- channels (Ca^{2+}/Cl^-). CFTR activates the outward-rectifying Cl^- channels (ORCC). The mechanism of interaction between CFTR and the other epithelial ion channels is not known. Direct protein-protein interaction through substances transported by CFTR is considered.

The mechanism of interaction between CFTR and other epithelial ion channels is not clear. Direct protein-protein interactions or modulation through substances transported by CFTR are considered most likely (reviewed in Stutts [48]). There is some evidence that CFTR transports adenosine-3′-phosphate-5′-phosphosulphate (PAPS) [49] and ATP out of cells [50], consistent with the observation that most members of this family of proteins actively transport substrates across the cell membrane. These findings have, however, been disputed by a number of studies [51].

Several studies have suggested that CFTR is also involved in a variety of intracellular processes such as membrane recycling [52], as well as the regulation of endocytosis and exocytosis [53]. In addition, it has been suggested that CFTR might be involved in regulating acidification within intracellular organelles [53], although this has been refuted by a number of subsequent studies [54].

5. Relationship of Basic Defect to Disease Pathology

How the clinical phenotype in CF lungs links with abnormalities in CFTR is unknown. One simplistic suggestion relates to impaired mucociliary clearance (MCC) in the airways, because efficient clearance of mucus and inhaled micro-organisms is likely to depend on an optimal volume of airway surface fluid in which the cilia involved in MCC beat. Thus, reduced Cl^- secretion onto, and increased Na^+ absorption from, the airway lumen may lead to a suboptimal volume of airway surface liquid and hence impaired MCC, increased bacterial colonization and repeated infection. However, other defects in host defence may also play a part, including increased bacterial adherence [55], reduced ingestion of bacteria by epithelial cells [56] and impaired antibacterial activity of surface defensins [57]. Recently, altered cytokine secretion has been detected in CF lungs and might in part explain the chronic inflammation seen in young CF patients in the absence of bacterial infection [3].

6. Animal Models

A gene homologous to CFTR has been identified in rodents [58, 59], cows, sheep and monkeys [60], dogfish [61] and *Xenopus laevis* [62]. A high degree of evolutionary conservation is seen in the nucleotide-binding folds and in membrane-spanning segments. This is not the case for the R-domain apart from the putative phosphorylation sites [60].

Over the past 5 years, several mouse models have been created through gene-targeting strategies, including mice carrying the ΔF508 mutation and the G551D mutation [63–71]. The phenotype of most mouse models is similar. Intestinal blockage caused by mucus accumulation and subsequent rupture of the intestines leads to premature death in 50–95% of mice. In contrast to the severe intestinal pathology, all mouse models fail to develop the severe lung pathology that is characteristic of CF patients. The presence of an alternative non-CFTR Cl^- channel in the lung, but not in the intestine, could explain these findings [72]. In addition, murine lungs largely lack submucosal glands, a major site of CFTR expression in humans, and do not demonstrate the characteristic increase in Na^+ absorption. Thus, a number of factors may be involved in this difference in phenotype.

Despite their limitations, the CF mouse models are valuable for electrophysiological, pharmacological and gene therapeutic research. Further, breeding studies using the $cftr^{tm1Hsc}$ mouse have identified a *CFTR* modifier locus on mouse chromosome 7 [65].

7. Therapy

7.1. Conventional Therapy

Conventional therapy for CF includes the use of physiotherapy, antibiotics and pancreatic supplements, the latter of which aid the malabsorption consequent on pancreatic damage. Many patients require treatment four times daily, including a considerable time spent on physiotherapy. This combination of treatment has helped increase life expectancy from about 1 year in the 1930s to the current 30 years of age.

Recently, studies have begun to address whether modulation of the ion transport abnormalities may provide a novel approach to treatment. The Na^+ channel blocker amiloride should theoretically reduce the hyperabsorption of sodium and hence improve MCC. Initial studies were encouraging, with nebulized amiloride producing an increase in MCC [73]. However, when amiloride was nebulized four times daily over 6 months in patients maintained on their usual medication, no benefit was seen in comparison to placebo [74].

More recently, activation of non-CFTR Cl^- channels in the apical membrane of airway epithelial cells has been suggested as another possible therapeutic option. Thus, both ATP and UTP increase Cl^- chloride transport *in vitro* [75] and *in vivo* [76] in CF patients. A clinical trial of UTP, in combination with amiloride, is currently under way. Extensive research is also under way to circumvent the processing defect of the ΔF508 mutant using chemical chaperones [77], as well as to up-regulate the function of residual CFTR by agents such as milrinone [78] or 8-cyclopentyl-1,3-dipropylxanthine (CPX) [79].

7.2. Gene Therapy

Although small further improvements in both quality of life and life expectancy are likely to occur from conventional therapy, gene therapy may provide an important next step up in clinical benefit. The lung is the obvious target organ for gene therapy. Pathology usually starts in the bronchioles, and eventually the more proximal airways are also affected, although the highest level of expression of CFTR occurs in the submucosal glands [80], which predominate in the more proximal airways. Expression is also seen in a subpopulation of both ciliated and non-ciliated cells more peripherally, although the precise cell types have not yet been identified [81]. The development of pathology in this region provides circumstantial evidence that these cells should be the target. Currently available nebulizer technology is able to reach this area of the lung, but a better knowledge of the cell type requiring transfection would undoubtedly by important. If, however, cells in submucosal glands play a role in initiating, or perhaps, exacerbating, existing pathology, topical administration is unlikely to be successful.

Overall expression of CFTR is very low in the lung [82]. This raises the question as to why CFTR malfunction is so important in this organ, and yet it is encouraging because only low levels of expression may be required for clinical benefit. The precise number of cells requiring transfection to demonstrate phenotypic correction is uncertain and much debated. Heterozygotes with 50% of normal CFTR levels demonstrate no lung pathology. The Cl^- conductance of R347P and R117 H mutant CFTR has been assessed *in vitro*, and has been suggested as being about 30% and 15% of normal levels, respectively [83]. Thus, patients who are R347P/ΔF508 or R117H/ΔF508 compound heterozygotes should demonstrate about 15% and 7.5% of normal CFTR function, respectively. Although, in the few such patients studied, lung disease is still a prominent feature. The $cftr^{m1HGU}$ CF mice demonstrate a range of approximately 2–10% of wild-type CFTR mRNA, but still demonstrate an airway cAMP-mediated Cl^- conductance that is reduced by about 50% compared with normal mice [84]. An *in vitro* study has shown that, if "corrected" and "uncorrected" CF cells are mixed within a monolayer, about 6–10% of the former produce the same effect as a monolayer of purely "corrected" cells [85]. Finally, interbreeding of compound heterozygote, wild-type and complete null CF mice has shown that the presence of 1–5% of normal *CFTR* mRNA within each cell is able to prevent the intestinal problems completely and to produce marked correction of the Cl^- defect [86]. These data start to suggest that only small increments in CFTR expression may be required in the airways to produce much larger changes in function.

As for any attempt at gene transfer, the requirements include the complementary DNA (cDNA) with appropriate promoter, linked to a gene transfer agent (GTA). Currently, most studies have used "ubiquitous" viral promoters such as simian virus 40 (SV40), cytomegalovirus (CMV) and respiratory syntial virus (RSV), although lung-specific promoters such as surfactant protein C and Clara cell (CC10) are available [87] and have been used in some studies [88]. Ideally, the endogenous CFTR promoter should be used to enusre tissue-specific regulation of the CFTR transgene, but a fully functional CFTR promoter has not yet been identified. Until the issue of which cell type to correct is resolved, and to a lesser extent until more cell-specific promoters are available, it is likely that most studies will use the more generalized promoters.

A number of GTAs are currently available [89, 90], the two main systems being adenoviruses and cationic liposomes, although adeno-associated viruses have recently emerged as further candidates. Each GTA has certain advantages and problems and future systems may combine the best features of each. Adenovirus has a natural tropism for the lungs and the relatively high efficiency of gene transfer can be demonstrated both *in vitro* [91] and *in vivo* [92]. However, points of concern are safety and efficacy on repeat administration. Viral coat proteins are likely to be immunogenic, and may be responsible for the immune or inflammatory reactions commonly seen with these viruses [93, 94]. Extensive deletions of the virus's own genome are being undertaken to make the virus less immunogenic and to enable the uptake of larger cDNA inserts [95, 96].

Cationic liposomes are less efficient at gene transfer *in vitro* in comparison with viral vectors, but have some major advantages. They have low toxicity and are unlikely to provoke inflammation or to initiate an immune reaction on repeat administration. However, their complex physicochemical properties with respect to combination with both DNA and the surrounding ionic environment are poorly understood, and this probably contributes to their variable transfection efficiency in gene transfer studies [88]. Nebulization is likely to be the most acceptable delivery system for routine repeat applications to the lower airway in humans. It has the advantage of widespread deposition, which can, to a limited extent, be controlled by varying droplet size. Reports of pulmonary epithelial gene transfer after intravenous injection of a liposome-reporter gene complex [97, 98] are tantalizing, and suggest the possibility of other gene transfer strategies. One potential disadvantage is widespread gene transfer to other organs, but organ- or cell-specific promoters, or targeted gene transfer, may help to overcome this difficulty.

7.2.1. In vitro *CFTR gene transfer*: The first reports of *in vitro* correction of the CF Cl^- channel defect came in 1990. Drumm et al. [99] used retroviral-mediated transfer of CFTR cDNA to correct the Cl^- defect in a CF pancreatic carcinoma cell line. The presence of normal CFTR mRNA was demonstrated and cAMP-mediated chloride movement induced as shown by patch clamp and radiolabelled efflux studies. This was followed by a second report in which vaccinia virus was used to transfect a CF airway epithelial cell line [100]. Again, Cl^- movement was restored, as shown by epifluorescence and patch clamping, after transfection with normal but not mutant CFTR cDNA. Subsequently, many other groups have repeated these findings in cell lines with a variety of GTAs. An interesting additional finding has been that restoration of the CFTR Cl^- defect after *CFTR* cDNA gene transfer is linked to correction of other CF ion transport defects, lending support to studies noted above which suggest that CFTR may have several functions [101].

7.2.2. CFTR gene transfer into animal models: A pioneering set of studies by Crystal and colleagues using gene transfer mediated by both adenoviruses [95] and liposomes [102] established that the *CFTR* gene could be expressed in the airways of mice *in vivo*. Instillation of the *CFTR* gene into the lungs was followed by the appearance of mRNA at day 1, which was sustained for up to 4 weeks. To extend these *in vivo* studies a number of useful animal models have been developed. Engelhardt et al. implanted human bronchial xenografts into immune-deficient mice and showed adenoviral-mediated gene transfer into the epithelium [103]. Whitsett et al. have generated transgenic mice incorporating the human *CFTR* gene under the control of a lung epithelial cell-specific promoter (surfactant protein C) [104]. Human CFTR was expressed in distal airway and alveolar cells with no adverse effects in terms of lung weight, morphology or somatic growth. These findings go some way to establishing that over-expression of CFTR is harmless, although recently both *in vivo* and *in vitro* data have suggested that this may not be so clear [105].

Transgenic CF mice, which have been generated by a number of laboratories, are now being used in the assessment of GTAs. Hyde et al. [106] instilled a liposome (DOTMA) complexed with CFTR cDNA into the trachea of cftr^{m1Cam} transgenic mice showing restoration of cAMP-stimulated Cl^- secretion. Alton et al. [88] nebulized a liposome (DC-Chol: DOPE) CFTR cDNA complex into the cftr^{m1HGU} mice and showed that correction of the CF Cl^- defect could be achieved by this method in some animals. However, the relatively large amount of DNA used and the variability of correction suggest that inefficient gene transfer may be a problem with liposome-based systems. Direct comparison of the efficiency of liposome and adenoviral-mediated gene transfer systems has not been done, nor has the duration of correction been studied in CF mice.

A number of studies using non-human primates have reported positive results, using both reporter genes and CFTR cDNA [107–109]. Expression was seen throughout the airways, including the alveoli, but was generally patchy in distribution. One report has suggested gene expression for up to 6 months in airways, including transfection of basal cells, using adeno-associated virus-mediated gene transfer [110].

7.2.3. Clinical trials: Human studies using both viral and non-viral systems have been carried out. Zabner et al. [111] studied adenovirus-mediated CFTR cDNA gene transfer to the nose of three CF volunteers. With respect to safety, a degree of localized inflammation around the site of application was seen, probably related to the method of delivery. CFTR mRNA could be demonstrated in two of the subjects. With respect to correction of the bioelectric abnormalities, baseline potential difference (PD) was reduced into the normal range in all three subjects, whereas a β-agonist (terbutaline) produced small changes, similar to those seen in non-CF subjects, after but not before gene transfer. These changes lasted up to 10 days after the single application, although the study was not designed to assess duration of expression. Although these data are encouraging, it is important to note that inflammation can itself reduce baseline PD and that such *in vivo* measurements are not well suited to assessment of small changes in PD.

Crystal et al. [112] administered an adenoviral vector containing normal CFTR cDNA to the nasal and bronchial epithelium of four CF patients and showed that the vector could express the CFTR cDNA *in vivo*. At 2×10^8 plaque-forming unit (pfu) there was no recombination/complementation or shedding of the vector or rise of neutralizing antibody titres. At 2×10^9 pfu, a transient systemic and pulmonary syndrome was observed in one subject, possibly mediated by IL-6. There were no long-term adverse effects.

Knowles et al. [113] administered four logarithmically increasing doses of a CFTR containing adenovirus or vehicle alone, to the nasal epithelium of 12 patients with CF in a randomized double-blind study. The vector was detected in nasal fluid by culture, polymerase chain reaction (PCR) or both for up to 8 days after administration. There was molecular evidence of gene transfer by reverse transcriptase PCR (RT-PCR) or *in situ* hybridization in five of six patients treated with the two highest doses. However, less than 1% of cells were transfected and no significant changes in electrophysiological measurements were detected. At the highest dose there was mucosal inflammation in two of three patients.

Finally, Bellon et al. [114] administered escalating doses of a replication-deficient adenovirus expressing the human CFTR protein to the nose (instillation) and to the lung (aerosolization) of six CF patients. No acute toxic side effects were observed. CFTR mRNA was detected in all nasal samples at day 15 after virus administration, but only in one of six bronchial brushing samples. Recombinant CFTR protein was also detectable in all nasal samples at day 15 after administration, but only in two of six bronchial brushing samples.

The results with non-viral systems are at least as promising as those using adenoviruses. Caplen et al. [115] reported a double-blind placebo-controlled trial of liposome-mediated CFTR cDNA gene transfer to the nasal epithelium in 15 ΔF508 homozygous CF patients (nine CFTR cDNA, six placebo). No safety problems were encountered, either in the routine clinical assessment or by a blinded, semi-quantitative analysis of nasal biopsies. Both plasmid DNA and CFTR mRNA were detected from the nasal biopsies in five of the eight treated patients. Chloride secretion, assessed by perfusion with a low Cl^- solution (see above), showed a significant 20% increase towards normal values, a change well outside the variation in these measurements. In two subjects, these Cl^- responses reached values within the non-CF range with the changes lasting for about 7 days.

In a similar double-blind randomized study, Porteous et al. [116] administered a single dose of a CFTR plasmid or buffer alone to 16 volunteers with CF. The plasmid contained a CMV promoter complexed with the cationic liposome DOTAP. There was no evidence of nasal inflammation on biopsy, circulating inflammatory markers or other adverse events related to active treatment. Transgene DNA was detected in seven of the eight treated patients up to 28 days after treatment and vector-derived CFTR mRNA in two of the seven patients 3 and 7 days after administration. Partial correction of CFTR-mediated chloride transport was detected in two treated patients, sustained for up to 4 weeks. These findings were considered to be comparable to those reported previously using adenoviral vectors or the liposome study outlined above.

A third double-blind placebo-controlled study was performed by Gill et al. [117] using a CFTR cDNA plasmid containing an RSV promoter. Eight patients received the plasmid complexed with DC-Chol/DOPE and four received buffer alone. Biopsies of the nasal epithelium taken 7 days after dosing were normal. No signiifcant changes in any clinical parameters were observed. Functional expression of CFTR assessed by *in vivo* nasal potential difference measurements showed transient correction of the CF Cl^- transport abnormality in two patients. Fluorescence microscopy showed evidence for CFTR function *ex vivo* in cells from nasal brushings in a further four patients. In total, evidence of functional CFTR gene transfer was obtained in six of the eight treated patients.

8. Conclusion

Cystic fibrosis is the most common lethal autosomal recessive disease in the caucasian population, with most patients dying as a result of lung obstruction. The CF gene was cloned through positional cloning and named the cystic fibrosis transmembrane conductance regulator. CFTR is a member of the ABC superfamily and expressed in the apical membrane of epithelial cells. Apart from its function as a Cl^- channel, CFTR also appears to regulate other ion channels. Current treatments include physiotherapy, administration of antibiotics and pancreatic supplements with a current life expectancy of about 30 years. New pharmacological treatments, as well as gene therapy using viral or non-viral vectors, may further increase quality of life as well as life expectancy in CF patients.

References

1 Welsh MJ, Tsui LC (1995) Cystic Fibrosis. In: CR Scriver, AL Beaudet, WS Sly, D Valle (eds): *The metabolic and molecular basis of inherited disease*. MacGraw-Hill Inc, New York, 3799–3876
2 Gilligan PH (1991) Microbiology of airway disease in patients with cystic fibrosis. *Clin Microbiol Rev* 4: 35–51
3 Bonfield TL, Konstan MW, Burfeind B, Panuska JR, Hilliard B, Berger M (1995) Inflamatory cytokines in cystic fibrosis lungs. *Am J Respir Cell Mol Biol* 13: 257–261
4 Durie PR (1992) Pathophysiology of the pancreas in cystic fibrosis. *Netherlands J Med* 41: 97–100
5 Kopelman H, Corey M, Gaskin K, Durie P, Weizman Z, Forstner G (1988) Impaired chloride secretion, as well as bicarbonate secretion underlies the fluid secretory defect in the cystic fibrosis pancreas. *Gastroenterology* 95: 349–355
6 Tanner MS, Taylor CJ (1995) Liver disease in cystic fibrosis. *Arch Dis Child* 72: 281–284
7 Oates RD, Amos JA (1993) Congenital bilateral absence of the vas deferens and cystic fibrosis. *World J Urol* 11: 82–88
8 Canny GJ, Corey M, Livingstone RA, Caroenter S, Green L, Levison H (1991) Pregnancy and cystic fibrosis. *Obstet Gynecol* 77: 850–853
9 Kopito LE, Kosasky HL, Shwachman K (1973) Water and electrolytes in cervical mucus from patients with CF. *Fertil Steril* 24: 512–516
10 Jarvi K, Zielenski J, Wischanski M, Durie P, Buckspan M, Tullis E, Markiewicz D, Tsui LC (1995) Cystic fibrosis transmembrane conductance regulator and obstructive azoospermia. *Lancet* 345: 1578
11 Webb S, Clark R (1996) Increased incidence of cystic fibrosis gene mutation in adults with brochiectasis [Abstract]. *Israel J Med Sci* 32 (suppl): S183
12 Riordan JR, Rommens JM, Kerem B, Alon N, Rozmahel R, Grzelczak Z, Zielenski J, Lok S, Plavisc N, Chou JL et al. (1989) Identification of the cystic fibrosis gene: cloning and characterisation of the complementary DNA. *Science* 245: 1066–1073
13 Rommens JM, Iannuzzi MC, Kerem B, Drumm ML, Melmer G, Dean M, Rozmahel R, Cole JL, Kennedy D, Hidaka N et al. (1989) Identification of the cystic fibrosis gene: chromosome walking and jumping. *Science* 245: 1059–1065
14 Heng HH, Shi XM, Tsui LC (1993) Fluorescence in situ hybridisation mapping of the cystic fibrosis transmembrane conductance regulator (CFTR) gene to 7q31.3. *Cytogenet Cell Genet* 62: 200–204
15 Zielenski J, Rozmahel R, Bozon D, Kerem B, Grzelczak Z, Riordan JR, Rommens JM, Tsui LC (1991) Genomic DNA sequence of the cystic fibrosis transmembrane conductance regulator (CFTR) gene. *Genomics* 10: 214–228
16 Chu CS, Trapnell BC (1992) Cystic fibrosis transmembrane conductance regulator (CFTR) gene transcripts. *EMBO J* 11: 379–385
17 Delaney SJ, Rich DP, Thomson SA, Hargrave MR, Lovelock PK, Welsh MJ, Wainwright BJ (1993) Cystic fibrosis transmembrane conductance regulator splice variants are not conserved and fail to produce Cl^- channels. *Nature Genet* 4: 426–431
18 Zielenski J, Tsui LC (1995) Cystic fibrosis: genotypic and phenotypic variations. *Annu Rev Genet* 29: 777–807
19 Knudson AGJ, Wagner L, Hallett WY (1967) On the selective advantage of cystic fibrosis heterozygotes. *Am J Hum Genet* 19: 388–392
20 Meindl RS (1987) Hypothesis: A selective advantage for cystic fibrosis heterozygotes. *Am J Phys Anthropol* 74: 39–45
21 Morral N, Bertranpetit J, Estivill X, Nunes V, Casals T, Gimeres J, Reis A, Varon-Mateeva R, Macek M Jr, Kalaydjieva L et al. (1994) The origin of the major cystic fibrosis mutation (ΔF508) in European populations. *Nature Genet* 7: 169–175
22 Super M (1979) Factors influencing the frequency of cystic fibrosis in south west Africa. *Monog Pediatr* 10: 106–113
23 Wilschanski M, Zielenski J, Markiewicz D, Tsui LC, Corey M, Levison H, Durie PR (1995) Correlation of sweat chloride concentration with classes of the cystic fibrosis transmembrane conductance regulator gene mutations. *J Pediatr* 127: 705–710

24 Denning GM, Ostedgaard LS, Anderson MP, Amara JF, Marshall J, Smith AE, Welsh MJ (1992) Processing of mutant cystic fibrosis transmembrane conductance regulator is temperature-sensitive. *Nature* 358: 761–764
25 Hyde SC, Emsley P, Harshorn MJ, Mimmack MM, Gileadi U, Pearce SR, Gallagher MP, Gill DR, Hubbard RE, Higgins CF (1990) Structural model of ATP-binding proteins associated with cystic fibrosis, multidrug resistance and bacterial transport. *Nature* 346: 362–365
26 Bremer S, Hoof T, Busche R, Scholte B, Riordan JR, Maass G, Tummler B (1992) Quantitative expression patterns of multidrug resistance P-glycoprotein (MDR1) and differentially spliced cystic fibrosis transmembrane conductance regulator mRNA transcripts in human epithelia. *Eur J Biochem* 206: 137–149
27 Ames GF, Lecar H (1992) ATP-dependent bacterial transporters and cystic fibrosis: analogy between channels and transporters. *FASEB J* 6: 2660–2666
28 Rommens JM, Dho S, Bear CE, Kartner N, Kennedy D, Riordan JR, Tsui LC, Foskett JK (1991) cAMP-inducible chloride conductance in mouse fibroblast lines stably expressing the human cystic fibrosis transmembrane conductance regulator. *Proc Natl Acad Sci USA* 88: 7500–7504
29 Cunningham SA, Worrell RT, Benos DJ, Frizzell RA (1992) cAMP-stimulated ion currents in *Xenopus* oocytes expressing CFTR cRNA. *Am J Physiol* 262: C783–C788
30 Bear CE, Duguay F, Naismith AL, Kartner N, Hanrahan JW, Riordan JR (1991) Cl^- channel activity in *Xenopus* oocytes expresing the cystic fibrosis gene. *J Biol Chem* 266: 19142–19145
31 Tabcharani JA, Chang XB, Riordan JR, Hanrahan JW (1991) Phosphorylation-regulated Cl^- channel in CHO cells stably expressing the cystic fibrosis gene. *Nature* 352: 628–631
32 Drumm ML, Wilkinson DJ, Smith LS, Worrell RT, Strong TV, Frizell RA, Dawson DC, Collins FS (1991) Chloride conductance expressed by ΔF508 and other mutant CFTRs in *Xenopus* oocytes. *Science* 254: 1797–1799
33 Dalemans W, Barbry P, Champigny G, Jallat S, Dott K, Dreyer D, Crystal RG, Pavirani A, Lecocq JP, Lazdunski M et al. (1991) Altered chloride ion channel kinetics associated with the delta F508 cystic fibrosis mutation. *Nature* 354: 526–528
34 Anderson MP, Greogry KJ, Thompson S, Souza DW, Paul S, Mulligan RC, Smith AE, Welsh MJ (1991) Demonstration that CFTR is a chloride channel by alteration of its anion selectivity. *Science* 253: 202–205
35 Bear CE, Li CH, Kartner N, Bridges RJ, Jensen TJ, Ramjeesingh M, Riordan JR (1992) Purification and functional reconstitution of the cystic fibrosis transmembrane conductance regulator (CFTR). *Cell* 68: 809–818
36 Gadsby DC, Nairn AC (1996) Regulation of CFTR channels activity. In: JA Dodge, DJH Brock, JH Widdicombe (eds): *Cystic fibrosis-current topics*. John Wiley & Sons, New York, 65–90
37 Gadsby DC, Nairn AC (1994) Regulation of CFTR channel gating. *Trends Biochem Sci* 19: 513–518
38 Chang XB, Tabcharani JA, Hou XY, Jenson TJ, Kartner N, Alon N, Hanrahan JW, Riordan JR (1993) Protein kinase A (PKA) still activates CFTR chloride channel after mutagenesis of all 10 PKA consensus phosphorylation sites. *J Biol Chem* 268: 11304–11311
39 Boucher RC, Stutts MJ, Knowles MR, Cantley L, Gatzby JT (1986) Na^+ transport in cystic fibrosis respiratory epithelia. Abnormal basal rate and response to adenylate cyclase activation. *J Clin Invest* 78: 1245–1252
40 Johnson LG, Boyles SE, Wilson J, Boucher RC (1995) Normalisation of raised sodium absorption and raised calcium-mediated chloride secretion by adenovirus-mediated expression of cystic fibrosis transmembrane regulator in primary human cystic fibrosis airway epithelial cells. *J Clin Invest* 95: 1377–1382
41 Canessa CM, Schild L, Buell G, Thorens B, Gautschi I, Horrisberger JD, Rossier BC (1994) Amiloride-sensetive epithelial Na^+ channel is made of three homologous subunits. *Nature* 367: 463–467
42 Stutts MJ, Canessa CM, Olson JC, Hamrich M, Cohn JA, Rossier BC, Boucher RC (1995) CFTR as a cAMP-dependent regulator of sodium channels. *Science* 269: 847–850
43 Chinet TC, Fullton JM, Yankaskas JR, Boucher RC, Stutts MJ (1994) Mechanism of sodium hyperabsorption in cultured cystic fibrosis nasal epithelium: a patch clamp study. *Am J Physiol* 266: C1061–C1068

44 Ward CL, Harris A (1992) Cystic fibrosis gene expression is not correlated with rectifying Cl^- channels. *Proc Natl Acad Sci USA* 88: 5277–5281
45 Gabriel SE, Clarke LL, Boucher RC, Stutts MJ (1993) CFTR and outward rectifying chloride channels are distinct proteins with a regulatory relationship. *Nature* 363: 263–268
46 Grubb BR, Vick RN, Boucher RN (1994) Hyperabsorption of Na^+ and raised Ca^{2+}-mediated Cl^- secretion in nasal epithelia of CF mice. *Am J Physiol* 266: C1478–C1483
47 McNicholas CM, Guggino WB, Schwiebert EM, Hebert SC, Giebisch G, Egan ME (1996) Sensitivity of a renal K^+ channel (ROMK2) to the inhibitory sulfonylurea compound glibenclamide is enhanced by coexpression with the ATP-binding cassette transporter cystic fibrosis transmembrane regulator. *Proc Natl Acad Sci USA* 93: 8083–8088
48 Stutts MR (1996) Regulation of other airway epithelial ion channels by CFTR. In: JA Dodge, DJH Brock, JH Widdicombe (eds): *Cystic fibrosis-current topics*. John Wiley & Sons, New York, 91–106
49 Pasyk EA, Foskett JK (1995) CFTR is permeable to adenosine 3′-phosphate 5′-phosphosulfate (PAPS) [Abstract]. *Pediatr Pulmonol* 12 (suppl): 187
50 Reisin IL, Prat AG, Abraham EH, Amara JF, Gregary RJ, Ausiello DA, Cantiello HF (1994) The cystic fibrosis transmembrane conductance regulator is a dual ATP and chloride channel. *J Biol Chem* 269: 20584–20591
51 Reddy MM, Ouinton PM, Haws C, Wine JJ, Grygorczk R, Tabcharani JA, Hanrahan JW, Gunderson KL, Kopito RR (1996) Failure of the cystic fibrosis transmembrane conductance regulator to conduct ATP. *Science* 171: 1876–1879
52 Bradbury NA, Jilling T, Berta G, Sorscher EJ, Bridges RJ, Kirk KL (1992) Regulation of plasma membrane recycling by CFTR. *Science* 256: 530–532
53 Barasch J, Kiss B, Prince A, Saiman L, Gruenert D, al-Awqati Q (1991) Defective acidification of intracellular organelles in cystic fibrosis. *Nature* 352: 70–73
54 Seksek O, Biwersi J, Verkman AS (1996) Evidence against defective acidification in cystic fibrosis. *J Biol Chem* 271: 15542–15548
55 Saiman L, Cacalano L, Gruenert D, Prince A (1992) Comparison of adherence of *Pseudomonas aeruginosa* to respiratory epithelial cells from cystic fibrosis patients and healthy subjects. *Infect Immun* 60: 2808–2814
56 Pier GB, Grout M, Zaidi TS, Olsen JC, Johnson LG, Yankaskas JR, Goldberg JB (1996) Role of mutant CFTR in hypersusceptibility of cystic fibrosis patients to lung infections. *Science* 271: 64–67
57 Smith JJ, Travis SM, Greenberg EP, Welsh MJ (1996) Cystic fibrosis airway epithelia fail to kill bacteria because of abnormal airway surface fluid. *Cell* 85: 229–236
58 Tata F, Stanier P, Wicking C, Halford S, Kruyer H, Lench NJ, Scambler PJ, Hansen C, Braman JC, Williamson R (1991) Cloning of the mouse homologue of the human cystic-fibrosis transmembrane conductance regulator. *Genomics* 10: 301–307
59 Trezise AE, Szpirer C, Buchwald M (1992) Localisation of the gene encoding the cystic fibrosis transmembrane regulator (CFTR) in rat to chromosome 4 and implications for the evolution of mammalian chromosomes. *Genomics* 14: 869–874
60 Diamond G, Scanlin TF, Zasloff MA, Bevins CL (1991) A cross species analysis of cystic fibrosis transmembrane conductance regulator. Potential functional domains and regulatory sites. *J Biol Chem* 266: 22761–22769
61 Marshall J, Martin KA, Picciotto M, Hochfield S, Nairn AC, Kaczmarek LK (1991) Identification and localisation of a dogfish homologue of human cystic fibrosis transmembrane regulator. *J Biol Chem* 266: 22749–22754
62 Tucker SJ, Tannahill D, Higgins CF (1992) Identification and developmental expression of the *Xenopus laevis* cystic fibrosis transmembrane conductance regulator gene. *Hum Mol Genet* 1: 77–82
63 Hasty P, O'Neal WK, Liu K, Morris A, Bebok Z, Shumyatsky GB, Jilling T, Sorscher EJ, Bradley A, Beaudet AL (1995) Severe phenotype in mice with termination mutation in exon 2 of the cystic fibrosis gene. *Somat Cell Mol Genet* 21: 177–187
64 Ratcliff R, Evans MJ, Cuthbert AW, Macvinish LJ, Foster D, Anderson JR, Colledge WH (1993) Production of a severe cystic fibrosis mutation in mice by gene targeting. *Nature Genet* 4: 35–41
65 Rozmahel R, Wilschanski M, Matin A, Plyte S, Olivier M, Auerbach W, Moore A, Forstner J, Durie P, Nadeau J, Bear C, Tsui LC (1996) Modulation of disease severity in cystic

fibrosis transmembrane conductance regulator deficient mice by a secondary genetic factor. *Nature Genet* 12: 280–287
66 Snouwart J, Brigman KK, Latour AM, Malouf NN, Boucher RC, Koller BH (1992) An animal model for cystic fibrosis made by gene targeting. *Science* 257: 1083–1088
67 Zeiher BG, Eichwald E, Zabner J, Smith JJ, Puga AP, McCray PB, Capecchi MR, Welsh MJ, Thomas KR (1995) A mouse model for the delta F508 allele of cystic fibrosis. *J Clin Invest* 96: 2051–2064
68 Dorin JR, Dickinson P, Alton EWFW, Smith SN, Geddes DN, Stevenson BJ, Kimber WL, Fleming S, Clarke AR, Hooper ML et al. (1992) Cystic fibrosis in the mouse by targeted insertional mutagenesis. *Nature* 359: 211–215
69 O'Neal WK, Hasty P, McCray PB, Casey B, Rivera-Perez J, Welsh MJ, Beaudet AL, Bradlet A (1993) A severe phenotype in mice with a duplication of exon 3 in the cystic fibrosis locus. *Hum Mol Genet* 2: 1561–1569
70 Colledge WH, Abella BS, Southern KW, Ratcliff R, Jiang C, Cheng SH, Macvinish LJ, Anderson JR, Cuthbert AW, Evans MJ (1996) Generation and characterisation of a delta F508 cystic fibrosis mouse model. *Nature Genet* 10: 445–452
71 Delaney SJ, Alton EWFW, Smith SN, Lunn DP, Farley R, Lovelock PK, Thomson SA, Hume DA, Lamb D, Porteous DJ et al. (1996) Cystic fibrosis mice carrying the missense mutation G551D replicate human genotype-phenotype correlations. *EMBO J* 15: 955–963
72 Clarke LL, Grubb BR, Yankaskas JR, Cotton CU, McKenzie A, Boucher R (1994) Relationship of a non-CFTR mediated chloride conductance to organ-level disease in cftr 9–/–) mice. *Proc Natl Acad Sci USA* 91: 479–483
73 App EM, King M, Helfesreider R, Kohler D, Matthys H (1990) Acute and long-term amiloride inhalation in cystic fibrosis lung disease. *Am Rev Respir Dis* 141: 605–612
74 Graham A, Hasani A, Alton EWFW, Martin GP, Marriott C, Hodson ME, Clarke SW, Geddes DM (1993) No added benefit from nebulized amiloride in patients with cystic fibrosis. *Eur Respir J* 6: 1243–1248
75 Mason SJ, Paradiso AM, Boucher RC (1991) Regulation of transepithelial ion transport and intracellular calcium by extracellular ATP in human and normal cystic fibrosis airways. *Br J Pharmacol* 103: 1649–1656
76 Knowles MR, Clarke LL, Boucher RC (1991) Activation by ectracellular nucleotides of chloride secretion in the airway epithelia of patients with cystic fibrosis. *N Engl J Med* 325: 533–538
77 Sato K, Ward CL, Krouse ME, Wine JJ, Kopito RR (1996) Glycerol reverses misfolding phenotype of the most common cystic fibrosis mutation. *J Biol Chem* 271: 635–638
78 Kelley TJ, Thomas K, Milgram LJ, Drumm ML (1996) *In vivo* activation of the cystic fibrosis transmembrane conductance regulator mutant delta F508 in murine nasal epithelium. *Proc Natl Acad Sci USA* 94: 2604–2608
79 Guay-Broder C, Jacobson KA, Barnoy S, Cabantchik Zi, Guggino WB, Zeitlin PL, Turner RJ, Vergara L, Eidelman O, Pollard HB (1995) Al receptor antagonist 8-cyclopentyl-1,3-dipropylxanthine selectively activates chloride efflux from human epithelial and mouse fibroblast cell lines expressing the cystic fibrosis transmembrane regulator delta F508 mutation. *Biochemistry* 34: 9079–9087
80 Engelhardt JF, Yankaskas JR, Ernst SA, Yang Y, Marino CR, Boucher RC, Cohn JA, Wilson JM (1992) Submucosal glands are the predominant site of CFTR expression in the human bronchus. *Nature Genet* 2: 240–248
81 Engelhardt JF, Zepeda M, Cohn JA, Xankaskas JR, Wilson JM (1994) Expression of the cystic fibrosis gene in adult human lung. *J Clin Invest* 93: 737–749
82 Crawford I, Maloney PC, Zeitlin PL, Guggino WB, Hyde SC, Turley H, Gatter KC, Harris A, Higgins CF (1991) Immunocytochemical localization of the cystic fibrosis gene product CFTR. *Proc Natl Acad Sci USA* 88: 9262–9266
83 Sheppard DN, Rich DP, Ostedgaard LS, Gregory RJ, Smith AE, Welsh MJ (1993) Mutations in CFTR associated with mild-disease-form Cl^- channels with altered pore properties. *Nature* 362: 160–164
84 Dorin JR, Stevenson BJ, Fleming S, Alton EW, Dickinson P, Porteous DJ (1994) Long-term survival of the exon 10 insertional cystic fibrosis mutant mouse is a consequence of low level residual wild-type Cftr gene expression. *Mammalian Genome* 5: 465–472

85 Johnson LG, Olsen JC, Sarkadi B, Moore KL, Swanstrom R, Boucher RC (1992) Efficiency of gene transfer for restoration of normal airway epithelial function in cystic fibrosis. *Nature Genet* 2: 21–25
86 Dorin JR, Farley R, Webb S, Smith SN, Farini E, Delaney SJ, Wainwright BJ, Alton EWFW, Porteous DJ (1996) A demonstration using mouse models that successful gene therapy for cystic fibrosis requires only partial gene correction. *Gene Therapy* 3: 797–801
87 Wert SE, Glasser SW, Korfhagen TR, Whitsett JA (1993) Transcriptional elements from the human SP-C gene direct expression in the primordial respiratory epithelium of transgenic mice. *Devel Biol* 156: 426–443
88 Alton EWFW, Middleton PG, Caplen NJ, Smith SN, Steel DM, Munkonge FM, Jeffery PK, Geddes DM, Hart SL, Williamson R (1993) Non-invasive liposome-mediated gene delivery can correct the ion transport defect in cystic fibrosis mutant mice. *Nature Genet* 5: 135–142
89 Coutelle C, Caplen N, Hart S, Huxley C, Williamson R (1993) Gene therapy for cystic fibrosis. *Arch Dis Child* 68: 437–443
90 Wilson J (1993) Vehicles for gene therapy. *Nature* 365: 691–692
91 Rosenfeld MA, Chu CS, Seth P, Danel C, Banks T, Yoneyama K, Yoshimura K, Crystal RG (1994) Gene transfer to freshly isolated human respiratory epithelial cells *in vitro* using a replication-deficient adenovirus containing the human cystic fibrosis transmembrane conductance regulator cDNA. *Hum Gene Therapy* 5331–5342
92 Zabner J, Petersen DM, Puga AP, Graham SM, Couture LA, Keyes LD, Lukason MJ, St George JA, Gregory RJ, Smith AE, Welsh MJ (1994) Safety and efficacy of repetitive adenovirus-mediated transfer of CFTR cDNA to airway epithelia of primates and cotton rats. *Nature Genet* 6: 75–83
93 Trapnell B (1993) Adenoviral vectors for gene transfer. *Adv Drug Deliv Rev* 12: 185–199
94 Simon RH, Engelhardt JF, Yang Y, Zepeda M, Weber-Pendleton S, Grossman M, Wilson JM (1993) Adenovirus-mediated transfer of the CFTR gene to lung of nonhuman primates: toxicity study. *Hum Gene Therapy* 4: 771–780
95 Rosenfeld MA, Yoshimuram K, Trapnell BC, Yoneyama K, Rosenthal ER, Dalemans W, Fukayama M, Bargon J, Stier LE, Stratford-Perricaudet L et al. (1992) *In vivo* transfer of the human cystic fibrosis transmembrane conductance regulator gene to the airway epithelium. *Cell* 68: 143–155
96 Yang Y, Nunes FA, Berencsi K, Gönczöl E, Engelhardt JF, Wilson JM (1994) Inactivation of *E2a* in recombinant adenoviruses improves the prospect for gene therapy in cystic fibrosis. *Nature Genet* 7: 362–369
97 Zhu N, Liggit D, Lui Y, Debs R (1993) Systemic gene expression after intravenous DNA delivery into adult mice. *Science* 261: 209–211
98 Griesenbach U, Chonn A, Cassady R, Hannam V, Ackerley C, Post M, Tanswell AK, Olek K, O'Brodovich H, Tsui LC (1998) Comparison of intratracheal and intravenous administration of liposome-DNA complexes for cystic fibrosis lung gene therapy. *Gene Therapy* 5: 181–188
99 Drumm M, Pope HA, Cliff WH, Rommens JM, Marvin SA, Tsui LC, Collins FS, Frizzell RA, Wilson JM (1990) Correction of the cystic fibrosis defect *in vitro* by retrovirus-mediated gene transfer. *Cell* 62: 1227–1233
100 Rich DP, Anderson MP, Gregory RJ (1990) Expression of cystic fibrosis transmembrane conductance regulator corrects defective chloride regulation in cystic fibrosis airway epithelial cells. *Nature* 347: 358–363
101 Egan M, Flotte T, Afione S, Solow R, Zeitlin PL, Carter BJ, Guggino WB (1992) Defective regulation of outwardly rectifying Cl^- channels by protein kinase A corrected by insertion of CFTR. *Nature* 358: 581–584
102 Yoshimura K, Rosenfeld MA, Nakamura H, Scherer EM, Pavirani A, Lecocq JP, Crystal RG (1992) Expression of the human cystic fibrosis transmembrane conductance regulator gene in the mouse lung after *in vivo* intratracheal plasmid-mediated gene transfer. *Nucleic Acids Res* 20: 3233–3240
103 Engelhardt JF, Yang Y, Stratford-Perricaudet LD, Allen ED, Kozarsky K, Perricaudet M, Yankaskas JR, Wilson JM (1993) Direct gene transfer of human CFTR into human bronchial epithelia of xenografts with E1-deleted adenoviruses. *Nature Genet* 4: 27–34
104 Whitsett JA, Dey CR, Stripp BR, Wikenheiser KA, Clark JC, Wert SE, Gregory RJ, Smith AE, Cohn JA, Wilson JM, Engelhardt J (1992) Human cystic fibrosis transmembrane con-

ductance regulator directed to respiratory epithelial cell of transgenic mice. *Nature Genet* 2: 13–20

105 Schiavi SC, Abelkader N, Reber S, Pennington S, Narayana R, McPherson JM, Smith AE, Hoppe H, Cheng SH (1996) Biosynthetic and growth abnormalities are associated with high-level expression of CFTR in heterologous cells. *Am J Physiol* 270: C341–C351

106 Hyde SC, Gill DR, Higgins CF, Treziser AE, MacVinish CJ, Cuthbert AW, Ratcliff R, Evans MJ, Colledge WH (1993) Correction of ion transport defect in cystic fibrosis transgenic mice by gene therapy. *Nature* 362: 250–255

107 Zabner J, Petersen DM, Puga AP, Graham SM, Couture LA, Keyes LD, Lukason MJ, St George JA, Gregory RJ, Smith AE, Welsh MJ (1994) Safety and efficacy of repetitive adenovirus-mediated transfer of CFTR cDNA to airway epithelia of primates and cotton rats. *Nature Genet* 6: 75–83

108 Engelhardt JF, Simon RH, Yang Y, Zepeda M, Weber-Pendleton S, Doranz B, Grossman M, Wilson JM (1993) Adenovirus-mediated transfer of the CFTR gene to lung of nonhuman primates: biological efficacy study. *Hum Gene Therapy* 4: 759–769

109 Bout A, Perricaudet M, Baskin G, Imler JL, Scholte BJ, Pavirani A, Valerio D (1994) Lung gene therapy: *in vivo* adenovirus-mediated gene transfer to rhesus monkey airway epithelium. *Hum Gene Therapy* 5: 3–10

110 Flotte TR, Afione SA, Solow R, Drumm ML, Markakis D, Guggino WB, Zeitlin RL, Carter BJ (1993) Expression of the cystic fibrosis transmembrane conductance regulator from a novel adeno-associated virus promoter. *J Biol Chem* 268: 378–390

111 Zabner J, Couture LA, Gregory RJ, Graham SM, Smith AE, Welsh MJ (1993) Adenovirus-mediated gene transfer transiently corrects the chloride transport defect in nasal epithelial of patients with CF. *Cell* 75: 207–216

112 Crystal RG, McElvaney NG, Rosenfeld MA, Chu C-S, Mastrangeli A, Hay JG, Broday SL, Jaffe HA, Eissa NT, Danel C (1994) Administration of an adenovirus containing the human *CFTR* cDNA to the respiratory tract of individuals with cystic fibrosis. *Nature Genet* 8: 42–51

113 Knowles MR, Hohneker KW, Zhou Z, Olsen JC, Noah TL, Hu P, Leigh MW, Engelhardt JR, Edwards LJ, Jones KR et al. (1995) A controlled study of adenoviral-vector-mediated gene transfer in the nasal epithelium of patients with cystic fibrosis. *N Engl J Med* 333: 823–831

114 Bellon G, Michel-Calemard L, Thouvenot D, Jagneaux V, Poitevin F, Malcus C, Nathalie A, Layani MP, Aymard M, Beron H et al. (1997) Aerosol administration of a recombinant adenovirus expressing CFTR to cystic fibrosis patients: a phase I clinical trial. *Hum Gene Therapy* 8: 15–25

115 Caplen NJ, Alton EWFW, Middleton PG, Dorin JR, Stevenson BJ, Gao X, Durham SR, Jeffery PK, Hodson ME (1995) Liposome-mediated CFTR gene transfer to the nasal epithelium of patients with cystic fibrosis. *Nature Med* 1: 39–46

116 Porteous DS, Dorin JR, McLachlan G, Davidson-Smith H, Davidson H, Stevenson BJ, Carothers AD, Wallace AJ, Moralle S, Hoenes C (1997) Evidence for safety and efficency of DOTAP cationic liposome mediated CFTR gene transfer to nasal epithelium of patients with cystic fibrosis. *Gene Therapy* 4: 210–218

117 Gill DR, Southern KW, Mofford KA, Seddon T, Huang L, Sorgi F, Thomson A, MacVinish LJ, Ratcliff R, Bilton D (1997) A placebo controlled study of liposome mediated gene transfer to nsasl epithelium of patients with cystic fibrosis. *Gene Therapy* 4: 199–209

Molecular Biology of the Lung
Vol. 1: Emphysema and Infection
ed. by R. A. Stockley

CHAPTER 12
Respiratory Bacterial Infections in Patients with Cystic Fibrosis: Pathogenicity and Implications for Serine Proteinase Inhibitor Therapy

Gerd Döring

Department of General and Environmental Hygiene, Hygiene-Institut, University of Tübingen, Tübingen Germany

1. Introduction

Cystic fibrosis (CF) is one of the most common genetic disorders affecting white European populations with autosomal-recessive inheritance. It is characterized by abnormal exocrine gland secretion [1] a. As a result of mutations in a single gene of chromosome 7 which encodes the CF transmembrane conductance regulator (CFTR). The CFTR protein is a membrane-bound cAMP-regulated chloride channel which is also thought to regulate other chloride (Cl^-) and sodium (Na^+) channels. More than 700 different mutations have been identified so far which affect epithelial ion and water transport mainly in cells in the respiratory, gastrointestinal, hepatobiliary and reproductive tracts. In CF airways intracellular chloride and water retention leads to viscous secretions and impaired mucociliary clearance (Figure 1 A).

A hallmark of CF is respiratory infection [1]. A variety of Gram-positive and Gram-negative bacteria and fungi can be isolated from CF sputum or bronchoalveolar lavage (BAL) samples. The predominant bacterial species colonizing the respiratory tract in people with CF, however, are *Pseudomonas aeruginosa*, *Staphylococcus aureus* and *Haemophilus influenzae* [1, 2]. Infections may start very early in the life of these patients and, up to the age of 5 years, about a quarter of CF patients are infected with *P. aeruginosa* [2], this increases steadily with age. A North American analysis includ-

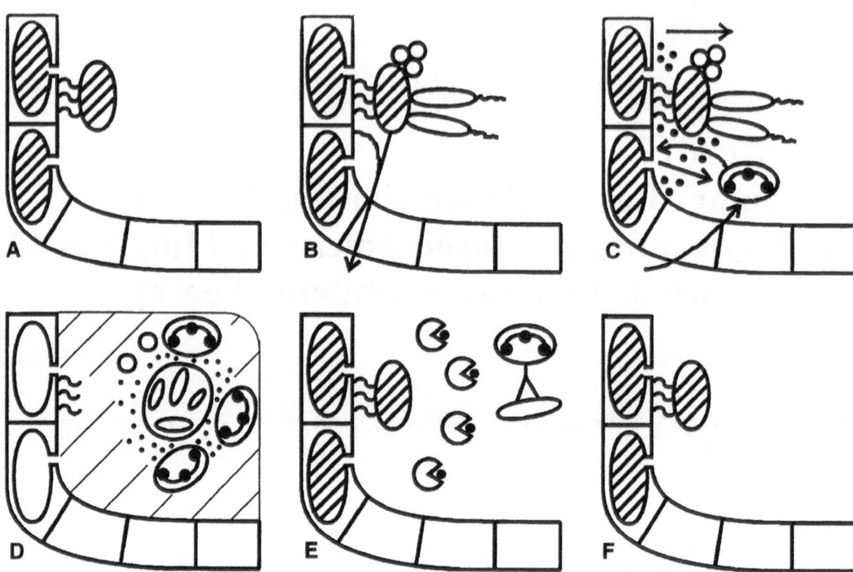

Figure 1. Schematic view of the development of bacterial lung infections in patients with cystic fibrosis. (A) As a result of abnormal viscous mucus, mucociliary clearance is impaired; (B) bacteria such as *Pseudomonas aeruginosa* and *Staphylococcus aureus* may colonize the CF airways by adhering to mucus components. Chemotactic factors for polymorphonucelar leukocytes (PMN) are generated from bacteria and host; (C) migrating PMNs become activated and secrete reactive oxygen species, antimicrobial peptides, enzymes and serine proteinases, the last stimulate mucus hypersecretion; (D) reactive oxygen species trigger the change of non-mucoid *P. aeruginosa* to a mucoid phenotype forming exopolysaccharide covered microcolonies, which survive by taking advantage of PMN proteinases; mucus hypersecretion removes bacteria from the epithelium into the airway lumen; (E) serine proteinase inhibitor therapy reduces mucus hypersecretion, restores PMN function and restricts bacterial survival conditions; (F) this leads to decreased numbers of bacterial pathogens in the airways and resolution of inflammation.

ing almost 20000 CF patients revealed that the percentage of *P. aeruginosa* infections rose from 16.2% in the age group of 0–1 years to 82% in the age group of 35–44 years. The percentage of CF patients infected with *S. aureus* (37%) and *H. influenzae* (15.4%), on the other hand, remains relatively constant in all age groups. These epidemiological data clearly reveal the importance of the *P. aeruginosa* lung infection in CF. Although several antibiotic regimens are used in CF, eradication of the infective pathogens from the airways is difficult to achieve. Antibiotic treatment early after onset of colonization/infection seems, however, to be successful: in an open study, the combined treatment with colistin and oral ciprofloxacin significantly reduced the onset of *P. aeruginosa* infection in treated compared with untreated patients (14% *vs.* 58%) [3]. A placebo-controlled, double-blind, randomized tobramycin inhalation study showed that the time of conversion to a *P. aeruginosa*-negative respiratory culture after onset of *P. aeruginosa* colonization was significantly shortened by active treatment, suggesting that early tobramycin inhalation may prevent *P. aeruginosa* pulmonary infection in CF [4].

When antibiotic therapy fails to eradicate the pathogens, chronic respiratory infection results. As a result of vigorous immune response of the immunocompetent CF patients, chronic inflammation leads to progressive obstruction and destruction of bronchioli and bronchi. The major cause of morbidity is loss of lung function and the 50% survival rate of patients in the US Registry was 31.3 years in 1996 [2]. The importance of the secondary acquired bacterial lung infections for the prognosis and life expectancy in CF has led to considerable research activities about the mechanisms of bacterial pathogenicity and host response in the last 25 years. Based on these results, several approaches to treat and to prevent lung infections in CF patients have been considered or applied. The purpose of this review is to summarize host–pathogen interactions in this context, emphasizing the role of bacterial and host proteinases and the therapeutic usefulness of proteinase inhibitors.

2. Bacterial Colonization

The exact route of entry of the bacteria into the lower airways of CF patients is not known. It is generally believed that the pathogens colonize the upper respiratory tract and thereafter reach the lower airways. For example, genotyping of *S. aureus* strains from infected CF patients [5] revealed a high degree of strain identity between nose and sputum isolates [6], suggesting that initial colonization of the nasal mucosa with *S. aureus* precedes the development of lower respiratory tract infection. Such a route of transmission has also been proposed for other types of *S. aureus* infection [7–9] and *P. aeruginosa* in the CF lung [10].

It is still uncertain whether bacterial pathogens, once having entered the airways, adhere to the epithelium or to components of the mucus. Using immunofluorescence, scanning and transmission electron microscopy, adherence of *S. aureus* to membranes of airway epithelial cells in CF patients was found to be negligible compared with adherence to components of the secreted mucous layer [11] (see Figure 1 B). Similarly, large numbers of *S. aureus* adhere to mucus on top of the cilia and overlying non-ciliated cells in a three-dimensional primary cell culture system, whereas only low numbers of *S. aureus* adhere to mucus-depleted vesicles (Figure 2). These data confirm results from previous *in vitro* and animal studies. Sanford et al. [12] demonstrated that *S. aureus* was associated with the mucus gel coating the upper respiratory tract of ferrets and that *S. aureus* bound to purified mucins *in vitro* [12, 13]. Also Shuter et al. [14] showed mucin binding of *S. aureus in vitro* and proved that adherence of *S. aureus* to mucus-coated cells was greater than to non-mucus-coated cells.

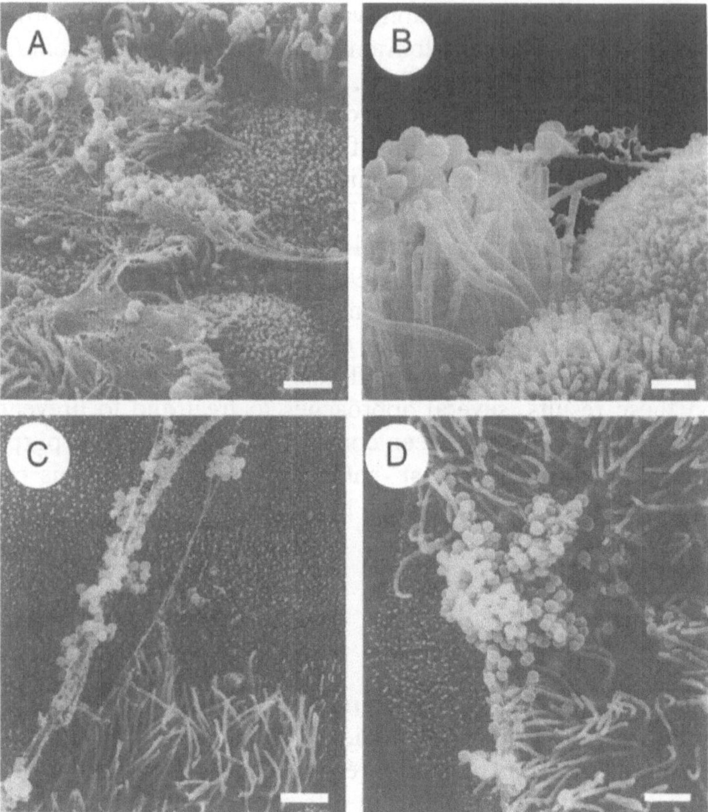

Figure 2. Scanning electron micrograph of primary nasal epithelial cells of a cystic fibrosis patient (A, C), and a healthy individual (B, D) grown as three-dimensional cell balls (A, B) or as monolayer on biocoat membranes (C, D). *S. Aureus* cells adhere to mucus on cell balls but not on cell membranes. Magnifications: (A) × 1750; (B) × 3500, (C) × 1750; (D) × 1750. Bars (A, C, D): 1.7 μm; (B): 0.84 μm. (Courtesy of Martina Ulrich, Hygiene-Institute, University of Tübingen, Germany).

Similarly, *P. aeruginosa*, the other major pathogen in CF patients, may also adhere to mucins of the respiratory tract rather than to the epithelial membrane of these patients *in vivo* and *in vitro* [15–17]. As binding of *S. aureus* to cell balls from CF patients or controls did not differ significantly [11], impaired mucociliary clearance may explain the cause of endobronchial bacterial infection in CF patients better than factors such as an increased sulphation or increased concentrations of asialoganglioside 1 of the glycocalix of epithelial cells [18]. As a result of mucus hypersecretion, bacteria are further removed from the epithelium (see Figure 1 C, D) (see below). It is possible that hypersecretion prevents tissue damage resulting from *S. aureus* toxins [19], as well as invasion and systemic infection with *S. aureus*, because *S. aureus* sepsis has never been described in CF patients.

3. Bacterial Persistence

The successful persistence of *P. aeruginosa* is the result of its ability to avoid the host immune response by changing its phenotype. Whereas mostly a non-mucoid *P. aeruginosa* is seen early after onset of infection (see Figure 1B, C), mucoid *P. aeruginosa*, characterized by the formation of exopolysaccharide-coated microcolonies [17, 20], is present in chronic infection (see Figure 1 D). A microcolony mode of growth has considerable advantages for the survival of *P. aeruginosa* in the hostile CF environment. As a consequence of the abundant production of exopolysaccharide, the surface enlargement prevents effective phagocytosis by alveolar macrophages or polymorphonuclear leukocytes (neutrophils) merely because of its size [21, 22]. Furthermore, reactive oxygen species such as the superoxide anion radical, hydrogen peroxide (H_2O_2) and the hydroxyl radical produced and secreted by stimulated neutrophils may be inactivated by mucoid *P. aeruginosa* exopolysaccharide [23–26], which displays a large negatively charged sugar matrix around single bacteria.

Also myeloperoxidase (MPO) could be trapped on the surface of the matrix; this is a cationic lysosomal enzyme that is released from activated neutrophils and transforms H_2O_2 into highly reactive oxygen metabolites [27]. In addition, catalase could be trapped – an enzyme that detoxifies H_2O_2 to oxygen and water. MPO and catalase are both present in high concentrations and are enzymatically active in CF airways [28, 29]. Matrix binding most probably also affects cationic antimicrobial peptides produced by neutrophils [30] and epithelial cells [31], thereby reducing their efficacy. Another major weapon of neutrophils, lysosomal serine proteinases, apparently do not harm *P. aeruginosa* but instead support its growth (see below). Thus, *P. aeruginosa* is sufficiently protected by its exopolysaccharide coat from the action of reactive oxygen species and other antimicrobial substances in the CF lung. Although a lot is known about alginate biosynthesis [32], the signals that trigger the mucoid phenotype of *P. aeruginosa* are largely unknown. Recently, H_2O_2 was shown to induce the mucoid phenotype of strain PAO1 [33] *in vitro* suggesting that factors in airway inflammation may actually be responsible. CF is not the only disease characterized by mucoid *P. aeruginosa* lung infection since Japanese patients with diffuse panbronchiolitis often harbour this bacterial phenotype [34].

In contrast to *P. aeruginosa*, *S. aureus* seems to pursue a different strategy in CF airways. Although the pathogen can produce several capsular polysaccharides, we recently demonstrated that *S. aureus* strains, producing capsular polysaccharide type 5 (CP5) *in vitro*, lack CP5 when directly examined by immunofluorescence in thin sections of airways from patients with CF and that CP5 was re-expressed when the isolates were grown under normal air conditions [35]. Addition of 1% CO_2 rendered the strains CP5 negative. As, in the bronchioli, the mean value of the inspiratory and expiratory CO_2 is about 4%, it is possible that CP5 expression *in vivo* may be inhibited as a result of the elevated pCO_2 (CO_2 partial pressure) compared with the pCO_2 in normal air. Although *P. aeruginosa* protects itself by a thick polysaccharide layer, *S. aureus* loses its micropolysaccharide capsule. Thus, secretion of teichoic acid or fixation of antibodies by protein A seems to be sufficient to enable the bacterium to persist in the CF airways.

4. *P. aeruginosa* Proteinases

The virulence of *P. aeruginosa* is multifactorial, for example, it may secrete the three extracellular proteinases, elastase (Ela) [36], alkaline proteinase (AP) [37, 38] and LasA protease [39, 40], in addition to other virulence factors [41–43]. Based on *in vitro* experiments, the detection of bacterial proteinases in bronchial secretions of CF patients [44] and experimental animal infection models [45–49], extracellular toxins and other bacterial virulence factors have been shown to play an important role in human infectious diseases including CF. For instance, *P. aeruginosa* proteases cleave fibronectin leading to greater bacterial cell adherence [50, 51], and increase airway secretion [52] causing obstruction of airways. The proteinases also induce lung tissue damage thereby reducing lung clearance in rats [53] and make iron (an essential bacterial growth factor) available for the pathogen [54–56]. Thus, proteases may provide locally preferential growth substances for the bacteria by cleaving a variety of proteins. In addition, *P. aeruginosa* proteases may interfere with host defence, particularly opsonophagocytosis by cleaving immunoglobulins [57], complement components [58, 59] and cell receptors [60–62], thereby supporting bacterial persistence in the CF airways.

During the chronic course of infection specific antibodies are, however, produced against a large number of bacterial antigens including *P. aeruginosa* proteinases [63], which neutralize their enzymatic activities in immune complexes [64]. Thus, the importance of *P. aeruginosa* proteinases in the pathogenicity of the chronic lung infection in CF patients *in vivo* may be minimal [65, 66]. Similarly, other bacterial protein toxins such as exotoxin A are neutralized, or protoelytically cleaved, by host serine proteinases [67], again raising doubts about their relevance *in vivo*. In summary, *P. aeruginosa* in CF is characterized by a non-motile phenotype that overexpresses exopolysaccharides and which survives "passively" in the obstructed airways, taking advantage of a highly proteolytically active environment provided by the host (see below). Provided that this hypothesis is correct, serine proteinase inhibitor therapy might also decrease bacterial growth.

5. Polymorphonuclear Leukocyte Proteinases

As mentioned earlier, neutrophils dominate the local inflammatory response to bacterial airway infection in CF. Recently, markers of inflammation were detected in some infants with CF as young as 4 weeks with negative bacterial cultures, suggesting that inflammation may actually precede infection in CF [68]. Neutrophils are attracted from the vascular space into the CF tissues by bacterial products [69], activated complement components [70], leukotriene B_4 [71–73], or interleukin-8 [68]. Binding of immune complexes (and other particles) to neutrophil surface receptors leads to cell stimulation, resulting in a fusion of intracellular granules or lysosomes with the neutrophil cell surface membrane [22]. Neutrophils contain many granules which can be differentiated into specific and primary (azurophilic) granules, the latter containing the serine proteinases elastase, cathepsin G and proteinase 3, as well as other enzymes involved in hydrolytic, proteolytic and oxidative breakdown of phagocytosed particles [74]. As a result of continuous neutrophil recruitment mainly caused by the inability of neutrophils to phagocytose the large mucoid phenotype of *P. aeruginosa*, considerable quantities of neutrophil lysosomal enzymes are found in CF airways. As a result of the broad substrate specificities of lysosomal proteinases (particularly neutrophil elastase), they have been implicated in the pathogenesis of CF (and other diseases characterized by type III hypersensitivity reactions) by causing tissue damage and decreasing lung functions [1]. Both *P. aeruginosa* and neutrophils are closely associated in the CF sputum at concentrations of about 10^7–10^8 cells/ml sputum or bronchial lavage [75].

The role of neutrophil serine proteinases in inflammation in general and in CF in particular is thought to be critical in pathogenesis [28, 73, 75–80]. All three proteinases (particularly elastase) damage various host structures including fibronectin [51], cilia [81] and elastin [75, 82], immunoglobulins [83], complement components [84–86], and cell receptors on neutrophils [62, 87, 88] and T cells [89]. This would clearly have a major effect on the normal surrounding tissue and the protein pattern of an inflammatory focus. Specifically, the reduction in opsonophagocytosis and killing of *P. aeruginosa*, as well as other pathogens related to CF such as *S. aureus*, *H. influenzae* and *Streptococcus pneumoniae* when neutrophils are pretreated with neutrophil elastase [62, 87], has led to the concept that, in CF, free serine proteinase activity is deleterious for the host and serine proteinase inhibitor therapy may be useful (see below). As *P. aeruginosa* proteinases are neutralized in immune complexes, as mentioned earlier, the pathogen may rely on the enzymatic activity of secreted neutrophil proteinases to colonize and persist in the respiratory tract. A comparison of substrates for host serine proteinases and *P. aeruginosa* proteinases showed that they are very similar [90]. For example, both the *P. aeruginosa* metalloproteases and the neutrophil serine proteinases have been shown to degrade and inactivate the host proteinase inhibitors α_1-proteinase inhibitor (α_1-PI) [28, 91, 92] and human bronchial mucosal proteinase inhibitor (synonym: secretory leukocyte protease inhibitor, SLPI) [93, 94] and *P. aeruginosa* metalloproteases also cleave α_1-antichymotrypsin [95]. During chronic *P. aeruginosa* lung infection in CF, sputum α_1-PI function is minimal (3.8%) [28, 96] and thus the activity of released lysosomal proteinases from neutrophils would remain less well controlled, supporting the survival of *P. aeruginosa* in CF airways. Nevertheless, the net effect may not be totally harmful to the patient.

The ability of neutrophil elastase as well as cathepsin G to stimulate airway gland secretion [97, 98] may lead to airway obstruction which is not necessarily deleterious (see Figure 1C, D). The mucus hypersecretion, as mentioned earlier, may remove bacterial pathogens from airway epithelium and thus reduce the likelihood of systemic infection. In addition, although cleavage of phagocytic receptors may suppress the process of antigen recognition, it would also reduce amplification of the immune response by other cells and therefore may be regarded as beneficial for the patient by reducing an ineffective but harmful inflammatory response [99].

Besides neutrophil serine proteinases, other host proteinases may play a pathogenic role in CF lung disease. Neutrophil collagenase [100], a metalloproteinase of specific granules [101], has been detected in sputum of CF patients [102]. In addition to other substrates, it also cleaves and inactivates α_1-PI [103]. Other potential active proteinases include: human interstitial collagenase (matrix metalloproteinase-1), an enzyme the synthesis of which is widely distributed among endothelial, epithelial and mesenchymal cells and which also cleaves serine proteinase inhibitors, including α_1-PI [104], macrophage-derived metalloproteinase [105], and cysteine proteinases [106]. However, as serine proteinase inhibitors largely inhibit proteolytic activity in sputum samples from patients with CF, the role of metalloproteinases in the pathogenicity of the CF lung inflammation of host or bacterial origin may (at best) be minimal and indirect. These concepts, and in particular the role of neutrophil elastase, are summarized in Figure 3.

6. α_1-Proteinase Inhibitor Therapy

To remove neutrophil-released elastase and other proteinases from the extracellular space, the host is provided with several receptor-mediated clearance mechanisms by the reticuloendothelial system. Alveolar macrophages are capable of binding and internalizing elastase by binding the elastase-α_2-macroglobulin complexes [107]. Human monocytes and hepatocytes have an abundant, high-affinity cell surface receptor that binds α_1-PI elastase complexes, mediates endocytosis and lysosomal degradation of the complexes, and induces an increase in synthesis of α_1-PI. A pentapeptide domaine in the carboxyl-terminal fragment of α_1-PI is sufficient

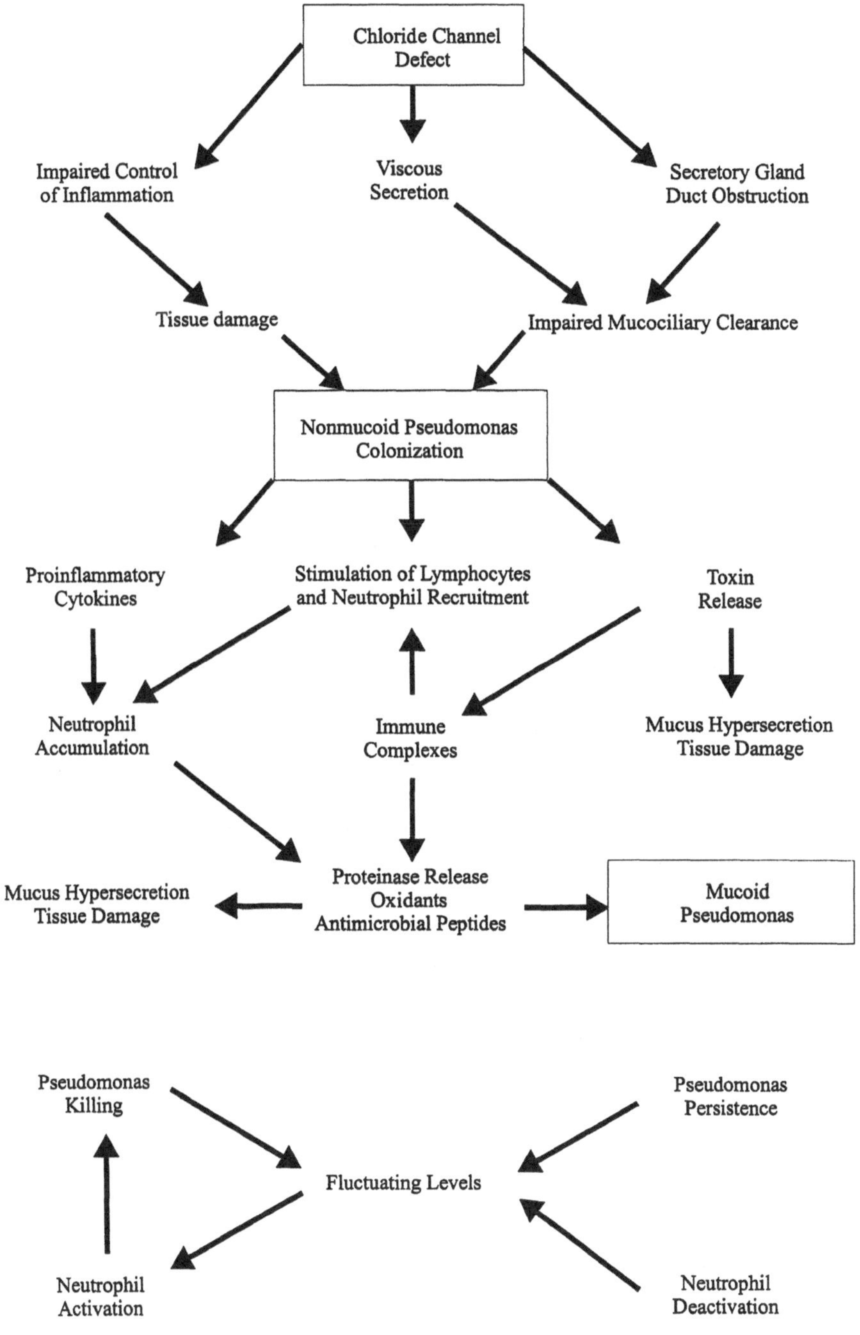

Chloride Channel Defect
Impaired Control of Inflammation
Viscous Secretion
Secretory Gland Duct Obstruction
Tissue damage
Impaired Mucociliary Clearance
Nonmucoid Pseudomonas Colonization
Proinflammatory Cytokines
Stimulation of Lymphocytes and Neutrophil Recruitment
Toxin Release
Neutrophil Accumulation
Immune Complexes
Mucus Hypersecretion Tissue Damage
Mucus Hypersecretion Tissue Damage
Proteinase Release Oxidants Antimicrobial Peptides
Mucoid Pseudomonas
Pseudomonas Killing
Pseudomonas Persistence
Fluctuating Levels
Neutrophil Activation
Neutrophil Deactivation

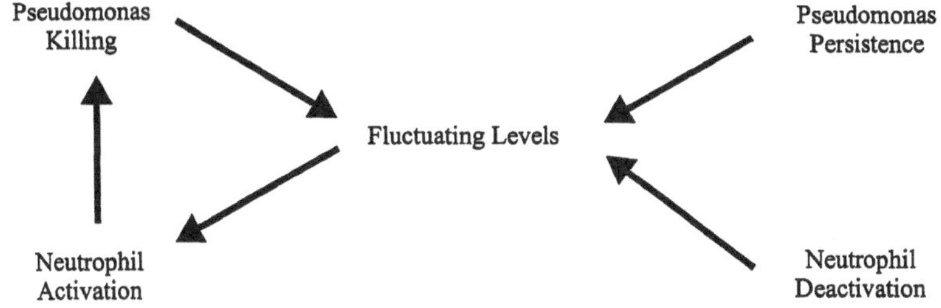

Figure 3. Pathogenesis of chronic *P. aeruginosa* infection in cystic fibrosis.

for binding to this receptor which was named SERPIN enzyme complex (SEC) receptor [108]. Furthermore, a common receptor for elastase, cathepsin G and lactoferrin exists on alveolar macrophages which binds elastase with no need for a previous interaction with a proteinase inhibitor [109]. Apparently, these mechanisms are insufficient in chronic inflammation in CF patients, because elastase activity is invariably present [28]. Therefore, α_1-PI administration by inhalation has been considered as a therapeutic strategy in CF to reduce elastase activity and, hence, its potentially deleterious effects on host defences.

α_1-PI is the most abundant of the plasma proteinase inhibitors (30–50-μmol/l) and the inactivation of neutrophil elastase by this inhibitor is one of the fastest biochemical reactions known [110]. Based on *in vivo* half-time inhibition data, α_1-antichymotrypsin rather than α_1-PI inhibits cathepsin G [110]. α_1-PI is produced by hepatocytes, but also in small amounts by alveolar macrophages [111] and neutrophils [112]. The function of the latter source is unknown, although it has been shown that elastase binds to CR3 (CD11b/CD18) on the surface of neutrophils and thus mediates detachment of CR3 from its ligand intercellular adhesion molecule 1 (ICAM-1) during diapedesis [113]; it is possible that α_1-PI secreted from neutrophils may modulate this migration process.

As mentioned above, blood-derived α_1-PI is mostly inactive in inflamed CF airways which may be the result of proteolytic cleavage by a surplus of neutrophil elastase [28] or other proteinases, as well as oxidation of the methionine residue in the active centre of the enzyme; Met-358 [114]. However, recently we have shown [29] that Met-358 oxidation by the MPO/H_2O_2/halide system does not occur in inflamed CF airways, even though considerable amounts of active MPO are present. Apparently, complexing of neutrophil elastase with α_1-PI (which renders Met-358 inaccessible for MPO-induced oxidation) is faster than MPO-induced oxidation of uncomplexed α_1-PI. The findings that MPO is rendered immobile by the negatively charged DNA or glycoprotein matrix in sputum [29] may help explain this fact. Furthermore, high concentrations of catalase detoxifying H_2O_2 are present in this sputum [29]. Thus, proteolytic cleavage rather than oxidation of α_1-PI is likely to be the major cause of inactivation in CF sputum. These findings may have considerable impact on trials of aerosol therapy with α_1-PI in CF: aerosolized α_1-PI may still actively complex with neutrophil elastase despite the presence of high concentrations and activities of MPO in CF airways.

Only a few trials with human plasma-derived α_1-PI have been carried out in CF patients mainly because of the shortage of available α_1-PI for this patient group [115]. McElvaney and colleagues showed convincingly that the active neutrophil elastase concentrations in the epithelial lining fluid of 12 CF patients were significantly reduced using 1.5–3.0 mg α_1-PI/kg body weight twice daily for one week. The use of transgenic α_1-PI produced in the milk of sheep may soon overcome the shortage of the inhibitor for clinical studies [116]. Inhibition of neutrophil serine proteinases may also restore neutrophil function, render bacterial survival more difficult and lastly reduce mucus hypersecretion. Decreasing sputum volumes may then enable antibiotics to kill pathogens more effectively. The success of such specific studies and, more importantly, the clinical, bacteriological and inflammatory response, will clarify the true role of neutrophil elastase in the pathogenesis of CF and pseudomonas colonization.

References

1 Hodson ME, Geddes D (eds) (1995) *Cystic fibrosis*. Chapman & Hall, London
2 Cystic Fibrosis Foundation (1997) Patient Registry 1996. *Annual Data Report*, Bethesda, MA
3 Valerius NH, Koch C, Høiby N (1991) Prevention of chronic *Pseudomonas aeruginosa* colonization in cystic fibrosis by early treatment. *Lancet* 338: 725–726
4 Wiesemann HG, Steinkamp G, Ratjen F, Bauernfeind A, Przyklenk B, Döring G, von der Hardt H (1998) Placebo controlled, double blind, randomized study of aerosolized tobramycin for early treatment of *Pseudomonas aeruginosa* colonization in patients with cystic fibrosis. *Pediatr Pulmonol* 25: 88–92
5 Schlichting C, Branger C, Fournier J-M, Witte W, Boutonnier A, Wolz C, Goullet P, Döring G (1993) Typing of *Staphylococcus aureus* by pulsed field gel electrophoresis, zymotyping, capsular typing, and phage typing: resolution of clonal relationships. *J Clin Microbiol* 31: 227–232
6 Goerke C, Brost I, Surrey K, Kraning K, Botzenhart K, Döring G, Wolz C (1996) *Staphylococcus aureus* in families with and without cystic fibrosis patients. *Monatsschr Kinderheilkd* 144: 1045
7 Luzar MA, Coles GA, Faller B, Slingeneyer A, Dah GD, Briat C, Wone C, Knefati Y, Kessler M, Peluso F (1990) *Staphylococcus aureus* nasal carriage and infection in patients on continuous ambulatory peritoneal dialysis. *N Engl J Med* 322: 505–509
8 Tuazon C, Sheagren JN (1975) Staphylococcal endocarditis in parenteral drug abusers: source of the organism. *Ann Intern Med* 82: 788–790
9 Yu VL, Goetz A, Wagener A, Smith PB, Rihs JD, Hancett J, Zuravleff JJ (1986) *Staphylococcus aureus* nasal carriage and infection in patients on hemodialysis. *N Engl J Med* 315: 91–96
10 Shapiro ED, Milmoe GJ, Wald ER, Rodnan JB, Bowen A (1982) Bacteriology of the maxillary sinuses in patients with cystic fibrosis. *J Infect Dis* 146: 589–593
11 Ulrich M, Herbert S, Berger J, Bellon G, Louis D, Münker G, Döring G (1998) Localization of *Staphylococcus aureus* in infected airways of patients with cystic fibrosis and in a cell culture model of *S. aureus* adherence. *Am J Respir Cell Mol Biol* 19: 83–91
12 Sanford BA, Thomas VL, Ramsay MA (1989) Binding of Staphylococci to mucus *in vivo* and *in vitro*. *Infect Immun* 57: 3735–3742
13 Thomas VL, Sanford BA, Ramsay MA (1993) Calcium- and mucin-binding proteins of staphylococci. *J Gen Microbiol* 139: 632–639
14 Shuter J, Hatcher VB, Lowy FD (1996) *Staphylococcus aureus* binding to human nasal mucin. *Infect Immun* 64: 310–318
15 Ramphal R (1990) The role of bacterial adhesion in cystic fibrosis including the staphylococcal aspect. *Infection* 18: 61–64
16 Baltimore RS, Christie CDC, Smith GJW (1989) Immunohistopathologic location of *Pseudomonas aeruginosa* in lungs of patients with cystic fibrosis. *Am Rev Respir Dis* 140: 1650–1661
17 Simel DL, Masten BS, Pratt PC, Wisseman CL, Shelburne JD, Spock A (1984) Scanning electron microscopic study of the airways in normal children and in patients with cystic fibrosis and other lung diseases. *Pediatr Pathol* 2: 47–64

18 Imundo L, Barasch J, Prince A, Al-Awqati Q (1995) Cystic fibrosis epithelial cells have a receptor for pathogenic bacteria on their apical surface. *Proc Natl Acad Sci USA* 92: 3019–3023
19 Arvidson S (1983) Extracellular enzymes from *Staphylococcus aureus*. In: CSF Easmon, C Adlam (eds) *Staphylococci and staphylococcal infections*. Academic Press, London, p 745–808
20 Lam J, Chan R, Lam K, Costerton JW (1980) Production of mucoid microcolonies by *Pseudomonas aeruginosa* within infected lungs in cystic fibrosis. *Infect Immun* 28: 546–556
21 Goldstein IM (1976) Polymorphonuclear leukocyte lysosomes and tissue injury. *Prog Allergy* 20: 301–340
22 Cabral DA, Loh BA, Speert DP (1987) Mucoid *Pseudomonas aeruginosa* resists nonopsonic phagocytosis by human neutrophils and macrophages. *Pediatr Res* 22: 429–431
23 Simpson JA, Smith SE, Dean RT (1989) Scavening by alginate of free radicals released by macrophages. *Free Radic Biol* 6: 347–353
24 Learn DB, Brestel EP, Seetharama S (1987) Hypochlorite scavenging by *Pseudomonas aeruginosa* alginate. *Infect Immun* 55: 1813–1818
25 Hassett DJ (1996) Anaerobic production of alginate by *Pseudomonas aeruginosa*: alginate restricts diffusion of oxygen. *J Bacteriol* 178: 7322–7325
26 Costerton JW, Lewandowski Z, deBeer D, Caldwell D, Korber D, James G (1994) Biofilms, the customized microniche. *J Bacteriol* 176: 2137–2142
27 Klebanoff SJ, Waltersdorph AM, Rosen H (1984) Antimicrobial activity of myeloperoxidase. *Methods Enzymol* 105: 399–403
28 Goldstein W, Döring G (1986) Lysosomal enzymes and proteinase inhibitors in the sputum of patients with cystic fibrosis. *Am Rev Respir Dis* 134: 49–56
29 Worlitzsch D, Herberth G, Ulrich M, Döring G (1998) Catalase, myeloperoxidase and hydrogen peroxide in cystic fibrosis. *Eur Respir J* 11: 377–383
30 Levy O (1996) Antibiotic proteins of polymorphonuclear leukocytes. *Eur J Haematol* 56: 263–277
31 Gabay JE, Almeida RP (1993) Antibiotic peptides and serine proteinase homologs in human polymorphonuclear leukocytes: defensins and azurocidin. *Curr Opin Immunol* 5: 97–102
32 Govan JRW, Deretic V (1996) Microbial pathogenesis in cystic fibrosis: mucoid *Pseudomonas aeruginosa* and *Burkholderia cepacia*. *Microbiol Rev* 60: 539–574
33 Mathee K, Sternberg C, Coifu O, Jensen P, Campbell J, Givskv M, Ohman D, Høiby N, Kharazmi A (1997) Oxygen radical induced phenotypic change from non-alginate producing to alginate-producing form of *Pseudomonas aeruginosa* in biofilms. Pseudomonas '97. VI International Congress on Pseudomonas: Molecular Biology and Biotechnology. Madrid A115
34 Homma H, Yamanaka A, Tanimoto S, Tamura M, Chijimatsu Y, Kira S, Izumi T (1983) Diffuse panbronchiolitis: a disease of the transitional zone of the lung. *Chest* 83: 63–69
35 Herbert S, Worlitzsch D, Dassy B, Boutonnier A, Fournier J-M, Bellon G, Dalhoff A, Döring G (1997) Regulation of the *Staphylococcus aureus* capsular polysaccharide type 5: CO_2 inhibition *in vitro* and *in vivo*. *J Infect Dis* 176: 431–438
36 Fukushima J, Yamamoto S, Morihara K, Atsumi Y, Takeuchi H, Kawamoto S, Okuda K (1989) Structural gene and complete amino acid sequence of *Pseudomonas aeruginosa* IFO 3455 elastase. *J Bacteriol* 171: 1698–1704
37 Guzzo J, Murgier M, Filloux A, Lazdunski A (1990) Cloning of the *Pseudomonas aeruginosa* alkaline protease gene and secretion of the protease into the medium by *Escherichia coli*. *J Bacteriol* 172: 942–948
38 Guzzo J, Duong F, Wandersman C, Murgier M, Lazdunski A (1991) The secretion genes of *Pseudomonas aeruginosa* alkaline protease are functionally related to those of *Erwinia chrysanthemi* proteases and *Eschericia coli* α-haemolysin. *Mol Microbiol* 5: 447–453
39 Gustin JK, Kessler E, Ohman DE (1996) A substitution at His-120 in the LasA protease of *Pseudomonas aeruginosa* blocks enzymatic activity without affecting propeptide processing or extracellular secretion. *J Bacteriol* 178: 6608–6617
40 Goldberg JB, Ohman DE (1987) Cloning and transcriptional regulation of the elastase LasA gene in mucoid and nonmucoid *Pseudomonas aeruginosa*. *J Bacteriol* 169: 1349–1351

41 Döring G, Holder IA, Botzenhart K (eds) (1987) *Basic Research and Clincial Aspects of* Pseudomonas aeruginosa. Karger, Basel
42 Høiby N, Pedersen SS, Shand SJ, Döring G, Holder IA (eds) (1989) Pseudomonas aeruginosa *infection*. Karger, Basel
43 Homma JY, Tanimoto H, Holder IA, Høiby N, Döring G (eds) (1991) *Basic Research and clinical aspects of* Pseudomonas aeruginosa *infection*. Karger, Basel
44 Döring G, Obernesser HJ, Botzenhart K, Flehmig B, Høiby N, Hofmann A (1983) Proteases of *Pseudomonas aeruginosa* in cystic fibrosis. *J Infect Dis* 147: 744–750
45 Pavlovskis OR, Wretlind B (1979) Assessment of protease (elastase) as a *Pseudomonas aeruginosa* virulence factor in experimental mouse burn infection. *Infect Immun* 24: 181–187
46 Holder IA, Haidaris CG (1979) Experimental studies of the pathogenesis of infections due to *Pseudomonas aeruginosa*: extracellular protease and elastase as *in vivo* virulence factors. *Can J Microbiol* 25: 593–599
47 Cicmanec JF, Holder IA (1979) Growth of *Pseudomonas aeruginosa* in normal and burned skin extract: role of ectracellular proteases. *Infect Immun* 25: 477–483
48 Döring G, Dalhoff A, Vogel O, Brunner H, Dröge U, Botzenhart K (1984) *In vivo* activity of proteases of *Pseudomonas aeruginosa* in a rat model. *J Infect Dis* 149: 532–537
49 Steuhl KP, Döring G, Henni A, Thiel H-J, Botzenhart K (1987) Relevance of host-derived and bacterial factors in *Pseudomonas aeruginosa* corneal infections. *Invest Ophtalmol Vis Sci* 28: 1559–1568
50 Woods DE, Straus DC Jr, Johansson WGR, Bass JA (1981) Role of salivary protease activity in adherence of gram-negative bacilli to mammalian buccal epithelial cells *in vivo*. *J Clin Invest* 68: 1435–1440
51 Suter S, Schaad UB, Morgenthaler JJ, Chevallier I, Schnebli H-P (1988) Fibronectin-cleaving activity in bronchial secretions of patients with cystic fibrosis. *J Infect Dis* 158: 89–100
52 Sommerville M, Richardson PS, Rutman A, Wilson R, Cole PJ (1991) Stimulation of secretion into human and feline airways by *Pseudomonas aeruginosa* proteases. *J Appl Physiol* 70: 2259–2267
53 Döring G, Dauner H-M (1988) Clearance of *Pseudomonas aeruginosa* in different rat lung infection models. *Am Rev Respir Dis* 138: 1249–1253
54 Döring G, Pfestorf M, Botzenhart K, Abdallah M (1988) Impact of proteases on iron uptake of *Pseudomonas aeruginosa* pyoverdin from transferrin and lactoferrin. *Infect Immun* 56: 291–293
55 Wolz C, Hohloch K, Acaktan A, Poole K, Evans RW, Rochel N, Albrecht-Gary A-M, Abdallah M, Döring G (1994) Iron release from transferrin by pyoverdin and elastase from *Pseudomonas aeruginosa*. *Infect Immun* 62: 4021–4027
56 Britigan BE, Edeker BL (1991) Pseudomonas and neutrophil products modify transferrin and lactoferrin to create conditions that favor hydroxyl radical formation. *J Clin Invest* 88: 1092–1102
57 Döring G, Obernesser HJ, Botzenhart K (1981) Extracellular toxins of *P. aeruginosa*. II. Effect of two proteases on human IgG, IgA and secretory IgA. *Zbl Bakt Mikrobiol Hyg 1 Abt Orig A* 249: 89–98
58 Schultz DR, Miller KD (1974) Elastase of *Pseudomonas aeruginosa*: inactivation of complement components and complement-derived chemotactic and phagocytic factors. *Infect Immun* 10: 128–135
59 Hong YQ, Ghebrehiwet B (1992) Effect of *Pseudomonas aeruginosa* elastase and alkaline protease on serum complement and isolated components C1q and C3. *Clin Immunol Immunopathol* 62: 133–138
60 Kharazmi A, Nielsen H (1991) Inhibition of human monocyte chemotaxis and chemiluminescence by *Pseudomonas aeruginosa* elastase. APMIS 99: 93–95
61 Ijiri Y, Matsumoto K, Kamata R, Nishino N, Okamura R, Kambara T, Yamamoto T (1994) Suppression of polymorphonuclear leucocyte chemotaxis by *Pseudomonas aeruginosa* elastase *in vitro*: a study of the mechanisms and the correlation with ring abscess in pseudomonal keratitis. *Int J Exp Pathol* 75: 441–451
62 Berger M, Sorensen RU, Tosi MF, Dearborn DG, Döring G (1989) Complement receptor expression on neutrophils at an inflammatory site, the Pseudomonas-infected lung in cystic fibrosis. *J Clin Invest* 84: 1302–1313

63 Döring G, Høiby N (1983) Longitudinal study of immune response to *Pseudomonas aeruginosa* antigens in cystic fibrosis. *Infect Immun* 42: 197–201
64 Döring G, Buhl V, Høiby N, Schiøtz PO, Botzenhart K (1984) Detection of proteases of *Pseudomonas aeruginosa* in immune complexes isolated from the sputum of cystic fibrosis patients. *Acta Pathol Microbiol* [*C*] 92: 307–311
65 Jaffar-Bandjee MC, Lazdunski A, Bally M, Carrere J, Chazalette JP, Galabert C (1995) Production of elastase, exotoxin A, and alkaline protease in sputa during pulmonary exacerbation of cystic fibrosis in patients chronically infected by *Pseudomonas aeruginosa*. *J Clin Microbiol* 33: 924–929
66 Cantin A, Bilodeau G, Bégin R (1989) Granulocyte elastase-mediated proteolysis of α_1-antitrypsin in cystic fibrosis bronchopulmonary secretions. *Pediatr Pulmonol* 7: 12–17
67 Döring G, Müller E (1989) Different sensitivity of *Pseudomonas aeruginosa* exotoxin A and diphtheria toxin to enzymes from polymorphonuclear leukocytes. *Microbiol Pathogen* 6: 287–295
68 Khan TZ, Wagener JS, Bost T, Martinez J, Accurso FJ, Riches DWH (1995) Early pulmonary inflammation in infants with cystic fibrosis. *Am J Respir Crit Care Med* 151: 1075–1082
69 Kharazmi A, Schiøtz PO, Høiby N, Baek L, Döring G (1986) Demonstration of neutrophil chemotactic activity in the sputum of cystic fibrosis patients with *Pseudomonas aeruginosa* infection. *Eur J Clin Invest* 16: 143–148
70 Fick RB Jr, Robbins RA, Squier SU, Schoderbek WE, Russ WD (1986) Complement activation in cystic fibrosis respiratory fluids: *in vivo* and *in vitro* generation of C5a and chemotactic activity. *Pediatr Res* 20: 1258–1268
71 Cromwell O, Walport MJ, Morris HR, Taylor GW, Hodson HR, Batten J, Kay AB (1981) Identification of leukotrienes D and B in sputum from cystic fibrosis patients. *Lancet* i: 16416–16425
72 Zakrzewski JT, Barnes NC, Costello JF, Piper PJ (1987) Lipid mediators in cystic fibrosis and chronic obstrucitve pulmonary disease. *Am Rev Respir Dis* 136: 779–782
73 Martin TR, Pistorese BP, Chi EY, Goodman RB, Mattay MA (1989) Effects of leukotriene B4 in the human lung. Recruitment of neutrophils into the alveolar spaces without a change in protein permeability. *J Clin Invest* 84: 1609–1619
74 Sandborg RR, Smolen JE (1988) Biology of disease. Early biochemical events in leukocyte activation. *Lab Invest* 59: 300–320
75 Bruce MC, Poncz L, Klinger JD, Stern RC, Tomashefski JF Jr, Dearborn DG (1985) Biochemical and pathological evidence for proteolytic destruction of lung connective tissue in cystic fibrosis. *Am Rev Respir Dis* 132: 529–535
76 Fick RB, Naegel GP, Squier SU, Wood RE, Gee BL, Reynolds HY (1984) Proteins of the cystic fibrosis respiratory tract. *J Clin Invest* 74: 236–248
77 Tournier JM, Jacquot J, Puchelle E, Bieth JG (1985) Evidence that *Pseudomonas aeruginosa* elastase does not inactivate the bronchial inhibitor in the presence of leukocyte elastase. *Am Rev Respir Dis* 132: 524–528
78 Meyer KC, Lewandoski JR, Zimmerman JJ, Nunley D, Calhoun WJ, Dopico GA (1991) Human neutrophil elastase and elastase/α-antiprotease complex in cystic fibrosis. *Am Rev Respir Dis* 144: 580–585
79 Jackson AH, Hill SL, Afford SC, Stockley RA (1984) Sputum sol-phase proteins and elastase activity in patients with cystic fibrosis. *Eur J Respir Dis* 65: 114–124
80 Suter S, Schaad UB, Roux L, Nydegger UE, Waldvogel FA (1984) Granulocyte neutral proteases and Pseudomonas elastase as possible causes of airway damage in patients with cystic fibrosis. *J Infect Dis* 149: 523–531
81 Smallman LA, Hill SL, Stockley RA (1984) Reduction of ciliary beat frequency *in vitro* by sputum from patients with bronchiectasis: A serine proteinase effect. *Thorax* 39: 663–667
82 Stone PJ, Konstan MW, Berger M, Dorkin HL, Franzblau C, Snider GL (1995) Elastin and collagen degradation products in urine of patients with cystic fibrosis. *Am J Respir Crit Care Med* 152: 157–162
83 Döring G, Goldstein W, Botzenhart K, Kharazmi A, Schiøtz PO, Høiby N, Dasgupta M (1986) Elastase from polymorphonuclear leucocytes – a regulatory enzyme in immune complex disease. *Clin Exp Immunol* 64: 597–605

84 Suter S, Schaad UB, Roux L, Nydegger UE, Waldvogel FA (1984) Granulocyte neutral proteases and Pseudomonas elastase as possible causes of airway damage in patients with cystic fibrosis. *J Infect Dis* 149: 523–531
85 Orr FW, Varani J, Kreutzer DL, Senior RM, Ward PA (1979) Digestion of the fifth component of complement by leukocyte enzymes. *Am J Pathol* 94: 75–84
86 Carlo R, Spitznagel JK, Studer EJ, Konrad DN, Ruddy S (1981) Cleavage of membrane bound C3bi, an intermediate on the third component of complement to C3c and C3d-like fragments by crude leucocyte elastase. *Immunology* 44: 381–391
87 Tosi MF, Zakem H, Berger M (1990) Neutrophil elastase cleaves C3bi on opsonized Pseudomonas as well as CR1 on neutrophils to create a functionally important opsonin receptor mismatch. *J Clin Invest* 86: 300–308
88 Häkansson H, Venge P (1982) Kinetic studies on neutrophil phagocytosis. V: Studies on the cooperation between the Fc and C3b receptors. *Immunology* 47: 687–694
89 Döring G, Frank F, Boudier C, Herbert S, Fleischer B, Bellon G (1995) Cleavage of lymphocyte surface antigens CD2, CD4, and CD8 by polymorphonuclear leukocyte elastase and cathepsin G in patients with cystic fibrosis. *J Immunol* 154: 4842–4850
90 Döring G (1997) The role of proteinases from *Pseudomonas aeruginosa* and polymorphonuclear leukocytes in cystic fibrosis. *Drugs Today* 33: 393–403
91 Morihara K, Tsuzuki H, Oda K (1979) Protease and elastase of *Pseudomonas aeruginosa*: inactivation of human plasma α_1-proteinase inhibitor. *Infect Immun* 24: 188–193
92 Suter S, Chevallier I (1991) Proteolytic inactivation of α_1-proteinase inhibitor in infected brochial secretions from patients with cystic fibrosis. *Eur Respir J* 4: 40–49
93 Johnson DA, Carter-Hamm B, Dralle WM (1982) Inactivation of human bronchial mucosal proteinase inhibitor by *Pseudomonas aeruginosa* elastase. *Am Rev Respir Dis* 126: 1070–1073
94 Vogelmeier C, Hubbard RC, Fells GA, Schnebli H-P, Thompson RC, Fritz H, Crystal RG (1991) Anti-neutrophil elastase defense of the normal human respiratory epithelial surface provided by the secretory leukoprotease inhibitor. *J Clin Invest* 87: 482–488
95 Catanese J, Kress LF (1984) Enzymatic inactivation of human plasma C1-inhibitor and α_1-antichymotrypsin by *Pseudomonas aeruginosa* proteinase and elastase. *Biochim Biophy Acta* 789: 37–43
96 Cantin AM, Lafrenaye S, Begin RO (1991) Antineutrophil elastase activity in cystic fibrosis serum. *Pediatr Pulmonol* 11: 249–253
97 Sommerhof CP, Nadel JA, Basbaum CB, Caughey GH (1990) Neutrophil elastase and cathepsin G stimulate secretion from cultured bovine airway gland serous cells. *J Clin Invest* 85: 682–689
98 Schuster A, Fahy JV, Ueki I, Nadel JA (1995) Cystic fibrosis sputum induces a secretory response from airway gland serous cells that can be prevented by neutrophil protease inhibitors. *Eur Respir J* 8: 10–14
99 Döring G (1994) The role of neutrophil elastase in chronic inflammation. *Am J Respir Crit Care Med* 150: S114–S147
100 Lazarus GS, Brown RS, Daniels JR, Fullmer HM (1968) Human granulocyte collagenase. *Science* 159: 1483–1485
101 Murphy G, Reynolds JJ (1977) Collagenase is a component of the specific granules of human neutrophil leukocytes. *Biochem J* 162: 195–197
102 Power C, O'Connor CM, Macfarlane D, O'Mahoney S, Gaffney K, Hayes J, Fitzgerald MX (1994) Neutrophil collagenase in sputum from patients with cystic fibrosis. *Am J Respir Crit Care Med* 150: 818–822
103 Vissers MCM, George PM, Bathurst IC, Brennan SO, Winterbourn CC (1988) Cleavage and inactivation of α_1-antitrypsin by metalloproteinases released from neutrophils. *J Clin Invest* 82: 706–711
104 Desrochers PE, Jeffrey JJ, Weiss SJ (1991) Interstitial collagenase (matrix metalloproteinase-1) expresses serpinase activity. *J Clin Invest* 87: 2258–2265
105 Welgus HG, Campbell EJ, Cury JD, Eisen AZ, Senior RM, Wilhelm SM, Goldberg GI (1990) Neutral metalloproteinases produced by human mononuclear phagocytes. Enzyme profile, regulation and expression during cellular development. *J Clin Invest* 86: 1496–1502
106 Reilly JJ Jr, Chen P, Sailor LZ, Mason RW, Chapman HA Jr (1990) Uptake of extracellular enzyme by a novel pathway is a major determinant of cathepsin L levels in human macrophages. *J Clin Invest* 86: 176–183

107 Campbell EJ, White RR, Senior RM, Rodriguez RJ, Kuhn C (1979) Receptor-mediated binding and internalization of leukocyte elastase by alveolar macrophages *in vitro*. *J Clin Invest* 64: 824–833
108 Joslin G, Fallon RJ, Bullock J, Adams SP, Perlmutter DH (1991) The SEC receptor recognizes a pentapeptide neodomain of α_1-antitrypsin-protease complexes. *J Biol Chem* 266: 11282–11288
109 Campbell EJ (1982) Human leukocyte elastase, cathepsin G and lactoferrin: family of neutrophil granule glycoproteins that bind to an alveolar macrophage receptor. *Proc Natl Acad Sci USA* 79: 6941–6945
110 Travis J, Salvesen GS (1983) Human plasma proteinase inhibitors. *Annu Rev Biochem* 52: 655–709
111 White R, Lee D, Habicht GS, Janoff A (1981) Secretion of α_1-proteinase inhibitor by cultured rat alveolar macrophages. *Am Rev Respir Dis* 123: 447–450
112 Pääkkö P, Kirby M, du Bois RM, Gillissen A, Ferrans VJ, Crystal RG (1996) Activated neutrophils secrete stored α_1-antitrypsin. *Am J Respir Crit Care Med* 154: 1829–1833
113 Cai T-Q, Wright SD (1996) Human leukocyte elastase is an endogenous ligand for the integrin CR3 (CD11b/CD18, Mac-1, $\alpha_M\beta_2$) and modulates polymorphonuclear leukocyte adhesion. *J Exp Med* 184: 1213–1223
114 Matheson NR, Wong PS, Travis J (1979) Enzymatic inactivation of human α_1-proteinase inhibitor by neutrophil myeloperoxidase. *Biochem Biophys Res Commun* 88: 402–409
115 McElvaney NG, Hubbard RC, Birrer P, Chernick MS, Caplan DB, Frank MM, Crystal RG (1991) Aerosol α_1-antitrypsin treatment for cystic fibrosis. *Lancet* 337: 392–394
116 Gershon D (1991) Biotechnology. Will milk shake up industry? *Nature* 353: 7

Index